Implementing Physical Activity Strategies

Put the
National Physical Activity Plan
into action with 42
proven programs

Russell R. Pate, PhD
University of South Carolina

David M. Buchner, MD, MPH
University of Illinois

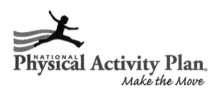

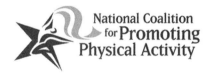

National Coalition for Promoting Physical Activity

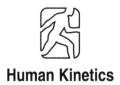

Human Kinetics

Library of Congress Cataloging-in-Publication Data

Implementing physical activity strategies / Russell R. Pate, David M. Buchner, editors.
  p. ; cm.
Includes bibliographical references and index.
ISBN-13: 978-1-4504-2499-8
ISBN-10: 1-4504-2499-6
I. Pate, Russell R. II. Buchner, David.
[DNLM: 1. Motor Activity--United States. 2. Exercise--United States. 3. Health Policy--United States. 4. Healthy People Programs--organization & administration--United States. 5. Physical Fitness--United States. 6. Sedentary Lifestyle--United States. WE 103]
RA781
613.7'1--dc23

                                2013005847

ISBN-10: 1-4504-2499-6 (print)
ISBN-13: 978-1-4504-2499-8 (print)

The web addresses cited in this text were current as of June 2013, unless otherwise noted.

Acquisitions Editor: Myles Schrag; **Developmental Editor:** Melissa J. Zavala; **Managing Editor:** Amanda S. Ewing; **Assistant Editors:** Amy Akin and Anne E. Mrozek; **Copyeditor:** Julie Anderson; **Proofreader:** Jim Burns; **Indexer:** Andrea J. Hepner; **Permissions Manager:** Dalene Reeder; **Graphic Designer:** Fred Starbird; **Graphic Artist:** Dawn Sills; **Cover Designer:** Keith Blomberg; **Photographer (cover):** Neil Bernstein; **Photo Production Manager:** Jason Allen; **Art Manager:** Kelly Hendren; **Associate Art Manager:** Alan L. Wilborn; **Printer:** Sheridan Books

Printed in the United States of America   10 9 8 7 6 5 4 3 2 1

The paper in this book is certified under a sustainable forestry program.

Human Kinetics
Website: www.HumanKinetics.com

United States: Human Kinetics
P.O. Box 5076
Champaign, IL 61825-5076
800-747-4457
e-mail: humank@hkusa.com

Canada: Human Kinetics
475 Devonshire Road Unit 100
Windsor, ON N8Y 2L5
800-465-7301 (in Canada only)
e-mail: info@hkcanada.com

Europe: Human Kinetics
107 Bradford Road
Stanningley
Leeds LS28 6AT, United Kingdom
+44 (0) 113 255 5665
e-mail: hk@hkeurope.com

Australia: Human Kinetics
57A Price Avenue
Lower Mitcham, South Australia 5062
08 8372 0999
e-mail: info@hkaustralia.com

New Zealand: Human Kinetics
P.O. Box 80
Torrens Park, South Australia 5062
0800 222 062
e-mail: info@hknewzealand.com

E5691

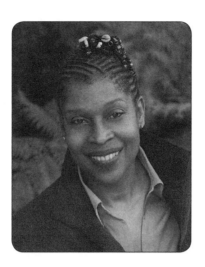

In memory of Antronette (Toni) K. Yancey, MD, MPH (1957–2013)

We dedicate this book to our colleague and friend, Toni Yancey. A pioneer in the field of physical activity and health, Toni brought energy and passion to a career that spanned research, teaching, and public health practice. Toni's commitment to social justice and promoting physical activity provided inspiration and leadership to a generation of public health professionals. She was an early advocate for promoting active lifestyles through evidence-based policy and environmental changes. She also touched the lives of children and adults through programs such as Instant Recess. She contributed to chapters 3, 22, and 24 of this book. We hope that this book embodies and honors her commitment to helping communities become more active.

Contents

Contributors

Eydie Abercrombie, MPH, CHES, PAPHS

Christiaan G. Abildso, PhD, MPH

Marice Ashe, JD, MPH

Birgitta L. Baker, PhD

Trever Ball, MS

Tara Ballard, CET, MES

Mary Balluff, MS, RD, LMNT

Adrian Bauman, PhD, FAFPHM

Bill Bellew, MPH, DPH

Megan Benedict, BS

Judy Berkowitz, PhD

Sarah Bilodeau, BSc

Terri Bopp, MPA

Ross C. Brownson, PhD

Sally Lawrence Bullock, MPH

Richard O. Burmeister, III, BAS

Rachelle Johnsson Chiang, MPH

Lesley Cottrell, PhD

Brian Coyle, MPH, PAPHS

Tiffany Creighton, MPH

Amber Dallman, MPH, PAPHS

Carolyn Dunn, PhD

Lillian Dunn, MPH

Eloise Elliott, PhD

Kelly R. Evenson, PhD

Amy A. Eyler, PhD, CHES

Guy Faulkner, PhD

Mark Fenton, MS

Melanie Goodell, MPH

Matthew Gurka, PhD

Melissa Hanson, BS, MBA

Peter Harnick, BA

Julie T. Harris, BS, MPA

Katherine Hebert, MCRP

Alison Herrmann, PhD

Ann-Hilary Heston, MPA

Marie-France Hivert, MD, MMSc

Nancy Huehnergarth

Marian Huhman, PhD

Lola Irvin, MED

Fik Isaac, MD, MPH, FACOEM

Portia Jackson, DrPH, MPH

Emily Jones, PhD

Elizabeth A. Joy, MD, MPH, FACSM

Haley Justice-Gardiner, MPH, CHES

Manel Kappagoda, JD, MPH

Abigail S. Katz, PhD

Suzanne P. Kelly, MS

Mary A. Kennedy, MS

Harold W. Kohl, III, PhD

Mariah Lafleur, MPH

Amy E. Latimer-Cheung, PhD

Kay Loughrey, MPH, MSM, RD, LDN

Jay Maddock, PhD

Andrew McGregor, MS

Grant McLean, BA(hons)

Whitney Meagher, MSW

Leslie A. Meehan, AICP

Andrew Mowen, PhD

Tinker D. Murray, PhD

Kelly Murumets

Jimmy Newkirk, Jr.

Donna C. Nichols, MSEd CHES

Cathy Nonas, MS, RD

Robert Ogilvie, PhD

Kara Peach, MA

Kerri R. Peterson, MS

Jill Pfankuch, MS, MCHES, PAPHS

Edward M. Phillips, MD

Martha M. Phillips, PhD, MPH, MBA

Amanda Philyaw-Perez, MPH

Katrina L. Piercy, PhD

Amber T. Porter, BS

Nicolaas P. Pronk, PhD

James M. Raczynski, PhD

Amy Rea, BA

Bill Reger-Nash, EdD

Lori Rhew, MA, PAPHS

Delia Roberts, PhD, FACSM

Candace Rutt, PhD

Robert Sallis, MD, FAAFP, FACSM

Sarah Samuels, DrPH

Andrew Scibelli, MBA, MA

Jennifer J. Selby, PE

Michael Seserman, MPH, RD

Ray Sharp, BA

Janet M. Shaw, PhD, FACSM

Trevor Shilton, MSc

Kindal A. Shores, PhD

Alice Silbanuz, BA

Stewart Sill, MS

Michael Skipper, AICP

Cathy Thomas, MAEd

Ian Thomas, PhD

Amber Vaughn MPH

Melinda Vertin, MSN, NP

Monica Hobbs Vinluan, JD

Sue Walker, PhD

Rhonda Walsh, MPH

Kristen Wan, MS

Dianne Ward, EdD

Jane D. Wargo, MA

Melicia C. Whitt-Glover, PhD

David Winfield, BA

Antronette (Toni) K. Yancey, MD, MPH

Joyce Young, MD, MPH

Sara Zimmerman, JD

Keith Zullig, PhD

Preface

Most Americans are not physically active at levels that will benefit their health, and many are completely inactive. A recent article in *The Lancet* described very low levels of physical activity, in the United States and worldwide, as a "pandemic, with far-reaching health, economic, environmental, and social consequences" (Kohl et al. 2012). In an effort to get Americans moving and reverse the tide of negative consequences, the U.S. Department of Health and Human Services released in 2008 the first federally approved guidelines: the 2008 *Physical Activity Guidelines for Americans*. The guidelines provide detailed recommendations on the types and amounts of physical activity that people should perform in order to gain important health benefits; specific guidance for youth, adults, older adults, and other demographic groups is provided. Clearly, issuing these guidelines was a major step forward in establishing physical activity as a public health priority in the United States.

Although the 2008 guidelines set the stage for increasing physical activity among Americans, guidelines alone are not enough to change people's health behaviors: The United States needed a clear and specific plan for helping all Americans become physically active. For that reason, representatives of leading health organizations and more than 300 physical activity experts began working in 2008 on the U.S. National Physical Activity Plan, which was released in 2010. The National Physical Activity Plan outlines a comprehensive strategy for changing America's communities in ways that will help many more people meet the Physical Activity Guidelines. The plan is organized around eight sectors of society (e.g.,

education, business and industry, health care) and includes more than 250 specific strategies and tactics. A key goal of the plan is to promote effective strategies to help Americans become more active, with an emphasis on policy and environmental approaches.

This book supports the implementation of the National Physical Activity Plan and showcases programs in all eight sectors that have implemented strategies outlined in the plan. By sharing examples and case studies of successful programs, the book serves as a resource for community organizations, schools, health care providers, nonprofits, political leaders, and other people and organizations that are working (or want to work) to promote physical activity.

We hope that readers will find the book to be both a useful resource for promoting physical activity and a tool for improving the quality of life in their communities. We also hope that readers will document and evaluate their own programs, so that they may be shared with others (possibly as case studies in future editions of this book*). Working together, we can move forward to achieve the vision established by the National Physical Activity Plan, that "one day, all Americans will be physically active, and they will live, work and play in environments that facilitate regular physical activity."

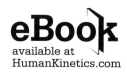
available at HumanKinetics.com

Reference

Kohl HW, Craig CL, Lambert EV, et al. 2012. The pandemic of physical inactivity: global action for public health. *Lancet* 380;294-305.

---

*Readers who wish to share with us information about their community programs to promote physical activity can visit www.physicalactivityplan.org/.

Acknowledgments

This book was produced to highlight the ways in which strategies included in the National Physical Activity Plan can be implemented. It was possible to produce this book only through the efforts of numerous talented and dedicated professionals. This project was undertaken as a partnership between the National Physical Activity Plan Alliance and the National Coalition for Promoting Physical Activity (NCPPA). NCPPA's support, provided through the contributions of Allison Topper-Kleinfelter and Cedric Bryant, was essential to the successful launch and completion of this project.

Central roles were played by the section editors, who provided wonderful leadership in identifying topics and authors who produced the core content of the book. The section editors, to a person, are exceptional professional leaders who have made enormous contributions to the National Physical Activity Plan and its goals. Clearly, this book could not have been produced without the contributions of the primary authors who committed their energies to explaining how the initiatives called for in the National Physical Activity Plan can be brought to life in our communities. The work of those authors gives us all hope that there is a more physically active population in America's future.

Finally, the contributions of three very special people must be recognized. Myles Schrag of Human Kinetics Publishers has been consistently and deeply supportive of this project from its inception. Janna Borden provided expert managerial support to the coeditors and section editors, and that support ensured that this project would come to a successful completion. Gaye Christmus, who edited the entire manuscript, is a remarkable professional whose expert editorial skills are reflected throughout this volume.

Sincerest thanks to all who made this book possible!

Education

Elizabeth Walker, MS

Association of State and Territorial Health Officials

The education setting provides an ideal environment in which to promote physical activity in preschoolers, children, and youth. With more than 54.9 million children under the age of 18 attending K-12 school in the United States (http://nces.ed.gov/fastfacts/display.asp?id = 65) and more than 60 percent of children attending early care and education settings (www.census.gov/prod/2010pubs/p70-121.pdf), implementing evidence-based and best practice programs and policies is critical to instilling physical activity habits early in life. The Community Guide, a publication of the Community Preventive Services Task Force, highlights a wide range of programs for which there is strong evidence of effectiveness at the school level, such as CATCH, Planet Health, and Spark Early Childhood; however, much has been written already about their results. This section focuses on how states and localities are able to implement evidence-based and best practice tools.

Chapters in this section highlight how policies are being implemented in Mississippi, North Carolina, Arkansas, West Virginia, and Tennessee. Agencies and organizations in these states are improving levels of physical activity by using evidence-based and best practices. Programs described in these chapters encourage physical activity throughout the day and, as the chapter authors highlight, improve children's focus and reduce sedentary behavior.

There is an increasing evidence base for improving physical activity in early care and education settings, and the case study of New York City described in chapter 4 highlights feasible programs as well as barriers to implementation in a challenging setting. Child care centers often have high staff turnover rates, employ teachers and paraprofessionals with varying education levels and ages, and serve children with a variety of cognitive and mobility ranges. The findings from this chapter describe the infrastructure, training, and resources that should be available to begin successful implementation.

CHAPTER 1

State Physical Activity Policies

Rachelle Johnsson Chiang, MPH
National Association of Chronic Disease Directors (NACDD)

Whitney Meagher, MSW
National Association of State Boards of Education (NASBE)

Kristen Wan, MS
Association of State and Territorial Health Officials (ASTHO)

NPAP Tactics and Strategies Used in This Program

Education Sector

STRATEGY 2: Develop and implement state and school district policies requiring school accountability for the quality and quantity of physical education and physical activity programs.

Regular physical activity is essential for children's health, including maintenance of a healthy weight. Beyond providing physical benefits, regular physical activity has been shown to improve academic achievement, cognitive functioning, and behavior in students (U.S. Department of Health and Human Services 2010). The school environment plays an important role in providing children and adolescents with daily, high-quality physical activity.

This chapter provides three examples of U.S. states that have taken the lead in enacting policies that support increased physical activity at school, at both the elementary and the secondary level. These states also have succeeded at perhaps the most challenging aspect of facilitating change through policy—implementation. The first example is Tennessee, which adopted a law requiring all local education agencies to integrate a minimum of 90 minutes of physical activity per week into the instructional school day for elementary and secondary students. The next example highlights Mississippi's experience adopting and implementing its Healthy Students Act, which included various requirements related to physical activity and physical education in the schools. The last example is from Texas, where a state mandate for physical activity enabled a local district to implement a strong physical activity program districtwide.

Although the states differed in their approach to policy making and implementation, all three succeeded in increasing physical activity in the school environment. They leveraged partnerships, involved stakeholders, engaged legislators, and allowed for flexibility, all while maintaining their objective of increasing physical activity in schools. Their experiences demonstrate that despite the challenges, it is possible to translate national recommendations into a strong physical activity policy that will work across an entire state and then implement the policy in a way that ensures success for individual districts and schools.

Evidence Base Used During Program Development

The 2008 Physical Activity Guidelines for Americans recommend that children engage in 60 minutes or more of physical activity daily, with most of the time focused on moderate to vigorous physical activity (U.S. Department of Health and Human Services 2008). However, a national study in the United States found that only 42 percent of children ages 6 to 11 meet the recommendation, and as students move into adolescence, their activity levels decrease dramatically, with just 12 percent of male and 3 percent of female adolescents achieving the recommendations (Troiano et al. 2008). Schools, which serve a large number of students for a substantial portion of each day, play a critical role in ensuring that children and adolescents are physically active. Consequently, the Institute of Medicine recommends that state and local education agencies and school districts ensure that all students in grades K-12 have adequate opportunities to engage in 60 minutes of physical activity per school day (Institute of Medicine 2012).

Research confirms that school-based physical activity interventions can increase the duration of physical activity, improve aerobic capacity, and reduce cholesterol in students (Dobbins et al. 2009). In addition, numerous studies have shown that students who are more physically active and fit achieve higher grades and test scores and have improved cognitive function, concentration during instruction time, classroom behavior, and attendance (Robert Wood Johnson Foundation 2007; U.S. Department of Health and Human Services 2010). Unfortunately, because of budgetary constraints and increased pressure for educators to improve standardized test scores, high-quality physical education and other physical activity programs are being reduced or eliminated completely by schools and school districts.

Recent research has demonstrated that state-level mandates such as the ones discussed in this chapter do make a difference, effectively increasing school-based physical activity opportunities for youth (Slater et al. 2012). Mandates for increased physical activity in school can help to ensure that children are getting the physical activity they need not only to lead healthier lives but also to achieve their fullest academic potential.

Tennessee: Physical Activity Law

In 2006, the General Assembly of the State of Tennessee passed the Physical Activity Law (T.C.A. § 49-6-1021) mandating that elementary and secondary schools provide a minimum of 90 minutes of physical activity each week for every student. In addition, to assist with the implementation of statewide Coordinated School Health (CSH), the CSH Expansion Law (T.C.A. § 49-6-1022) was passed, creating positions for a physical education specialist and a coordinator of school health within the Department of Education.

Program Description

In 2000, the Tennessee General Assembly passed the CSH Improvement Act (T.C.A. § 49-1-1002) to address the increasing rate of childhood obesity in the state. This made Tennessee the only state in the United States with a legislative mandate to implement the Centers for Disease Control and Prevention's CSH model; in addition, the State Board of Education created CSH standards and guidelines. The CSH Improvement Act provided state funding to start 10 CSH pilot sites. The aim of the CSH initiative was to improve the health of Tennessee public school children.

By 2005, key infrastructure for CSH was in place across the state and key stakeholders were actively engaged, including physical education teachers; the American Heart Association; the Tennessee Association for Health, Physical Education, Recreation and Dance; and other state and local school-related organizations. In 2006, with widespread support, the legislature passed the Physical Activity Law. This law required all local education agencies to integrate a minimum of 90 minutes of physical activity per week into the instructional school day for elementary and secondary students in all public and charter schools. Implementation of the Physical Activity Law began in 2007. This requirement aligns with Strategy 2 of the Education Sector of the National Physical Activity Plan: *Develop and implement state and school district policies requiring school accountability for the quantity and quality of physical education and physical activity programs.*

At the same time, the legislature passed the CSH Expansion Law, creating the position of school health coordinator within the Department of Education. Under the new law, each district was required to create an action plan to describe how it planned to incorporate the 90 minutes of physical activity into the school week and to outline the steps it would take. In addition, the Office of Coordinated School Health in the Department of Education and district CSH coordinators provided training, professional development, and ongoing refresher courses to ensure that all programs were being implemented with fidelity.

Implementation of the 90 minutes of physical activity has varied by school and by grade level. Because schools are allowed to choose what works best for their staff and students, Tennessee schools have seen success at all grade levels.

• Elementary school—Each school works closely with its CSH coordinator to integrate classroom-based physical activity (e.g., the

Take 10! program) into lesson plans. Schools provide daily physical education and morning activities and look for opportunities to add more recess time.

• Middle school—Schools use their exploratory class period for physical activity time by offering a variety of activities (e.g., walking, yoga, basketball) throughout the week. They also have implemented schoolwide activities and intramural programs.

• High school—Despite the challenges that exist with older students, schools are finding creative ways to integrate physical activity, such as having the entire school participate in a walking program, developing intramural programs, and creating team-building activities. CSH coordinators motivate students and staff through consistent messaging and reminders of the positive effects of physical activity on academic achievement.

Program Evaluation

The Physical Activity Law addressed a tactic of Strategy 2 of the Education Sector: *Develop and implement state and school district policies requiring school accountability for the quantity and quality of physical education and physical activity programs.*

In Tennessee, teacher, school, and district reporting has been built into the physical activity policy to increase compliance. Teachers are required to document the number of minutes of physical activity offered during each school day. A school is considered compliant with the law when every student receives a minimum of 90 minutes of physical activity per week. If students in one class or one grade do not receive the mandated minimum amount of physical activity, the school is considered noncompliant. Each school works closely with its district CSH coordinator to collect the necessary data, which is then reported to the State Department of Education Office of Coordinated School Health, to document compliance quarterly and at year-end. Coordinators also conduct occasional site visits to ensure compliance with the law.

All 95 counties in the state have accepted the law, and participation rates are high, with 78 percent of school systems reporting

Tennessee Physical Activity Handbook
Pre K - 12

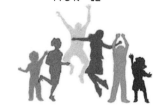

Healthy Students
Healthy Schools
Healthy Tennessee

Reprinted, by permission, from the Tennessee Department of Education.

implementation in 2010-2011 (98 percent at the elementary level, 90 percent middle school, and 69 percent high school). In 2011, the legislature passed a new amendment requiring the Office of Coordinated School Health to report to the General Assembly on the implementation of the 90-minute physical activity requirement for public schools. With the new amendment in place, it is expected that the number of schools reporting compliance will increase each year. School staff and students across the state have reported a positive response to the requirement and related activities.

The Physical Activity Law initially was passed to help combat childhood obesity (and there has been a 2 percent reduction since 2006), but other benefits have occurred. Truancy and the number of visits to school nurses have decreased, and student alertness, positive feelings, and positive behavior have increased. Most notably, academic performance has improved in all grade levels across the state, which has encouraged and motivated school districts to continue looking for opportunities to integrate physical activity throughout the school day.

Mississippi: The Healthy Students Act

In 2007, the Mississippi Legislature passed the Healthy Students Act, with the goal of strengthening physical activity, nutrition, and health education in public schools. The act included several mandates related to physical activity and physical education that align with Strategy 2 of the Education Sector of the National Physical Activity Plan: *Develop and implement state and school district policies requiring school accountability for the quantity and quality of physical education and physical activity programs.*

- A requirement of 150 minutes of activity-based instruction per week for grades K-8. A minimum of 50 of the minutes must be fulfilled with physical education.
- Creation of the position of physical activity coordinator at the Mississippi Department of Education, along with an appropriation of funds to support the position.

- A requirement that the physical activity coordinator monitor districts for implementation of the physical education curriculum.
- A requirement that school wellness plans promote increased physical activity.

Program Description

The Healthy Students Act was adopted in response to legislators' concern about the increasing problem of childhood obesity in Mississippi. In 2007, 44 percent of youth ages 10 to 17 were overweight or obese, the highest rate in the United States. During the policy-making process, there was broad consensus in the state legislature that action needed to be taken. However, many stakeholders were concerned about the burden that the policy would impose on schools. In addition to creating the physical activity and physical education requirement, the act required 45 minutes per week of health education instruction for grades K-8, bringing the total minutes required to 195 per week. In response to concerns about scheduling and not competing with other tested subject areas, the policy was written to provide schools flexibility in how the requirements could be met.

Implementation of the Healthy Students Act began in 2008. That year, the Mississippi State Board of Education adopted regulations (policy 4012) defining physical education, physical activity, and activity-based instruction and providing guidance to schools on implementation of the act. This included sample schedules for elementary, middle, and high school; recommendations for class size; guidance on waivers and exemptions; and a requirement for fitness testing in fifth grade and in one year of high school. The regulations also specified that physical education could be provided by a certified classroom teacher in grades K through 8 and a certified physical education teacher in grades 9 through 12. This last requirement aligns with one of the tactics of Strategy 1 regarding binding requirements for the employment of certified, highly qualified physical education teachers in accordance with U.S. national standards and guidelines.

The act addressed a tactic of Strategy 2: *Provide local, state and national funding to ensure that schools have the resources (e.g., facilities, equipment, appropriately trained staff) to provide high-quality physical education and activity programming. . . .* At the state level, the Office of Healthy Schools (OHS) in the Department of Education has worked diligently to provide technical assistance to districts and schools regarding implementation of the act. The state physical activity coordinator plays a key role in organizing training across the state. During the first year of implementation, the OHS provided more than 10 regional training programs to physical education teachers, classroom teachers, administrators, and other school staff. The initial trainings focused on the policy requirements, health education and physical education, and physical activity lessons and activities that could be integrated in the classroom. The OHS provides extensive resources to schools, including access to Health in Action (http://activities. healthyschoolsms.org/), a one-stop website that includes more than 1,400 web-based lesson plans for physical education, physical activity,

and health, with a primary focus on integrating movement into the classroom. The development of Health in Action was made possible by a local funder, the Bower Foundation.

From the beginning, partnerships with other state agencies and organizations have played a key role in the implementation of the Healthy Students Act. The Bower Foundation, Centers for Disease Control and Prevention, Center for Mississippi Health Policy, Robert Wood Johnson Foundation, National Association of State Boards of Education, National Association of Sport and Physical Education, Mississippi Community Education Center, Blue Cross Blue Shield Foundation of Mississippi, Mississippi School Boards Association, and others have lent their support through training, funding, and evaluation. These partnerships have ensured continued support, providing a mechanism for ongoing training, grants to districts, and valuable information regarding the impact of the act. During the 2010-2011 school year alone, OHS and partner organizations provided more than

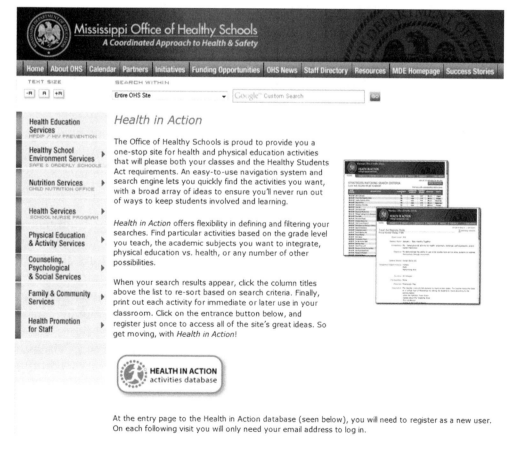

Reprinted, by permission, from The Bower Foundation.

25 training programs on integrating physical activity into the classroom.

Implementation of the physical education and physical activity requirements has varied significantly between schools, primarily because of the flexibility of the policy and state board regulations. At the elementary level, schools have modified schedules and trained classroom teachers in physical education in order to provide every student with 50 minutes of physical education per week. Schools have used recess, morning walks, and schoolwide activity breaks and have integrated physical activity into academic lessons to reach the additional 100 minutes of physical activity per week. At the middle school level, the challenges to implementation have been greater. Many schools have focused on boosting athletics and intramurals as a way to meet the requirements, because the state board regulations allow extracurricular activities such as sports, marching band, show choir, and cheerleading to be substituted for physical education. Other schools have chosen to build 150 minutes per week of physical education into the schedule or have adopted a schoolwide morning exercise routine.

Program Evaluation

One of the tactics for Strategy 2 is to develop and implement a measurement and reporting system to determine the progress of states toward meeting the strategy. In Mississippi, monitoring of the physical activity and physical education requirements is incorporated into the OHS coordinated school health monitoring tool. Each year, OHS selects schools in various districts to monitor for compliance. Each district is monitored once every five years. The primary focus of the OHS monitoring is not to chastise noncompliant schools but to assist them in implementation, and the monitoring tool helps to identify areas for improvement.

The Center for Mississippi Health Policy conducted a comprehensive two-year evaluation of the Healthy Students Act. The evaluation demonstrated significant increases in a variety of measures after the adoption of the Healthy Schools Act, including the percentage of students receiving a physical education curriculum, the percentage of schools adopting policies to promote physical activity, and the percentage of schools conducting fitness testing. The evaluation showed strong, continued support among lawmakers and district health and education officials for the Healthy Schools Act and motivation to continue improving on the groundwork that has been laid.

Texas: Physical Activity Law

Concerned about the growing problem of childhood obesity, the Texas Legislature amended the Education Code in 2005 to require 30 minutes of moderate to vigorous daily physical activity for students in grades K through 5. In 2009, the legislature strengthened the requirement by extending it into middle school, requiring 30 minutes of moderate to vigorous daily physical activity for students in grades 6 through 8 for at least four semesters.

Additional aspects of the laws include the following:

- Elementary schools unable to schedule daily physical activity may meet the requirement with 135 minutes of physical activity per week.

- Middle schools unable to schedule daily physical activity for four semesters may provide students with 225 minutes over the course of two weeks.

- School districts may provide an exemption for middle school students who participate in a structured extracurricular activity with a moderate to vigorous physical activity component.

- Local school health advisory councils are required to make recommendations to districts regarding the importance of daily recess.

- The physical activity requirement was accompanied by a requirement that schools conduct an annual fitness assessment for students in physical activity-based classes and activities in grades 3 through 12 using the Fitnessgram program.

The requirements of the policy are in alignment with Strategy 2 of the Education Sector of the National Physical Activity Plan: *Develop and implement state and school district policies requiring school accountability for the quantity and quality of physical education and physical activity programs.* In addition, the policy aligns with the tactic that requires school districts to annually collect, monitor, and track student-related fitness data, including body mass index.

The legislative process required flexibility. The legislation began as a physical education requirement, initially requiring 30 minutes of physical education every day with a qualified physical education instructor. This was eventually changed to a physical activity requirement to provide schools more flexibility in implementing the mandate. Under the final policy, schools are allowed to count the time that students are at recess and to integrate physical activity into other classroom activities, as long as the activity is structured and provides for moderate or vigorous intensity. In addition, the fitness assessment requirement began as an annual requirement for all students grades 3 through 12. However, in 2011, the requirement was changed to include only those students in physical education classes or their substitutes, rather than all students. The change was in response to economic concerns and a desire to minimize fiscal impact of an unfunded mandate on school districts. The biggest impact of this change is at the middle and high school levels, since most elementary students have physical education throughout the year.

Despite economic concerns and ever-increasing academic pressures, the Austin Independent School District has found innovative ways not only to fulfill the physical activity requirement but also to strengthen it with physical education. In fact, the program has been so successful that school board members have been reluctant to relax the school health policies, even in the face of economic concerns. Data collection has reinforced the belief that Austin has created a model program that has consistently led to improvements in students' Fitnessgram scores (table 1.1). By requiring that the program be a part of each school's strategic planning process, the school board has ensured that schools consistently look for ways to improve student health.

- At the elementary level, students have physical education classes every third day on a rotation with music and art class. This provides them physical education twice for the first two weeks of the rotation (90 minutes) and only once in the third week (45 minutes). Classroom teachers are required to provide physical activity to make up the additional 45 or 90 minutes each week.

- At the middle school level, most students take a year of physical education in sixth grade and one semester in seventh and eighth grades. The program is designed to teach lifelong enjoyment of exercise by focusing on lifetime recreation such as yoga, weightlifting, and circuit training. Students also learn about places in the community where they can participate in those activities.

- At the high school level, the physical education requirement for high school graduation was kept at 1.5 credits, even

Table 1.1 Austin Independent School District Fitnessgram Results and Goals: Percentage of Third to Twelfth Grade Students in the Healthy Fitness Zone

Year	Body mass index	Aerobic capacity	Curl-up	Push-up	Sit and reach	Trunk lift
2007-2008	60%	60%	85%	75%	73%	85%
2008-2009	60%	62%	85%	74%	73%	80%
2009-2010	60%	65%	86%	74%	74%	80%
2010-2011	61%	71%*	86%	75%	73%	82%

*New aerobic capacity criterion.

Reprinted, by permission, from Austin Independent School District. Available: www.austinschools.org/curriculum/pe_health/fitnessgram/dis_results.html

though it was reduced to 1 credit statewide in 2009. Students also are required to take 0.5 credits of health, even though the state dropped this requirement as well. This demonstrated the Austin School Board's commitment to student health.

An important tactic of Strategy 2 is to ensure that schools have the resources to provide high-quality physical education and physical activity programming. One way that elementary schools supplement the physical education curriculum with physical activity to reach the 135-minute requirement is by scheduling classroom physical activity time. All elementary schools are required to schedule 20-minute segments of structured physical activity time, called Working Out for Wellness (WOW). *Structured* means that the activity must be based on the physical education standards set by the Texas Education Agency. Each school determines how to schedule its WOW time each week. Classroom teachers are provided with a menu of grade-appropriate games that either are similar to what students do in physical education classes or have a component that reinforces classroom lessons (table 1.2). Health lessons are often integrated into WOW time.

Other initiatives include a pilot project for third grade students focused on training for leading WOW activities. By rotating through different roles, all students try positions such as leader, encourager, or referee. A few schools also have started marking playgrounds and sidewalks to encourage students to use their imaginations to create their own games. At these schools, students may play on giant times tables or jump rope down specially marked paths during recess. Administrators have provided teachers with training in using Brain Break activities as a way to provide students with short activity breaks throughout the day.

Lessons Learned

The experiences of these three states demonstrate that when it comes to policy making, you have to start somewhere. Tennessee and Texas started by creating statewide coordinated school health programs and later went on to pass physical activity policies. In Texas, officials initially proposed a physical education requirement, which was changed to a physical activity requirement during negotiations. It is important to be patient and strategic in the policy-making process and to recognize that there might be several unanticipated steps before reaching the ultimate goal. At the same time, it is also important to not wait until decisions are being made to become engaged in the legislative process. Advocates need to take the time to let the decision makers know their opinions. Most of decision makers will value knowing how current policies are being implemented and what changes should be considered. Being proactive and engaging with representatives during quieter times in the legislative cycle allows advocates to establish a relationship with decision makers and increases the likelihood that they will reach out to advocates when making key decisions.

It is essential to engage a diverse network to support and create a policy. Mississippi and Tennessee used a wide network of stakeholders at every stage of the policy-making process. Their experiences highlight how important it is, in the early stages of policy creation, to involve key advocates and the leaders of groups that will be involved with implementation (such as membership associations for teachers, principals, and other school staff and administrators). Support from stakeholders helps the process go more smoothly, and they can offer diverse perspectives and feedback that may help to create a stronger policy. Similarly, in each case discussed here, advocates cast a wide net and built strong relationships with school staff and others who were doing the work. There are many levels of authority between those who make policies and those who implement them. Teachers, principals, and others who work directly with students can be the most vocal critics or supporters of a new policy, and understanding this can make the difference between meeting minimum expectations and exceeding them. Strong relationships all the way down to the school level can help policy makers understand the impact of their decisions. Strong relationships all the way up to the state level can help schools feel supported and more willing to find ways to overcome challenges in order to comply.

Table 1.2 Working Out for Wellness (WOW) Activities for Third Grade

Math	Science	Social studies
Counting and exploring numbers Mingle, mingle Jump rope math It's in the cards	Healthy heart relay	**Citizenship and social studies skills** Independence Day tag Dice-R-Cise Texas symbols memory game American symbols memory game
Money and addition number sense Mingle, mingle Go for the dough	Mingle, mingle	Mingle, mingle
Adding and rounding Ocean exploration 1	**Properties of matter** Free radical attack!	**Celebrate Freedom Week; Constitution Day** Columbus tag Nineteenth amendment Historical figures memory game
Adding larger numbers Ready, set, show	**States of matter** Free radical attack!	**Community location and maps; chronology; analyzing sources** Vocabulary dribble
Subtraction Ocean exploration 1	**Force and motion** Do you know your facts?	**Diverse communities and influential heroes of society** historical figures memory game
Subtracting larger numbers Ready, set, show	**Vibration is a push and pull** Do you know your facts?	**How people learn about themselves** Countries memory game
Multiplication fact strategies (patterns) **Multiplication fact strategies (using unknown facts)** Ready, set, show Ocean exploration 1 Mingle, mingle Ice on the pond	**Magnets and magnetism** Cone crazy Magnetism	**Structure and responsibility of government; map skills** Fancy feet rock-paper-scissors (local) Fancy feet rock-paper-scissors (state) Fancy feet rock-paper-scissors (national)
Multiplication patterns and number sense Know your facts!	**Static electricity** Do you know your facts?	**National government and citizens** Fancy feet rock-paper-scissors (local) Fancy feet rock-paper-scissors (state) Fancy feet rock-paper-scissors (national)
Division meanings and facts Ocean exploration 1 Do you know your facts?	**Current electricity** Do you know your facts?	**Lewis and Clark** Historical figures memory game

(continued)

Table 1.2 *(continued)*

Math	Science	Social studies
Fraction concepts Crows and cranes Ocean exploration 1 Mingle, mingle The fraction fold	**Conductors and insulators** Vocabulary dribble	**Women's history; primary resources** Historical figures memory game
Whole numbers and fractions on the number line Number scramble	**The planets** Solar system scramble Vocabulary dribble	**Cinco de Mayo** Mexico's victory
Congruency and symmetry Jump rope math	**Sun's effect on earth's water and weather** Do you know your facts?	
Estimating and measuring length Air math Jump rope math	**Sun's effect on planet earth** Do you know your facts?	
Volume, capacity, weight, and mass Time and temperature Crows and cranes	**Structures of plants** Vocabulary dribble	
Time and temperature data, graphs, and probability Crows and cranes Smarty pants	**Germination of seeds** Vocabulary dribble	
	Life cycles Fish gobbler/shark attack Vocabulary dribble	
	Habitats Fish gobbler/shark attack Oyster tag	
	Food chains and webs Fish gobbler/shark attack Oyster tag Predator prey	

WOW games should last 15 to 20 minutes. Objectives are in bold type.

Reprinted, by permission, from Austin Independent School District. Available: www.austinschools.org/curriculum/pe_health/fitnessgram/dis_results.html

Mississippi leveraged the power of data to help drive policy-related decision making. Policy makers were motivated to take action when they were shown, through data, that there was a need to strengthen school health policies. In addition, they kept data central to the policy-making process and used it as the basis for making decisions. Requiring schools to collect and publicly share data from year to year can demonstrate the impact of policies and strengthen arguments for their existence in the face of difficult circumstances. Policymakers also understood the need to think creatively about framing the link between physical activity and academic achievement. It can be challenging to get school administrators and policy makers to understand that healthy, more physically active students are better learners.

This makes it all the more important to use the powerful research available to focus on the "wins" for the educators: Healthy students attend school more often, are better able to pay attention in class, and perform better on achievement tests.

In the area of policy implementation, Tennessee and Mississippi helped to ensure success by creating positions in the state departments of education that were responsible, in part, for implementation and monitoring of the policy. The Austin Independent School District hired new staff members to help ensure compliance with the state's coordinated school health laws. Implementation-focused employees are important to the long-term sustainability of a policy because they are able to collect and disseminate data to support the program, provide training and technical assistance, and create and disseminate resources. In addition, in all three cases discussed in this chapter, school and district-level staff received support through training and resources. An intensive training schedule may be needed at the initial stages of policy implementation. But after everyone is more comfortable with a policy and has created a routine for its implementation, web-based resources and shorter refresher courses can be adequate to support those who are implementing a policy.

The experiences of these states demonstrate the importance of seeking additional resources and partners to strengthen implementation, monitoring, and evaluation. Private funders who view increasing physical activity among youth as a priority can often provide additional resources to strengthen professional development and training efforts. Partnerships with universities can provide expertise and resources for monitoring and evaluation. The cases discussed here highlight the importance of approaching each district and school with an open mind, a flexible agenda, and a positive approach. Every district or school will start the policy implementation process in a different place and with a different set of supports and obstacles. A universally successful approach is to consider school officials as partners and find ways to assist them rather than tell them how things need to be done.

The adoption and implementation of physical activity policy in schools is a challenging endeavor that can have a powerful, positive impact on students and the school environment. That said, significant policy changes often take a long time, and it can be hard to maintain motivation throughout the process. Recognizing the smaller victories along the way can help provide energy and encouragement to continue the process. It is also important to remember why policy is important. Establishing a baseline ensures that every school provides some opportunity for physical activity. Even if sufficient resources are not provided to implement the policy, pointing to its existence can encourage some reluctant school administrators to comply. In the end, a strong physical activity policy serves to lay a foundation. Some schools will far exceed that foundation, and others will just meet the minimum expectations. But without the policy, far fewer schools would ever have endeavored on their own to make physical activity an important part of the school day.

Summary

The experiences of Tennessee, Mississippi, and Texas provide excellent examples of successful policy creation and implementation related to increasing physical activity in the schools. They also provide valuable lessons about the process, challenges, and barriers. Recognizing the key actions that were critical to accomplishing policy change in these states can help others replicate their success in ways that are suitable to their own states and communities.

Additional Reading and Resources

Active Living Research. 2009. Active education: Physical education, physical activity and academic performance. http://activelivingresearch.org/files/ALR_Brief_ActiveEducation_Summer2009.pdf.

Center for Mississippi Health Policy. 2011. Year two report: Assessing the impact of the Mississippi Healthy Students Act. www.rwjf.org/content/dam/farm/reports/evaluations/2011/rwjf402274.

Institute of Medicine. 2012. Accelerating progress in obesity prevention: Solving the weight of the nation. www.iom.edu/Reports/2012/Accelerating-Progress-in-Obesity-Prevention.aspx.

Kelder, S.H., A.S. Springer, C.S. Barroso, C.L. Smith, E. Sanchez, N. Ranjit, and D.M. Hoelscher. 2009. Implementation of Senate Bill 19 to increase physical activity in elementary schools. *J. Public Health Policy* 30(1 Suppl.):S221-47.

Robert Wood Johnson Foundation. 2007. Active education: physical education, physical activity and academic performance. www.rwjf.org/content/dam/web-assets/2007/11/active-education.

Tennessee Department of Education. 2010. Tennessee coordinated school health 2008-09: Executive summary. http://campaignforhealthykids.org/resources/TennesseeCoordinatedSchoolHealthExecutiveSummary20082009%20(2).pdf.

U.S. Department of Health and Human Services. 2010. The association between school-based physical activity, including physical education, and academic performance. www.cdc.gov/healthyyouth/health_and_academics/pdf/pa-pe_paper.pdf.

References

Dobbins, M., K. DeCorby, P. Robeson, H. Husson, and D. Tirilis. 2009. School-based physical activity programs for promoting physical activity and fitness in children and adolescents aged 6-18. *Cochrane Database Syst. Rev.* (1):CD007651.

Institute of Medicine. 2012. Accelerating progress in obesity prevention: Solving the weight of the nation. www.iom.edu/Reports/2012/Accelerating-Progress-in-Obesity-Prevention.aspx.

Robert Wood Johnson Foundation. 2007. Active education: Physical education, physical activity and academic performance. www.rwjf.org/content/dam/web-assets/2007/11/active-education.

Slater, S.J., L. Nicholson, J. Chiriqui, L. Turner, and F. Chaloupka. 2012. The impact of state laws and district policies on physical education and recess practices in a nationally representative sample of US public elementary schools. *Arch. Pediatr. Adolesc. Med.* 166(4):311-6.

Troiano, R., et al. 2008. Physical activity measured in the United States by accelerometer. *Med. Sci. Sports Exerc.* 40(1):181-8.

U.S. Department of Health and Human Services. 2008. Physical activity guidelines for Americans. www.health.gov/paguidelines/.

U.S. Department of Health and Human Services. 2010. The association between school-based physical activity, including physical education, and academic performance. www.cdc.gov/healthyyouth/health_and_academics/pdf/pa-pe_paper.pdf.

CHAPTER 2

Public School Physical Activity Legislative Policy Initiatives
What We Have Learned

Martha M. Phillips, PhD, MPH, MBA
Fay W. Boozman College of Public Health, University of Arkansas for Medical Sciences

Amanda Philyaw-Perez, MPH
Fay W. Boozman College of Public Health, University of Arkansas for Medical Sciences

Melanie Goodell, MPH
Fay W. Boozman College of Public Health, University of Arkansas for Medical Sciences

James M. Raczynski, PhD
Fay W. Boozman College of Public Health, University of Arkansas for Medical Sciences

NPAP Tactics and Strategies Used in This Program

Education Sector

STRATEGY 1: Provide access to and opportunities for high-quality, comprehensive physical activity programs, anchored by physical education, in Pre-kindergarten through grade 12 educational settings. Ensure that the programs are physically active, inclusive, safe, and developmentally and culturally appropriate.

STRATEGY 2: Develop and implement state and school district policies requiring school accountability for the quality and quantity of physical education and physical activity programs.

As noted elsewhere in this volume, the importance of physical activity (PA) to healthy growth and development in childhood is well established (Borms 1986; Chakravarthy and Booth 2004; Mein and Oseid 1982; Tomporowski et al. 2008). Most children spend a large portion of their waking hours in schools; thus, schools are an important venue for promoting PA, by teaching children about the relationship between PA and health and by providing opportunities for them to be physically active during the school day (Story et al. 2009). Those who guide schools in our communities (i.e., state and federal policy makers, state and local boards of education, state departments of education, school district superintendents, and principals) can promote children's PA in two primary ways: first, by providing programs, including physical education (PE), intramural and extramural sports, and PA programs before and after school, and second, by implementing policies that modify school PA practices and environments. A wide range of options exist for school-based PA policy interventions, including requiring (1) adequate time spent in PE; (2) adequate time spent in physical activity during PE classes;

Acknowledgments: This work was supported by the Robert Wood Johnson Foundation (grant numbers 30930, 51737, 60284, 61551). The preparation of this chapter has also been supported by the Arkansas Prevention Research Center (U48 DP001943). The authors acknowledge the assistance of Sherri Morris, Heather Johnston, Blake Talbot, Jennifer Montgomery, and Jada Walker in the preparation of this chapter.

(3) PE teacher certification; (4) staff development for PE teachers; (5) appropriate student to teacher ratios in PE classes; (6) time for physical activity outside of formal PE classes; and (7) modifications to school environments to promote physical activity.

This chapter explores the implementation of school policies designed to enhance school-based PA opportunities, focusing on the content and effect of federal and state efforts to influence school policies and lessons learned from those efforts. Legislative initiatives in three states—Arkansas, West Virginia, and Mississippi—are presented as examples of the efforts, challenges, and outcomes associated with efforts to change school policies to promote physical activity.

Federal Policy Initiatives

Control of schools is largely a state function, and thus most school policy initiatives arise from state legislatures and departments of education rather than federal initiatives. However, the Child Nutrition and WIC Reauthorization Act of 2004 included a requirement that all local education agencies participating in the federal school meals programs establish local wellness policies by the 2006-2007 school year, with the goal of improving PA and nutrition in schools. These policies were to be developed and implemented by local school wellness committees, with documented involvement of parents, students, school representatives, and members of the public. These requirements were continued in the most recent reauthorization, the Healthy, Hunger-Free Kids Act of 2010.

Unfortunately, research has indicated that PA policies promulgated by these committees have been neither strong nor comprehensive. A review of a national sample of district policies for the 2006-2007 and 2007-2008 school years, completed by Chriqui and associates (2009), found that the policies frequently were weak and fragmented and failed to include adequate plans for implementation and evaluation. The majority of policies did not meet evidence-based recommendations for PA (e.g., daily recess) or PE (e.g., time devoted to moderate to vigorous activity) (Chriqui et al. 2009). Further, by instituting policies that required a specific amount of time for PA but not PE, a number of school districts actually made it harder for schools to meet expert recommendations for time spent in PE (Chriqui et al. 2009). State-based reviews of district policies have yielded similar results. In general, state evaluators have found policies to be framed as recommendations rather than requirements (Metos and Nanney 2007; Molaison et al. 2011; Probart et al. 2008) and to lack specification and rigor in implementation and evaluation of their impact (Metos and Nanney 2007; Probart et al. 2008). Further, it has been reported that although district plans generally meet the minimum requirements to include goals related to both nutrition and PA, most address nutrition more extensively and comprehensively than PA (Brener et al. 2011; Harris and Bradlyn 2009).

State Legislative Initiatives

A second avenue for influencing schools is through policy made by state legislative bodies, a popular approach in the past decade. Boehmer and colleagues (2007) identified more than 1,000 pieces of legislation, including bills and resolutions, introduced in the 50 states during three years, 2003 through 2005. Approximately 25 percent of those legislative initiatives involved PA or PE policy changes in schools, and 28 percent addressed safe routes to schools (Boehmer et al. 2007). A similar review of legislative initiatives related specifically to PE identified approximately 780 bills introduced between 2001 and 2007, of which only 21 percent were enacted (Eyler et al. 2010). Eight-five percent of PE bills enacted contained strong language requiring action; however, only 23 percent were funded mandates and only 30 percent included a requirement that the bill's impact be evaluated (Eyler et al. 2010).

Program Description

Three state legislative approaches to reduce childhood obesity, in Arkansas, West Virginia, and Mississippi, are noteworthy in that they mandated multicomponent policy approaches to affect both nutrition and PA. In all three cases, the Robert Wood Johnson Foundation funded university-based research teams to evaluate the process, impact, and outcomes associated with the legislation.

Arkansas: Act 1220 of 2003 to Combat Childhood Obesity

In 2003, the Arkansas General Assembly enacted Arkansas Act 1220 to combat childhood obesity. Heralded as one of the earliest comprehensive approaches to reducing childhood obesity, this legislation contained only two specific immediate mandates for schools: (1) restricting student access to vending machines during the school day in elementary schools; and (2) measuring body mass index (BMI) for all public school students, with reports sent to parents. The act went further, however, to (1) establish a statewide panel of experts and advocates, the Child Health Advisory Committee, to make recommendations regarding nutrition, PA, and PE policies and standards for schools in a variety of areas; (2) require that the Department of Health hire health promotion specialists to assist schools; (3) require schools to report publicly the revenues and expenditures from competitive food and beverage contracts; and (4) require that each school district convene a nutrition and PA advisory committee to assist in the development of local policies for implementing nutrition and PA standards.

The rules and regulations promulgated by the State Board of Education, based on the recommendations made by the Child Health Advisory Committee, modified substantially the existing nutrition and PE and PA policies and practices required of schools. In terms of PE and PA, the new rules required that public schools establish strategies to achieve 30 minutes of PA daily for all students, kindergarten through 12th grade, and begin to implement those strategies before the end of the 2005-2006 school year. Further, the rules specified that (1) a maximum student to adult ratio of 30:1 would be maintained in grades kindergarten through 6, beginning in 2006-2007; (2) all students would receive 150 minutes of PA per week, with 60 minutes of that time being PE in grades kindergarten through 6, beginning in 2007-2008; (3) each school district would employ at least one certified PE teacher for each 500 students, beginning in 2008-2009; and (4) all personnel teaching PE in grades kindergarten through 12 would be certified to teach PE by the 2012-2013 school year.

West Virginia: The Healthy Lifestyles Act

In 2005, West Virginia passed the Healthy Lifestyles Act (HB 2816), which was more prescriptive than Arkansas Act 1220, in that the Healthy Lifestyles Act (1) restricted the sale of soft drinks during the school day in elementary and middle schools; (2) restricted beverage sales to water, 100 percent fruit and vegetable juices, low-fat milk, and juice beverages with at least 20 percent juice; (3) allowed the sale of soft drinks outside of meal periods if the local board of education specifically permitted it and if 50 percent of the beverage offerings were healthy beverages; (4) required a minimum time for PE instruction for all elementary students (90 minutes per week) and middle school students (2,700 minutes per year); (5) required one PE course credit for high school graduation; (6) required that high school students be offered instruction in physical activities likely to be maintained over one's lifetime; (7) required fitness testing and reporting for students in fourth through eighth grades and in the required high school course; (8) required the collection of BMI data for a scientifically drawn sample of students and reporting of findings to state agencies; (9) required that schools teach the importance of healthy eating and PA to maintain a healthy weight; and (10) required that health education assessment be conducted to measure student knowledge and program effectiveness. The State Department of Education responded by promulgating rules and regulations to operationalize the mandates, for example, specifying the use of Fitnessgram for fitness testing and the Health Education Assessment Project to measure knowledge gained in health education classes. Implementation of the school-based components of the Healthy Lifestyles Act began in August 2006.

Mississippi: The Healthy Students Act

In 2007, the Mississippi legislature passed the Mississippi Healthy Students Act (SB 2369) to improve nutrition, PA, and health education in public schools, with the goal of reducing childhood obesity. Described in more detail elsewhere in this volume, the act required the development of local school wellness plans, beginning with the 2008-2009 school year, to promote increased PA, healthy eating habits, and tobacco and drug abstinence. It further directed the State Board of Education to adopt regulations addressing school nutrition and specified the appointment of a committee to advise the board on the development of these rules and regulations. The bill also appropriated state funds for the hiring of a PA coordinator within the state's Department of Education. The required rules and regulations regarding PE and health education adopted by the State Board of Education went into effect in fall 2008.

Program Evaluation

The Arkansas evaluation was initially funded in 2004 to assess baseline policy levels prior to policy implementation; annual data collection concluded in spring 2012. In West Virginia, the evaluation spanned two consecutive years, with data collected in the 2007-2008 and 2008-2009 school years. The five-year Mississippi evaluation began in 2007 and concluded in 2012. Methods used in each of these comprehensive evaluations have been described in detail elsewhere (Harris and Bradlyn 2009; Phillips et al. 2010; Center for Mississippi Health Policy 2010). Each evaluation included surveys of school principals and school district superintendents, interviews with parents of students attending the state's public schools, and surveys or interviews of other key stakeholders (e.g., school nurses, PE teachers, health care providers, policy makers, and others). Although the research questions were state-specific, addressing the key issues of relevance to each state's stakeholders and the nuances of each state's law, there was substantial overlap across the three states in methods and variables, reflecting the common features of the three pieces of legislation and associated rules and regulations.

Lessons Learned

The three evaluations found that efforts to increase PA and PE for students received widespread endorsement by parents and school personnel. PE teachers (Harris and Bradlyn 2009), principals (Harris and Bradlyn 2009), and parents (Harris and Bradlyn 2009; Phillips et al. 2010; Center for Mississippi Health Policy 2010) in the three states reported that they wanted students to have more, even daily, opportunities to be physically active in school. However, in general, the state-based evaluations indicated that schools have had difficulty implementing the mandated increases in time devoted to PE and PA. The West Virginia researchers found, for example, that even though 85 percent of the principals viewed the PE time mandates favorably after two years of implementation, 31 percent of elementary schools and 8 percent of middle schools did not meet the specified requirements (Health Research Center 2005). In Arkansas, after rules and regulations specified increased PE time in all grades, school personnel appealed to the Arkansas legislature to intervene. Thus, in the 2007 legislative session, the Arkansas Department of Education rules were modified by law to specify that elementary students would receive 60 minutes of PE and 90 minutes of PA each week, middle school students would receive 60 minutes of PE instruction with no additional requirement for PA, and high school students would have no requirement for PA beyond the 1/2 unit of PE required for graduation (Phillips et al. 2008).

Many Arkansas schools have, however, voluntarily changed other PE and PA policies and practices over time. For example, in 2010, 70 percent of school districts reported that they required regularly scheduled recess in elementary schools, compared with only 58 percent in 2004. Other policies established by schools or school districts included the following (Phillips et al. 2011):

- Requiring regular assessment of student fitness (44 percent of schools in 2010, up from 26 percent at baseline in 2004)

- Forbidding the use of PA as punishment in PE classes (83 percent of schools, compared with 77 percent in 2004)
- Forbidding the punishment of bad behavior by excluding students from PE (93 percent, up from 84 percent in 2004) or recess (54 percent, up from 42 percent in 2004)
- Requiring that lifetime physical activity be included in PE instruction in elementary schools (55 percent, compared with 39 percent in 2004)
- Requiring that newly hired PE teachers in elementary schools be certified in PE (89 percent, up from only 69 percent in 2004)

Barriers to PA and PE Policy Change

Although national, state, and local legislative panels have focused on the need for comprehensive obesity reduction efforts, it appears that schools are more likely to make changes to nutrition policies and practices than to PA and PE policies (Harris and Bradlyn 2009; Phillips et al. 2010; Center for Mississippi Health Policy 2010). This difference in policy implementation is likely related to the real and perceived barriers to PA and PE policy change. For example, principals, superintendents, and PE teachers interviewed in Arkansas and West Virginia cited (1) lack of adequate facilities, with PE often taught in multiuse rooms that also served as cafeterias and music rooms; (2) lack of resources, with finances insufficient to hire enough certified teachers to serve all schools and reduce PE class sizes; and (3) lack of time, given substantial pressures placed on schools to focus on academic instruction and improve test scores. Belansky and colleagues (2009), investigating barriers to PA and PE policy change in Colorado schools, noted a failure to ensure accountability as a potential barrier to the effectiveness of policy initiatives.

Specific barriers arise when attempts are made to implement certain policies. For example, the likelihood that schools will implement joint use agreements that allow community groups to use school facilities outside of the school day may be reduced by concerns over liability and costs associated with security and staffing the facilities after school hours (Phillips et al. 2010). Similarly, walking and cycling to school have been affected by school attendance zoning (e.g., school choice, school consolidations, busing) and may be reduced by early school start times, lack of crossing guards, lack of storage for coats and helmets, policies requiring bikers and walkers to leave after car riders, and routing of cars and buses in drop-off and pick-up zones (Ahlport et al. 2008).

Impact on PA Among Students and Their Families

The impact of the changes to school PA and PE policies and practices on PA among students and their families appears to have been minimal. For example, in Arkansas, no significant changes in the frequency of child or adolescent physical activity (e.g., walking, playing games with family or friends, playing sports) have been noted since 2004 (Phillips et al. 2011). A change in parental appreciation for physical activity has been noted, however. Although the proportion of parents who indicated that they were trying to limit their children's sedentary activity (i.e., screen time) did not change significantly over time (73 percent in 2004; 71 percent in 2010), the reason for making that effort did change. The percentage of parents reporting that they wanted to give more time for physical activity rose steadily from 33 percent at baseline (in 2004) to a high of 49 percent in 2009 (Phillips et al. 2011). Similarly, the percentage of parents who required their children to stay inside after school rather than play outside dropped from a high of 11 percent at baseline to a low of 7 percent in 2009, and the percentage of parents who reported enrolling their children in sports or exercise activities rose from 42 percent in 2004 to a high of 53 percent in 2009 (Phillips et al. 2011).

Linkage to the National Physical Activity Plan

These three statewide school policy initiatives support the National Physical Activity Plan's Education Sector Strategies 1 and 2. Implementation of Strategy 1, which pertains to providing access to high-quality PA and PE programs at all grade levels from prekindergarten to grade 12, is particularly reflected in Mississippi's efforts to provide guidance and training for teachers in state-of-the art, age-appropriate physical activities and in how to incorporate PA into the academic curriculum. All three states addressed Strategy 2, which is concerned with developing and implementing state and district policies regarding the quality and quantity of PA and PE programs. The states achieved this by addressing class size, certification of teachers providing PE instruction, quantity of time to be allotted to PA and PE at various grade levels, and fitness or BMI testing.

Summary

Experts and policy makers recognize the opportunity to address childhood obesity by modifying school policies and environments related to PA and PE. Evaluations of recent legislative initiatives, however, suggest that even popularly supported changes are difficult for school districts and schools to implement. Barriers to change, particularly financial barriers and scheduling issues, must be addressed if such policy changes are to be implemented effectively. Further, although changes to school policies and practices related to PA and PE may increase PA during the school day, data suggest that those changes alone may not translate into behavior change for students and families at home. Efforts to change PA and PE policies in schools must be combined with efforts to engage families in behavior change for maximum effect and benefit on child health.

References

Ahlport, K.N., L. Linnan, A. Vaughn, K.R. Evenson, and D.S. Ward. 2008. Barriers to and facilitators of walking and bicycling to school: Formative results from the non-motorized travel study. *Health Educ. Behav.* 35(2):221-44.

Belansky, E.S., N. Cutforth, E. Delong, et al. 2009. Early impact of the federally mandated Local Wellness Policy on physical activity in rural, low-income elementary schools in Colorado. *J. Public Health Policy.* 30(Suppl. 1):S141-60.

Boehmer, T.K., R.C. Brownson, D. Haire-Joshu, and M.L. Dreisinger. 2007. Patterns of childhood obesity prevention legislation in the United States. *Prev. Chronic Dis.* 4(3):A56.

Borms, J. 1986. Children and exercise: An overview. *J. Sports Sci.* 4:3-20.

Brener, N.D., J.F. Chriqui, T.P. O'Toole, M.B. Schwartz, and T. McManus. 2011. Establishing a baseline measure of school wellness-related policies implemented in a nationally representative sample of school districts. *J. Am. Diet. Assoc.* 111(6):894-901.

Center for Mississippi Health Policy. 2010. *Year One— Assessing the Impact of the Mississippi Healthy Students Act.* Center for Mississippi Health Policy, Jackson, MS.

Chakravarthy, M., and F. Booth. 2004. Eating, exercise and "thrifty" genotypes: Connecting the dots toward an evolutionary understanding of modern chronic diseases. *J. Appl. Physiol.* 96:3-10.

Chriqui, J., L. Schneider, F. Chaloupka, K. Ide, and O. Pugach. 2009. *Local Wellness Policies: Assessing School District Strategies for Improving Children's Health. School Years 2006-07 and 2007-08.* Chicago: Bridging the Gap, Health Policy Center, Institute for Health Research and Policy, University of Illinois at Chicago.

Child Nutrition and WIC Authorization Act of 2004 [S. 2507]. www.govtrack.us/congress/bill.xpd?bill = s108-2507.

Eyler, A.A., R.C. Brownson, S.A. Aytur, et al. 2010. Examination of trends and evidence-based elements in state physical education legislation: a content analysis. *J. Sch. Health.* 80(7):326-32.

Harris, C., and A. Bradlyn. 2009. *West Virginia Healthy Lifestyles Act: Year One Evaluation Report.* Morgantown, WV: West Virginia University.

Health Research Center. 2010. *Year Two Evaluation West Virginia Healthy Lifestyles Act of 2005 Executive Summary.* West Virginia University, Morgantown, West Virginia

Healthy, Hunger-Free Kids Act of 2010 [S. 3307]. www.govtrack.us/congress/billtext.xpd?bill = s111-3307.

Mein, J., and S. Oseid. 1982. Physical activity in children and adolescents in relation to growth and development. *Scand. J. Soc. Med.* 9(Suppl. 2):121-34.

Metos, J., and M.S. Nanney. 2007. The strength of school wellness policies: One state's experience. *J. School Health* 77(7):367.

Molaison, E.F., S. Howie, J. Kolbo, K. Rushing, L. Zhang, and M. Hanes. 2011. Comparison of the local wellness policy implementation between 2006 and 2008. *J. Child Nutr. Manag.* 35(1):9.

Phillips, M., J. Raczynski, J. Walker, Act 1220 Evaluation Team. 2008. *Year Four Evaluation: Arkansas Act 1220 of 2003 to Combat Childhood Obesity.* Little Rock, AR: Fay W. Boozman College of Public Health, University of Arkansas for Medical Sciences.

Phillips M, Raczynski J, Walker J, Act 1220 Evaluation Team. 2010. *Year Six: Evaluation: Act 1220 of 2003 of Arkansas to Combat Childhood Obesity.* Little Rock, AR: University of Arkansas for Medical Sciences.

Phillips, M., J. Raczynski, J. Walker J, Act 1220 Evaluation Team. 2011. *Year Seven: Evaluation: Act 1220 of 2003 of Arkansas to Combat Childhood Obesity.* Little Rock, AR: Fay W. Boozman College of Public Health, University of Arkansas for Medical Sciences.

Probart, C., E. McDonnell, J.E. Weirich, L. Schilling, and V. Fekete. 2008. Statewide assessment of local wellness policies in Pennsylvania public school districts. *J. Am. Diet. Assoc.* 108(9):1497-1502.

Story, M., M.S. Nanney, and M.B. Schwartz. 2009. Schools and obesity prevention: creating school environments and policies to promote healthy eating and physical activity. *Milbank Q.* 87(1):71-100.

Tomporowski, P., C. Davis, P. Miller, and J. Naglieri. 2008. Exercise and children's intelligence, cognition, and academic achievement. *Educ. Psychol. Rev.* 20:111-31.

CHAPTER 3

Role of Recess and Physical Activity Breaks During the School Day

Antronette K. (Toni) Yancey, MD, MPH
*UCLA Kaiser Permanente
Center for Health Equity*

Amber T. Porter, BS
Gramercy Research Group

Melicia C. Whitt-Glover, PhD
Gramercy Research Group

Alison Herrmann, PhD
*UCLA Kaiser Permanente
Center for Health Equity*

NPAP Tactics and Strategies Used in This Program

Education Sector

STRATEGY 1: Provide access to and opportunities for high-quality, comprehensive physical activity programs, anchored by physical education, in Prekindergarten through grade 12 educational settings. Ensure that the programs are physically active, inclusive, safe, and developmentally and culturally appropriate.

STRATEGY 2: Develop and implement state and school district policies requiring school accountability for the quality and quantity of physical education and physical activity programs.

STRATEGY 3: Develop partnerships with other sectors for the purpose of linking youth with physical activity opportunities in schools and communities.

Research has established the contribution of regular physical activity to key health outcomes, such as obesity prevention and musculoskeletal development, and to educational outcomes, such as attentiveness, cognitive processing, discipline, and academic performance (USDHHS 2008). However, American children's physical activity levels have been declining during the past several decades (Knuth and Hallal 2009; Sturm 2005; Sturm 2008) and many children and youth are not active at recommended levels. Young people spend approximately half of their waking hours in school settings, and recent studies have demonstrated a positive contribution of school-based physical activity to children's overall physical activity levels and to weight management (Fernandes and Sturm 2011; Jackson et al. 2010; Wu et al. 2011). Hence, schools are prime targets for interventions that increase children's physical activity levels (Gonzalez-Suarez et al. 2009; Naylor and McKay 2009). A Cochrane review of school-based physical activity programs showed that such interventions have resulted in increased physical activity, decreased television viewing time, and improved aerobic capacity and blood cholesterol levels (Dobbins et al. 2009).

Physical activity during the school day has traditionally come in the form of recess, a supervised but unstructured time for free play, imagination, movement, stress relief, enjoyment, rest, and socialization, with demonstrated physical, social, emotional, cognitive, and organizational benefits (Beighle 2012; Ramstetter et al. 2010). However, because of an increased emphasis on standardized testing, time allotted to recess during the elementary school day is decreasing (Lee et al. 2007; Pressler 2006; UCLA and

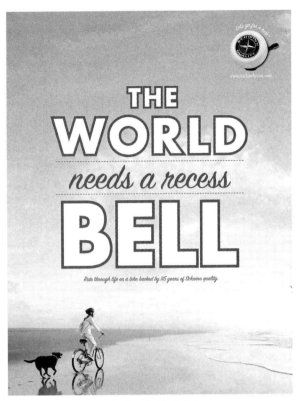

Schwinn® is used by permission from Pacific Cycle Inc.

Samuels and Associates 2007). (Time devoted to physical education is decreasing too, for the same reason; Henley et al. 2007; McKenzie and Kahan 2008). Some schools have banned traditional vigorous recess activities such as playing tag, climbing monkey bars, and running, because of fear of liability for injury (e.g., Bazar 2006), despite case law that makes this unlikely (Spengler et al. 2010).

Ridgers and colleagues (2011) observed significant decreases in recess and lunchtime moderate and vigorous physical activity, with commensurate increases in sedentary time, during the periods 2001-2006 and 2003-2008; these changes were magnified in older children. Similarly, data from the 2003-2004 National Health and Nutrition Examination Survey (NHANES) demonstrated that although approximately half (40-50 percent) of 6- to 11-year-old youth were active at levels that met current Centers for Disease Control and Prevention (CDC) recommendations (i.e., more than 60 minutes of at least moderate-intensity physical activity on five or more days per week), only 6 to 11 percent of 12- to 15-year-old youth achieved this level of activity (Whitt-Glover et al. 2009). In addi-

tion, 6- to 11-year-olds spend an average of 5.9 hours per day in sedentary behaviors, whereas 12- to 15-year-olds spend 7.8 hours per day in sedentary behaviors (Whitt-Glover et al. 2009).

In fact, studies in the emerging field of inactivity physiology have demonstrated the adverse consequences of prolonged sitting, independent of failure to achieve recommended levels of moderate to vigorous intensity physical activity (MVPA) (Dunstan et al. 2011; Owen et al. 2010). The sharp decline in physical activity and increase in sedentary behaviors during the ages of transition to adolescence suggest that the period between childhood and adolescence may be a critical time for intervening regarding physical activity. This may be an especially important period for children from racial and ethnic minority backgrounds, given data showing that teachers whose students were predominantly black or from low-income households reported less time allocated for recess than did teachers of white and more affluent students (Barros et al. 2009).

A number of strategies can be used to increase children's physical activity levels during recess. These strategies, which are particularly effective in combination, include providing inexpensive playground equipment (e.g., plastic hoops, jump ropes, and bean bags), training recess supervisors to organize or teach games and interact with students, painting playground surfaces with lines for games or murals, and designating playground "activity zones" (Beighle 2012; Stratton and Leonard 2002; Taylor et al. 2011; Verstraete et al. 2006).

The private sector is responding to the recess deficit. One notable example is PlayWorks, a nonprofit group that serves 129,000 students in 320 schools across the United States by structuring recess using trained adult coaches and student coach assistants (Robert Wood Johnson

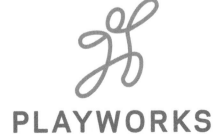

Reprinted, by permission, from Playworks.

Foundation 2007). Another is the Dannon company's Danimals Rally for Recess campaign, an online contest to encourage schools to resurrect recess, offering prizes for meeting certain benchmarks and lottery drawings to win construction of a playground. Many corporations and foundations provide play equipment to schools.

Despite the role of recess as a venerable and cherished school institution and recent efforts to increase the amount of energy children expend during recess (e.g., Morabia and Costanza 2009), little rigorous research has evaluated efforts to stem the erosion of recess. Considerable debate exists about the benefits of free play versus structured play, duration and timing of breaks, optimal supervision and monitoring arrangements, and changing needs as children age (Ramstetter et al. 2010; Robert Wood Johnson Foundation 2007). For example, a recent study found that permanent school playground facilities were associated with children's physical activity levels, but school physical activity policies were not. Two clear messages emerging from the sparse literature, and from practice-based evidence, are that recess should be considered children's personal time and should not be withheld for academic or punitive reasons and that physical activity (e.g., running, calisthenics) should not be used as a punishment (Ramstetter et al. 2010)

Program Description

Physical activity breaks, opportunities to incorporate physical activity into the school day, can supplement the levels of activity obtained through recess and physical education classes (Barr-Anderson et al. 2011; Katz et al. 2010; Trost 2007; Trost, Fees, and Dzewaltowski 2008; Weeks et al. 2008). Unlike recess, a topic on which research has been scarce, physical activity breaks have been the subject of a number of recent studies. These breaks, which incorporate short, structured, group physical activities into the school routine, are an environmental intervention that requires minimal upfront or ongoing costs and offers ready exportability and cultural adaptability. The White House Childhood Obesity Task Force Report identified activity breaks as a key secondary school

strategy, because recess is seldom an option for older students (United States White House Task Force on Childhood Obesity 2010). Research has demonstrated improvements in individual behaviors and health outcomes (e.g., increased MVPA, attenuated excess weight gain, lowered blood pressure, increased bone density) as well as organizational benefits (improved academic performance, longer attention spans, fewer disciplinary problems) among students participating in classroom physical activity breaks (Barr-Anderson et al. 2011; Murray et al. 2008). Furthermore, classroom physical activity breaks have been shown to improve students' attention and behavior, whereas breaks without physical activity do not (CDC 2010). An additional benefit of classroom-based physical activity interventions is that teachers and other school personnel may be engaged as active role models for students (Alexander et al. 2012; Donnelly et al. 2009; Erwin et al. 2011; Institute of Medicine 2006, 2009; Kibbe et al. 2011; Sibley et al. 2008; Woods 2011).

Take 10! (T10) and Instant Recess (IR) are examples of school-based physical activity break interventions with demonstrated success in increasing students' physical activity levels and improving academic engagement. In contrast to recess or physical education class, in which students are required to exit the classroom to engage in physical activity, these interventions bring physical activity into the classroom in order to increase children's physical activity during the school day. The two programs take different approaches: T10 incorporates brief bouts of physical activity into students' academic lessons, whereas IR is intended as a mental respite for students and teachers. The programs are similar in that both align with a number of the Education Sector strategies endorsed by the National Physical Activity Plan (NPAP). This chapter provides a review of T10 and IR, including an overview of how they relate to those NPAP strategies.

Take 10! (T10)

Introduced in 1999, T10 is a school-based program that has demonstrated the feasibility and utility of using 10-minute physical activity breaks in the elementary school classroom setting. Studies have shown that these breaks engage students in exercise of sufficient intensity and duration to count toward CDC-recommended levels: for example, average MET levels of 5 to 7 for first, third, and fifth graders, with commensurate caloric expenditures of 27 to 36 calories and step counts of 600 to 1,400 per 10-minute session (Kibbe et al. 2011; Lloyd et al. 2005; Stewart et al. 2004). (One MET is the metabolic equivalent equal to 3.5 milliliters of oxygen consumed per kilogram and per minute.) The breaks also improve on-task time, particularly in students who are easily distracted (Mahar et al. 2006; Mahar 2011). With its grade-level targeted curriculum, T10 provides an example of Strategy 1 of the Education Sector of the NPAP: *Provide access to and opportunities for high-quality, comprehensive physical activity programs, anchored by physical education, in prekindergarten through grade 12 educational settings. Ensure that the programs are physically active, inclusive, safe, and developmentally and culturally appropriate.*

Whereas T10 emphasizes being active while learning (Kibbe et al. 2011), Physical Activity Across the Curriculum (PAAC), a federally funded study of a variation of T10 that is being conducted at the University of Kansas, focuses on making physical activity integral to the lesson (DuBose et al. 2008). Research findings demonstrate that PAAC engaged 60 to 80 percent of elementary school non–physical education teachers in conducting T10 breaks in 24 low- to moderate-resource public schools in three eastern Kansas cities (Donnelly et al. 2009; Honas et al. 2008). Study staff provided teacher training in a six-hour, off-site in-service session at the beginning of each school year. The gradual increase in the number of teachers engaged each year and the number of minutes provided reflected a progressive cultural norm change (an average of 70 minutes a week of activity was offered, and nearly 50 percent of teachers achieved the goal of 90-100 minutes a week after two years).

PAAC increased children's physical activity levels, in school and outside of school and on both weekdays and weekend days, suggesting that children do not offset increases in school-based physical activity with decreases in out-of-school physical activity. PAAC also improved reading, math, spelling, and composition scores. In the intervention schools that averaged more than 75 minutes of active lessons weekly, students gained less weight than those in control schools.

Instant Recess (IR)

IR, previously known as Lift Off!, consists of 10-minute themed physical activity breaks, usually performed to music, with simple movements based on sports or ethnic dance traditions. IR is scientifically designed to engage major muscle groups, maximizing energy expenditure, enjoyment, and engagement of individuals of varying ability levels while minimizing perceived exertion and injury risk. IR began as a worksite wellness project of the Chronic Disease Prevention division of the Los Angeles County Department of Health Services in 1999 and expanded as a partnership between state and local health agencies, universities, foundations, corporations, and nonprofit groups (Yancey 2010; Yancey et al. 2004a, 2004b, 2006). Involvement with professional sports teams in 2006 led to the adaptation of IR for the school setting. In contrast to T10, in which the onus generally is on teachers to determine how best to incorporate activity into their lesson plans and to lead the physical activities themselves, IR is an extracurricular turnkey or "plug and play" intervention that is usually technology mediated (Yancey et al. 2009). IR breaks may be distributed as DVDs or CDs, streamed from the Internet, or uploaded as electronic files to district servers accessed by teachers through intranet "smart boards" or closed-circuit TV.

Linkage to the National Physical Activity Plan

Now in its 13th year, IR includes a library of more than 50 CDs and DVDs, with different target audiences from preschoolers to seniors; topics include American Indian powwow, Latin salsa, cumbia, reggae, hip hop, and line and African dance, along with basketball, baseball, football, boxing, and soccer moves. The physical activity breaks are in keeping with the Education Sector strategies of the NPAP, in that breaks are designed to be safe, inclusive, and developmentally and culturally appropriate (Strategy 1) and represent successful partnerships with other sectors (e.g., professional basketball and baseball teams) (Strategy 3). Funded in part by the California state health department's USDA-funded Network for a Healthy California, the program has been disseminated to thousands of schools.

Consistent with Education Sector Strategy 2, *Develop and implement state and school district policies requiring school accountability for the quality and quantity of physical education and physical activity programs*, a randomized controlled trial of policy implementation, funded by the Robert Wood Johnson Foundation, was conducted in eight elementary schools in Winston-Salem/Forsyth County, North Carolina. The study engaged high school athletes in peer modeling for younger students and encouraged students to develop their own breaks, for example, Got Moves? contests. This one-year evaluation, which used environmental audits in a sample of classrooms, demonstrated that IR not only increased activity minutes during the school day but also improved on-task time (Whitt-Glover et al. 2011). Because of the elementary school findings, the school superintendent mandated daily IR breaks in all 16 district middle schools (N = 12,000 students) during an eight-week pilot test of the impact of IR on the NC Healthy Active Children Policy (HSP-S-000) (Alexander et al. 2012). An online student survey (N = 1,553) found that 77 percent had participated, 56 percent participated daily, and 73 percent participated first thing in the morning. Environmental audits of 75 classrooms demonstrated that IR breaks delivered a mean of 8.0 ± 3.4 minutes of physical activity each day, including 3.9 ± 3.0 minutes of MVPA. However, on-task time was not affected in middle school students. A study in six Los Angeles Unified School District elementary schools (N = 647 students across 68 classrooms) showed a 1,910-step increase in students' daily activity levels after four to six weeks (Woods 2011). In this case, steps were measured across the entire school day, not just during the breaks.

Lessons Learned

Through efforts to promote physical activity breaks in schools, researchers and practitioners who use activity break programs have identified important lessons that are informing dissemination and implementation efforts:

- Support from key decision makers, including school administrators and faculty leaders, is crucial to the acceptance of activity breaks during the school day.

- Effective teacher training is important. Teachers who understood the instructions for activity breaks and felt comfortable and prepared to lead breaks were more likely to implement breaks than were teachers who were not comfortable with the content. Teacher enthusiasm influences student enthusiasm, and conversely, reluctance feeds reluctance—the more reluctant teachers are to implement exercise breaks, the more reluctant students are to participate, which then exacerbates teacher reluctance. A T10 study found that when teachers were active with the students, student physical activity levels were significantly higher (Donnelly et al. 2009). A study of IR found an association between teacher engagement and activity levels and students' MVPA levels during breaks (Alexander et al. 2012).

- Permitting teachers to space or vary the timing of activity breaks throughout the school day may allay concerns or resentment over having classroom time interrupted or controlled by administrators.

- Exercise breaks during the first and last 10 minutes of the school day could lead to lower participation in middle schools. In qualitative evaluations of IR, adolescents were reluctant to exercise at the beginning of the school day because they did not want to ruin their hairstyles or clothing; students were reluctant to participate at the end of the last period because they were ready for the school day to end (Alexander et al. 2012).

- Including students in the development of activity break content may be important for acceptability and engagement, particularly among older children and adolescents. In the case of IR, this has led to the creation of faster-paced, less-instructional activity breaks, similar to dance videos.

- Data on the organizational benefits of activity breaks to schools (e.g., better discipline and academic performance) are more persuasive than exhortations to enhance student health.

Summary

Classroom-based physical activity breaks are a promising means of increasing children's physical activity levels both inside and outside of the classroom. Evidence suggests that these breaks may also convey added benefits in the form of enhanced educational outcomes.

This chapter provides examples of two types of physical activity breaks that have been used successfully in classroom settings. One approach (T10) directly incorporates physical activity into academic lessons, which may be appealing in selling the strategy to administrators desperate to maintain instructional minutes. The other approach (IR) promotes culturally relevant physical activity breaks as a brief mental break and may not be directly related to classroom content, which enhances the feasibility of implementation in low-resource schools with overcrowded classrooms and fewer teacher specialists. Both approaches have merits and are in keeping with a number of the Education Sector strategies outlined in the NPAP. Given the demonstrated, independent successes of each approach, both should be included in the menu of intervention offerings that increase physical activity among school children.

References

Alexander, R., M.C. Whitt-Glover, S. Ham, N.P. Sutton, J.M. Belnap, and T. Yancey. 2012. Impact of physical activity breaks on Healthy Active Children Policy (HSP-S-000): Adherence in middle schools. Poster presented at the American College of Sports Medicine annual conference, San Francisco, CA, May 29, 2012.

Barr-Anderson, D., M. AuYoung, M. Whitt-Glover, B. Glenn, and A. Yancey. 2011. Structural integration of brief bouts of physical activity into organizational routine: A systematic review of the literature. *Am. J. Prev. Med.* 40:76-93.

Barros, R., E. Silver, and R. Stein. 2009. School recess and group classroom behavior. *Pediatrics.* 123:431-6.

Bazar, E. 2006, June 27. Not it! More schools ban games at recess. *USA Today.* Available at: http://usatoday30.usatoday.com/news/health/2006-06-26-recess-bans_x.htm. Retrieved August 1, 2013.

Beighle, A. 2012, January. *Increasing Physical Activity Through Recess. Research Brief.* Active Living Research Program. Princeton, NJ: Robert Wood Johnson Foundation.

Centers for Disease Control and Prevention. 2010. *The association between school-based physical activity, including physical education, and academic performance.* Atlanta, GA: U.S. Department of Health and Human Services.

Dobbins, M., K. De Corby, P. Robeson, H. Husson, and D. Tirilis. 2009. School-based physical activity programs for promoting physical activity and fitness in children and adolescents aged 6-18. Cochrane Database of Systematic Reviews , Issue 1. Art. No.: CD007651. DOI: 10.1002/14651858.CD007651.

Donnelly, J.E., J.L. Greene, C.A. Gibson, et al. 2009. Physical Activity Across the Curriculum (PAAC): A randomized controlled trial to promote physical activity and diminish overweight and obesity in elementary school children. *Prev. Med.* 49:336-41.

DuBose, K.D., M.S. Mayo, C.A. Gibson, et al. 2008. Physical activity across the curriculum (PAAC): Rationale and design. *Contemp. Clin. Trials* 29:83-93.

Dunstan D.W., A.A. Thorp, and G.N. Healy. 2011. Prolonged sitting: Is it a distinct coronary heart disease risk factor? *Curr. Opin. Cardiol.* 26:412-9.

Erwin, H., A. Beighle, C. Morgain, and M. Noland. 2011. Effect of a low-cost, teacher-directed classroom intervention on elementary students' physical activity. *J. Sch. Health* 81:455-61.

Fernandes, M.M., and R. Sturm. 2011. The role of school physical activity programs in child body mass trajectory. *J. Phys. Act. Health* 8(2):174-81.

Gonzalez-Suarez, C., A. Worley, K. Grimmer-Somers, and V. Dones. 2009. School-based interventions on childhood obesity: A meta-analysis. *Am. J. Prev. Med.* 37:418-27.

Henley, J., J. McBride, J. Milligan, and Nichols, J. 2007. Robbing elementary students of their childhood: The perils of No Child Left Behind. *Education*. 128(1): 56-63.

Honas, J., R. Washburn, B. Smith, J. Greene, and J. Donnelly. 2008. Energy expenditure of the physical activity across the curriculum intervention. *Med. Sci. Sports Exerc.* 40:1501-5.

Institute of Medicine, *Progress in Preventing Childhood Obesity: How Do We Measure Up?* 2006.

Institute of Medicine, *Local Government Actions to Prevent Childhood Obesity.* 2009.

Jackson, P., J. Hopkins, and A. Yancey. 2010. Individual and environmental interventions to prevent obesity in African-American children and adolescents. Childhood Obesity Prevention—International Research, Controversies and Interventions. Oxford, UK: Oxford University Press.

Katz, D.L., D. Cushman, J. Reynolds, V. Njike, J.A. Treu, J. Walker, et al. 2010. Putting physical activity where it fits in the school day: Preliminary results of the ABC (Activity Bursts in the Classroom) for fitness program. *Prev. Chronic Dis.* 7(4):A82.

Kibbe, D.L., J. Hackett, M. Hurley, A. McFarland, K.G. Schubert, A. Schultz, and S. Harris. 2011. Ten years of TAKE 10!®: Integrating physical activity with academic concepts in elementary school classrooms. *Prev. Med.* 52(Suppl. 1):S43-50.

Knuth, A.G., and P.C. Hallal. 2009. Temporal trends in physical activity: A systematic review. *J. Phys. Act. Health* 6(5):548-59.

Lee, S., C. Burgeson, J. Fulton, and C. Spain. 2007. Physical education and physical activity: Results from the SHPPS 2006. *J. Sch. Health* 77:435-63.

Lloyd, L.K., C.L. Cook, and H.W. Kohl. 2005, Spring. A pilot study of teachers' acceptance of a classroom-based physical activity curriculum tool: Take 10! *Texas Assoc. Health Phys. Educ. Rec. Dance J.* pp. 8-11.

Mahar, M.T., S.K. Murphy, D.A. Rowe, J. Golden, A.T. Shields, and T.D. Raedeke. 2006. Effects of a classroom-based program on physical activity and on-task behavior. *Med. Sci. Sports Exerc.* 38:2086-94.

Mahar, M. 2011. Impact of short bouts of physical activity on attention-to-task in elementary school children. *Prev. Med.* 52:S60-4.

McKenzie, T., and D. Kahan. 2008. Physical activity, public health and elementary schools. *Elem. Sch. J.* 108:171-80.

Morabia, A., and M.C. Costanza. 2009. Active encouragement of physical activity during school recess. *Prev. Med.* 48(4):305-6.

Murray, N., J. Garza, P. Diamond, D. Hoelscher, S. Kelder, and J. Ward. 2008. PASS and CATCH: Fitness and academic achievement among 3rd and 4th grade students in Texas. Presentation at the ACSM Annual Conference, Indianapolis, IN, May 30, 2008.

Naylor, P.J. and H.A. McKay. 2009. Prevention in the first place: Schools a setting for action on physical inactivity. *Br. J. Sports Med.* 43:10-3.

Owen, N., G.N. Healy, C.E. Matthews, and D.W. Dunstan. 2010. Too much sitting: The population health science of sedentary behavior. *Exerc. Sport Sci. Rev.* 38:105-13.

Pressler, M.W. 2006, June 1. Schools pressed to achieve put the squeeze on recess. *Washington Post.* Available at www.washingtonpost.com/wp-dyn/content/article/2006/05/31/AR2006053101949.html. Retrieved August 2, 2013.

Ramstetter, C., R. Murray, and A. Garner. 2010. The crucial role of recess in schools. *J. Sch. Health* 80:517-26.

Ridgers, N., A. Timperio, D. Crawford, and J. Salmon. 2011. Five-year changes in school recess and lunchtime and the contribution to children's daily physical activity. *Br. J. Sports Med.* 46(10):741-6.

Robert Wood Johnson Foundation. 2007. *Recess Rules: Why the Undervalued Playtime May Be America's Best Investment for Healthy Kids and Healthy Schools Report.* Princeton, NJ: Robert Wood Johnson Foundation.

Sibley, B.A., R.M. Ward, T.S. Yazvac, K. Zullig, and J.A. Potteiger. 2008. Making the grade with diet and exercise. *AASA Journal of Scholarship and Practice* 5:38-45.

Spengler, J.O., M.S. Carroll, D.P. Connaughton, and K.R. Evenson. 2010. Policies to promote the community use of schools: A review of state recreational user statutes. *Am. J. Prev. Med.* 39:81-8.

Stewart, J.A., D.A. Dennison, H.W. Kohl, and J.A. Doyle. 2004. Exercise level and energy expenditure in the TAKE 10! in-class physical activity program. *J. Sch. Health* 74:397-400.

Stratton, G., and J. Leonard 2002. The effects of playground markings on the energy expenditure of 5-7 year old school children. *Pediatr. Exerc. Sci.* 14:170-80.

Sturm, R. 2005. Childhood obesity—What we can learn from existing data on societal trends, part 2. *Prev. Chronic Dis.* 2(2):A20.

Sturm, R. 2008. Stemming the global obesity epidemic: What can we learn from data about social and economic trends? *Public Health* 122(8):739-46.

Taylor, R.W., V.L. Farmer, S.L. Cameron, K. Meredith-Jones, S.M. Williams, and J.I. Mann. 2011. School playgrounds and physical activity policies as predictors of school and home time activity. *Int. J. Behav. Nutr. Phys. Act.* 8:38.

Trost, S. 2007. *Active Education.* Oakland, CA: Active Living Research, The California Endowment.

Trost, S.G., B. Fees, and D. Dzewaltowski. 2008. Feasibility and efficacy of a "move and learn" physical activity curriculum in preschool children. *J. Phys. Act. Health* 5(1):88-103.

UCLA and Samuels and Associates. 2007. *Failing Fitness.* Oakland, CA: The California Endowment.

United States White House Task Force on Childhood Obesity. 2010. Solving the problem of childhood obesity within a generation. White House Task Force on Childhood Obesity Report to the President. Washington, DC: Executive Office of the President of the United States.

U. S. Department of Health and Human Services. 2008. 2008 physical activity guidelines for Americans: be active, healthy, and happy (ODPHP Publication No. U0036). Retrieved August 1, 2013 from www.health.gov/paguidelines/pdf/paguide.pdf.

Verstraete, S., G. Cardon, D. DeClercq, et al. 2006. Increasing children's physical activity levels during recess periods in elementary schools: The effects of providing game equipment. *Eur. J. Public Health* 16:415-9.

Weeks, B.K., C.M. Young, and B.R. Beck. 2008. Eight months of regular in-school jumping improves indices of bone strength in adolescent boys and girls: The POWER PE study. *J. Bone Miner. Res.* 23:1002-11.

Whitt-Glover, M., S.A. Ham, and A. Yancey. 2011. Instant Recess®: A practical tool for increasing physi-cal activity during the school day. *Prog. Community Health Partnersh.* 5(3):289-97.

Whitt-Glover, M.C., W.C. Taylor, M.F. Floyd, M.M. Yore, A.K. Yancey, and C.E. Matthews. 2009. Disparities in physical activity and sedentary behaviors among US children and adolescents: Prevalence, correlates, and intervention implications. *J. Public Health Pol.* 3:S309-34.

Woods, D. 2011, May. Implementation an evaluation of Instant Recess® in elementary school children (Dissertation). University of California Los Angeles.

Wu, S., D. Cohen, Y. Shi, M. Pearson, and R. Sturm. 2011. Economic analysis of physical activity interventions. *Am. J. Prev. Med.* 40(2):149-58.

Yancey, A.K., W.J. McCarthy, W. Taylor, A.M. Raines, C. Gewa, M. Weber, and J.E. Fielding. 2004b. The Los Angeles Lift Off: A sociocultural environmental change intervention to increase workplace physical activity. *Prev. Med.* 38;848-56.

Yancey, A.K., L.B. Lewis, D.C. Sloane, J.G. Guinyard, A.L. Diamant, L.M. Nascimento, W.J. McCarthy, and the REACH Coalition. 2004a. Leading by example: Process evaluation of a local health department-community collaboration to change organizational practice to incorporate physical activity. *J Public Health Manag. Prac.* 10(2):116-23.

Yancey, A.K., L.B. Lewis, J.J. Guinyard, D.C. Sloan, L.M. Nascimento, L. Galloway-Gilliam, A. Diamant, and W.J. McCarthy. 2006. Putting promotion into practice: The African Americans Building a Legacy of Health organizational wellness program. *Health Promot. Prac.* 7(3):233S-246S.

Yancey, A., D. Winfield, J. Larsen, et al. 2009. "Live, learn and play": Building strategic alliances between professional sports and public health. *Prev. Med.* 49:322-5.

Yancey, T. 2010. *Instant Recess: Building a Fit Nation 10 Minutes at a Time.* Berkeley, CA, UC Press.

CHAPTER 4

Physical Activity in Early Childhood Centers

New York City as a Case Study

Cathy Nonas, MS, RD
NYC Department of Health and Mental Hygiene

Lillian Dunn, MPH
NYC Department of Health and Mental Hygiene

Rhonda Walsh, MPH
NYC Department of Health and Mental Hygiene

NPAP Tactics and Strategies Used in This Program

Education Sector

STRATEGY 1: Provide access to and opportunities for high-quality, comprehensive physical activity programs, anchored by physical education, in Pre-kindergarten through grade 12 educational settings. Ensure that the programs are physically active, inclusive, safe, and developmentally and culturally appropriate.

STRATEGY 2: Develop and implement state and school district policies requiring school accountability for the quality and quantity of physical education and physical activity programs.

STRATEGY 4: Ensure that early childhood education settings for children ages 0 to 5 years promote and facilitate physical activity.

O ver the last 30 to 40 years, childhood obesity has increased to epidemic proportions, causing global concern for the increased health risks it confers on our children. Obesity in children is associated with type 2 diabetes, nonalcoholic fatty liver disease, high blood pressure, and dyslipidemia, among other risks. In 2006, the New York City Department of Health and Mental Hygiene (DOHMH) published a study (Young et al. 2006) examining obesity rates in early childhood group centers in New York City. Shockingly, more than 42 percent of the more than 16,000 young children enrolled in the study were overweight or obese. This chapter describes how the DOHMH responded, specifically highlighting its work to increase physical activity in early childhood through regulation and technical support.

Program Description

The goal of the DOHMH regulations on physical activity was to establish minimum amounts of time children were active in the group child care setting.

Establishing Regulations for Early Child Care

Group child care centers were a natural target for obesity interventions. National U.S. data from 2005 show that approximately 69 percent of four-year-olds spend time in child care facilities. In New York City, more than 130,000 children ages three to five years spend at least some of their time in group child care centers licensed by the DOHMH. These centers are visited regularly by DOHMH sanitarians and early childhood education consultants, who could be engaged to support efforts to improve the health of these children. The New York City Charter empowers the New York Board of Health to amend and create regulations in the city's health code that pertain to the health of all New Yorkers. In other words, when it comes to the city's health, the Board of Health has the rule of law within the areas over which its jurisdiction extends, including child care centers. The DOHMH proposes regulations to the Board of Health, and after a public comment period, the board then votes on whether to approve or reject those regulations as law. The laws are enforced by the DOHMH. All of these factors combined to make policy changes an attractive—and potentially very powerful—intervention to address obesity.

In 2006, the DOHMH proposed new regulations to the Board of Health that established a minimum amount of time during which group child care centers were required to provide physical activity, restricted sugary drinks from being served by centers, limited the amount of 100 percent juice that centers could provide to children, and required water to be made available to children at all times. In June 2006 the Board of Health modified the health code to include these obesity-focused regulations. The new regulations took effect on January 1, 2007.

Implementing Regulations

After the modifications to the health code were approved, the DOHMH took several actions to ensure that child care center directors were informed of and supported through the changes. First, the DOHMH provided training regarding the new regulations for all internal staff members who regularly visited the centers. These staff members were encouraged to talk to center directors about the goals of the new rules, the exact language of each statute, and the importance of physical activity and proper nutrition in early childhood. Second, the Bureau of Child Care (housed within the DOHMH) held six open meetings for center directors during which the new provisions were discussed in detail. Third, a letter announcing the changes

was sent to all early child care centers that the changes affected.

Although implementation of each regulation change required some education on the part of child care center staff, the DOHMH believed that the regulation on physical activity was the most challenging for centers to implement. This rule required all centers to provide their full-day three- to five-year-old classrooms with at least 60 minutes of physical activity per day, 30 minutes of which had to be structured and led by teachers. The city council provided funding to the DOHMH to help support centers' efforts to increase structured physical activity time, particularly in the neighborhoods with the highest rates of poverty and obesity-related disease. DOHMH released a request for proposal to identify a curriculum with which to train staff working in early childhood centers on ways to provide physical activity in the classroom. Shortly thereafter, the city council significantly increased funding to enable the program to expand citywide.

Training and Technical Assistance to Support Compliance

SPARK! (Sports, Play, and Active Recreation for Kids!) won the contract and DOHMH provided child care center staff with a one-day workshop on a modified SPARK!, a structured physical activity curriculum. Attendees received professional development credit for the workshop and were provided with a manual that detailed structured physical activity lessons and an equipment kit that contained spot markers, bean bags, scarves, and two music CDs (all of which were used in lessons demonstrated at the training). The day included a number of hours of practicing lessons with the help of a trainer. In addition, in three targeted neighborhoods where rates of obesity were highest, on-site follow-up support was provided to teachers after training.

The SPARK! curriculum had many strengths: Its lessons encouraged all children in the classroom to participate in movement, it emphasized noncompetitive play, and it taught teachers how to manage a classroom through physical activity. It also stressed the importance of teachers' role modeling of healthy behaviors for their students.

However, there were a few drawbacks for New York City. Many of the lessons in the manual required more space than most child care centers could access. Some lessons used equipment that the Physical Activity Program did not provide because those materials required large amounts of classroom or storage space (e.g., parachutes, large balls). Finally, the SPARK! manual was so large, including more than 100 lessons, that it intimidated many child care center staff.

Additionally, trainings and on-site support continued to shed light on how physical activity was actually implemented in the NYC group child care context. Program staff noticed that teachers were modifying lessons to make them work better for their classrooms. For example, teachers created stories that included the physical activity lessons so that children could relate better to certain kinds of movement. Teachers tended to repeat the same lessons over and over, generally leading children in no more than 20 activities all year long. Finally, teachers relied heavily on the music that was provided.

In 2009, contractual complications required the DOHMH to look for a new physical activity curriculum. The Physical Activity Program investigated other existing curricula but did not find an adequate replacement that was focused on early childhood, provided small classroom-based activities, and was offered by a nonprofit organization (a funding requirement). Therefore, in 2009, the program leaders decided to create a new curriculum, building on the knowledge gathered from five years of training early childhood staff. In this way, the DOHMH was able to create a program that was less expensive to administer and more tailored to its needs.

Learning from its experience, the Physical Activity Program created the Move-to-Improve Early Childhood Program. Activities in this curriculum were designed for the small spaces typical of classrooms in New York City. Each lesson was embedded within a story, so that children were not simply moving but were engaging in physical activity as an experience.

For example, one yoga lesson called Nature Walk encouraged children to do yoga by taking them on an imaginary walk through nature and asking them to hold their bodies in yoga positions that resemble mountains, butterflies, and grass in the wind. Because teachers seemed to use the same lessons over and over, the Move-to-Improve manual was shorter and included just 30 lessons. When possible, the program included music to match the exercises. Program staff created equipment kits to match the lessons in the manual and included two CDs, one with songs that guided children through physical activities and another that provided background music for lessons in the manual.

Demand for physical activity training among child care centers has always been high. Staff generally enjoy the experience of the workshop and often declare it to be the best professional development workshop they have ever attended. Since the program began in 2004, more than 15,000 child care center staff members from more than 1,200 centers across New York City have been trained in either SPARK! or Move-to-Improve.

Although the trainings are currently only funded for elementary school teachers, program challenges remained among early childcare staff, despite all of the efforts to hone the experience for participants. Because center directors did not always know who could attend workshops until the day of training, equipment kits were not sent to centers until after a workshop training was completed. Delivery of these kits could take a month or more. In addition, the staff at child care centers tends to be very transient. Ongoing training, therefore, is required to make sure that new staff members learn how to provide structured activity for their children. Because of limited budgets, DOHMH could only provide a one-day training to participants, despite requests from child care center staff for onsite follow-up and a second full-day workshop. Finally, budget constraints made it impossible to provide the workshop or manuals in other languages. Although most center staff members are conversant in English, many would benefit from materials in Spanish or other languages.

Program Evaluation

Traditionally, child care centers have not been cited for violations in physical activity regulations. When DOHMH staff members conduct site visits, they review each classroom's daily schedule (when available), discuss the importance of physical activity with center staff, and determine whether adequate time is allotted to physical activity. However, the regulatory staff members do not have time to observe every classroom in every center. All of these factors make it difficult to determine whether each classroom is providing the required amount of physical activity. Cited violations, then, are not a sufficient way of assessing impact of the regulations or training on the quantity of physical activity children receive in the group child care setting.

However, some data exist to suggest that training in SPARK! or Move-to-Improve improves a center's capacity to comply with health code regulations on physical activity. Because of funding constraints, evaluations of the Physical Activity Program in early childhood have been limited to self-reported data. In the 2006-2007 school year, the program conducted pre- and postprogram surveys with trained child care center staff to examine the impact of training on structured physical activity. Teachers in full-day classrooms stated that the number of minutes of structured physical activity they provided rose from 78 minutes per week before training to 100 minutes per week after training. Teachers used the SPARK! curriculum for a median of 75 minutes per week. This evaluation suggests that teacher training significantly increases activity in early childhood classrooms but also suggests that centers do not provide enough structured physical activity time. These results are limited, however, by the self-reported nature of the evaluation.

In 2008, the Robert Wood Johnson Foundation (RWJ) and the Centers for Disease Control and Prevention began an evaluation of the New York City regulations governing group child care centers, including those on physical activity. This evaluation collected self-reported, observed, and accelerometry-based physical activity data. Results of the RWJ-funded evaluation will be published elsewhere.

Programmatically, observational data have proven the most useful for New York City. To date, the DOHMH has used observational data to assess the impact of Move-to-Improve training in other age groups. These evaluations provided qualitative data on how structured physical activity actually happens in the classroom setting and resulted in a significant difference between trained and untrained classrooms in number of minutes dedicated to physical activity. Although an observational study in early childcare centers was begun, it was not completed due to budget cuts.

Linkage to the National Physical Activity Plan

The regulations and technical support address three strategies of the Education Sector of the National Physical Activity Plan:

- Strategies 1 and 2 call for states and school districts to develop policies that require comprehensive physical activity programs and include mechanisms for monitoring implementation. DOHMH, the agency that oversees child care centers in New York City, requested, implemented, and is monitoring regulations that require centers to provide young children with 60 minutes of physical activity per day.

- Strategy 4 entails ensuring that early childhood education settings for children ages 0 to 5 years promote and facilitate physical activity. The DOHMH health care regulations require all city-regulated child care centers to provide regular physical activity for all children 12 months and older, but include structured physical activity for three- to five-year-old children.

Evidence Base Used During Program Development

The National Association for Sport and Physical Education (NASPE) guidelines for early childhood state that toddlers should engage in at least 60 minutes of unstructured activity daily and 30 minutes of structured activity (NASPE 2013). Recommendations released by the Institute of Medicine (IOM) in June 2011 state that child care regulatory bodies should require centers to provide opportunities for physical activity throughout the day (IOM 2011).

Populations Best Served by the Program

The policy changes and associated technical support created by the DOHMH are appropriate for children two to five years old.

Lessons Learned

The DOHMH has learned a great deal about implementing regulations on physical activity. First, having a policy in place to establish a minimum amount of physical activity is an important foundation from which to begin working with child care centers. Although everyone agrees that physical activity is important for children, having an established policy elevates the discussion: Compliance with this law becomes a part of each center's legal requirements and places physical activity on an equal level of importance as protections against infectious diseases through immunizations.

Second, enforcing policies can be very challenging without requirements for centers to post daily classroom schedules. Although posting physical activity schedules does not promise compliance, it is one way to begin planning for physical activity in each classroom. This would also make it easier for inspectors to visit centers to see the activities underway.

Third, technical assistance for physical activity is welcomed by most child care centers. Nobody understands the need for children to move better than do the people who work with young children all day long. However, many staff members are daunted by or uncomfortable with leading activities in a room full of three-year-olds. Technical assistance that dem-

onstrates ways to manage a classroom through these activities is pragmatic and necessary.

Fourth, technical assistance does not have to be expensive. Lessons should be short, and CDs and a manual are the most important parts of the training. Currently, the Move to Improve curriculum can be downloaded for free at the DOHMH's website.

Fifth, evaluation of physical activity can be very challenging. Observational data are credible but expensive to gather. If possible, government agencies should provide evaluation funds when they enact new policies to ensure that the evaluation will take place.

Ultimately, the goals of DOHMH's changes to the health code and the technical assistance directed to support implementation have been well received. Informal feedback from center directors and staff indicates that regulations concerning physical activity tend to be the most challenging to implement. Ongoing support of these efforts may be necessary to ensure that rules governing physical activity time are translated into action in child care centers.

Tips for Working Across Sectors

Although DOHMH played the lead role in implementing these regulations and associated technical support, the NYC Administration for Child Services was a key partner in promoting compliance among group child care centers and encouraging participation in the physical activity trainings. Partnering with that organization helped ensure that centers were aware of the regulations and DOHMH technical support.

Additional Reading and Resources

Additional reading on the regulations affecting group child care centers in New York City, as well as DOHMH's policy guide recommending additional policies that promote physical activity and healthy eating, can be found at www.nyc.gov/html/doh/html/living/phys-move.shtml.

References

Dunn L.L., J.A. Venturanza, R.J. Walsh, and C.A. Nonas. 2012. An Observational Evaluation of Move-To-Improve, a Classroom-Based Physical Activity Program, New York City Schools, 2010. Prev Chronic Dis 9:120072.

Institute of Medicine of the National Academies. 2011. *Early Childhood Obesity Prevention Policies: Goals, Recommendations and Potential Actions*. Washington, DC: The National Academic Press.

National Association for Sport and Physical Education. 2013. Active Start: A statement of physical activity guidelines for children from birth to age 5. 2nd ed. www.aahperd.org/naspe/standards/nationalGuidelines/ActiveStart.cfm.

Young C.R., P. Peretz, R. Jaslow, S. Chamany, D. Berger, et al. 2006. Obesity in Early Childhood: More Than 40% of Head Start Children in NYC Are Overweight or Obese. NYC Vital Signs 5(2): 1-2.

CHAPTER 5

After-School Programs and Physical Activity

Submitted by the Afterschool Alliance
(www.afterschoolalliance.org)

NPAP Tactics and Strategies Used in This Program

Education Sector

STRATEGY 5: Provide access to and opportunities for physical activity before and after school.

Years ago, physical education—PE—was a routine part of American schoolchildren's day. But in the nation's efforts to focus classroom instruction on topics that standardized tests measure, physical education has received less time and attention. Until recently, physical education classes in schools could be relied on to engage children in a half hour or more of physical exercise or health instruction each day. But the increasing focus on test scores in the nation's public schools has rendered physical education a luxury in many school districts and has trimmed or reduced recess time in some elementary schools (Fletcher 2010). One study found that in 2006, only 7.9 percent of middle schools provided students with daily physical education (Lee et al. 2007).

Although schools have deemphasized physical activity and fitness, there is little evidence that children are compensating in other settings. According to the Centers for Disease Control and Prevention, 61.5 percent of children do not participate in any organized physical activity outside of school hours (Centers for Disease Control and Prevention 2002). Thus, after-school hours have become a focus of efforts to ensure the healthy development of children and youth. It is a challenge that the nation's after-school programs have embraced eagerly.

After-school programs that focus on positive physical outcomes, in addition to positive academic outcomes, are an invaluable resource for alleviating the health crisis facing American youth. These programs allow schools and community organizations to encourage involvement in physical activity, as well as to encourage sound nutrition. With 8.4 million children participating in after-school programs and a staggering 18.5 million more who would likely enroll given the opportunity, after-school programs have the potential to affect the fitness of a large portion of the nation's youth (Afterschool Alliance 2009).

After-school programs can be a particularly valuable physical activity resource because they

- serve children most at risk for being overweight, including minorities and those from lower socioeconomic strata;

- operate during a time of the day when many children would otherwise be sedentary and not likely to participate in physical activity;

- provide staff members who understand children's needs and can promote active lifestyles and healthy eating (Afterschool Investments Project 2006); and

- provide an opportunity for young people to interact with role models who display the habit of regular physical activity.

The Afterschool Alliance has established a goal of promoting physical activity before school, after school, and during the summer (collectively known as *after-school*).

Program Description

A number of national organizations are working to help after-school programs build physical activity and fitness into their daily offerings. One such effort, a set of health-focused standards for after-school programs, is a result of the Healthy Out-of-School Time (HOST) coalition, led by the National Institute on Out-of-School Time at the Wellesley Centers for Women, the University of Massachusetts College of Nursing and Health Sciences, and the YMCA. With funding from the Robert Wood Johnson Foundation, HOST developed practical standards for healthy eating and physical activity in programs held outside of school time. The standards subsequently were adopted by the National AfterSchool Association (2011).

The standards focus on evidence-based, practical steps aimed at fostering the best possible nutrition and physical activity outcomes for K-12 children in programs held outside of school hours. The best practices

- dedicate at least 20 percent or at least 30 minutes of morning or after-school program time to physical activity (60 minutes for a full-day program);
- provide physical activities in which students are moderately to vigorously active for at least 50 percent of the physical activity time;
- ensure that daily physical activity time includes aerobic activities and age-appropriate muscle- and bone-strengthening activities;
- offer noncompetitive activities; and
- conduct physical activities that are integrated with enrichment, academic, or recreation content and are goal-driven,

sequential, safe, inclusive, developmentally appropriate, and success oriented.

The standards also offer a series of best practices for staff training, social supports intended to encourage children to enjoy and participate in physical activity, program supports, and environmental supports related to physical fitness equipment and facilities.

Linkage to the National Physical Activity Plan

After-school programs support a key strategy of the Education Sector of the National Physical Activity Plan:

Strategy 5: Provide access to and opportunities for physical activity before and after school. For many children, after-school programs provide the best (and often only) opportunity to participate in fun, health-promoting physical activity after school. Increasingly, after-school organizations and providers are working to ensure that children who attend after-school programs have opportunities every day to enjoy physical activities and develop skills that promote lifelong physical activity.

Evidence Base Used During Program Development

The research to date indicates that programs that take advantage of out-of-school-time hours to create opportunities for children to enjoy physical activity and learn about healthy lifestyles can improve student health outcomes.

- A study that measured the health and social benefits of after-school programs found that after investigators controlled for baseline obesity, poverty status, and race and ethnicity, the prevalence of obesity was significantly lower for after-school program participants (21 percent) compared with nonparticipants (33 percent) (Mahoney and Heather 2005).
- A report by the U.S. Department of Education found that 10- to 16-year-olds who

have a relationship with a mentor are less likely to engage in unhealthy behaviors. Forty-six percent are less likely to start using drugs and 27 percent are less likely to start drinking alcohol (Riley et al. 2000).

- Active adolescents are more likely than their sedentary peers to use contraception during sexual intercourse and to delay the initiation of first sexual intercourse (Miller et al. 1998).

- A recent evaluation of after-school programs in California found that youth reached federally recommended levels of moderate to vigorous physical activity for an average of 24.4 minutes daily when they participated in structured activities. By contrast, students participated in only 13 minutes through unstructured activities (CANFit 2009).

- A study reported in the *Journal of Adolescence* found that youth whose summer arrangements involved regular participation in organized activities showed significantly lower risk for obesity than did other youth. This was most evident during early adolescence—the middle school years. Youth whose regular summer arrangement was primarily parent care without organized activity participation showed the greatest risk for obesity (Mahoney 2011).

Population Best Served by the Program

After-school programs often serve children most at risk for being overweight, including minorities and children of low socioeconomic status. After-school programming is particularly important to the development of elementary and middle school children, who are at critical points in their physical, social, and emotional development. Elementary students need opportunities to develop the habits of physical activity and to hear and absorb messages about its importance. Middle school students are fueled by a desire to find a place to belong and therefore are at risk of making decisions that

negatively affect their health. As a result, they can benefit greatly from the increased opportunities for physical activity that after-school programs can provide. Accordingly, after-school programs across the United States offer youth a mix of academic and physical enrichment that promotes positive physical, emotional, and social development.

Lessons Learned

After-school programs offer countless health benefits, but efforts to include a focus on fitness and well-being often face challenges. However, programs across the United States are implementing innovative strategies that allow them to include health and wellness activities in after-school offerings. Following are some examples of the challenges programs face and the solutions they have developed:

- Funding is a universal concern for after-school programs, and inadequate funding for staffing, professional development, and equipment is a particular problem for physical activity efforts.

  The San Antonio Youth Centers (SAYC) are nine after-school programs in Texas that address the funding challenge by using funds from the federal- and state-supported Carol M. White Physical Education Program to implement a physical education and youth development curriculum. The centers seek to promote healthy lifestyles, improve academic achievement, and foster and develop positive youth self-esteem. Middle school students at SAYC participate in at least 45 minutes of structured daily physical activities that are both fun and vigorous, including karate, swimming, cheerleading, and rock-climbing. Additionally, the centers educate youth about the dangers of smoking, alcohol, and drugs and promote healthy decision making. The programs offer weekly family "boot camp" sessions to cultivate parental involvement and help ensure that healthy living extends into the home.

- Physical activity is not always perceived as an essential need, particularly when concerns about test scores pit physical activity and academics in competition for after-school time.

Children participating in the Ed Snider Youth Hockey Foundation (ESYHF) in Philadelphia enjoy a host of positive youth development outcomes that stem from one basic hook: playing hockey. Developed by former Philadelphia Flyers and 76ers owner Ed Snider, ESYHF programs target youth from inner-city neighborhoods who otherwise would not have an opportunity to participate in an after-school program. In an effort to tackle the barrier of pitting academic support against physical activity, the program goes beyond on-the-ice physical development and promotes increased school attendance, provides homework help, and offers a life skills curriculum that encourages healthy habits and smart choices.

- For many programs, the absence of shared-use or joint-use agreements between schools and the community-based organizations that operate after-school programs is a significant problem, leaving programs unable to access facilities. In some locations, physical space is limited for after-school programs' physical activity programming, sometimes because sports leagues have rented out available fields or facilities.

The main goal of the School Health Interdisciplinary Program (SHIP) in Gainesville, Florida, is to combat childhood obesity through a combination of age-appropriate physical fitness, nutrition, and science- and math-related educational activities. In addition to teaching children about the water cycle and food pyramid, SHIP dedicates time to an array of active outdoor pursuits, such as endurance running, aerobics, and energetic games. Using local community-based organizations and undergraduate and graduate student volunteers from the University of Florida,

the program offers 90 minutes of weekly mentoring opportunities for students at two middle schools and a host of other beneficial health education activities.

- High staff turnover limits the ability of programs to train staff to provide high-quality physical activity.

The Ohio Afterschool Network received funding from the Ohio Department of Health to address the challenge of finding qualified after-school program staff trained in physical activity instruction. A diverse group of providers, educators, funders, health professionals, and other experts created guidelines that addressed types of activities; time and intensity; curriculum; qualified staff; ratio; staff policies and administration; evaluation; facilities; equipment; and family, school, and community connections. The guidelines were disseminated in fall 2011. The guidelines have been presented at state and regional conferences and trainings, and the network is working to have the guidelines included in the state's quality rating system for child care.

Paying the Bill: Sustainability and After-School Physical Activity

Funding for after-school programs is almost universally tight, but a number of funding streams are available to support fitness activities:

- The U.S. Department of Education's Carol M. White grants. In fiscal year 2013, the department planned to award 95 grants ranging from $100,000 to $750,000 to local education agencies and community-based organizations to support programs designed to develop, expand, or improve physical education programs for K-12 students. The estimated average size of the grants was $375,000. The program is not specific to after-school programs (U.S. Department of Education n.d.). The future of the Carol M. White program is cloudy, as some in Congress have targeted it for elimination.

- The Centers for Disease Control and Prevention (CDC) state-based Nutrition and

Physical Activity Program to Prevent Obesity and Other Chronic Diseases funds 25 states to address obesity and other chronic diseases with statewide efforts that draw in multiple partners (CDC 2012).

• The 21st Century Community Learning Centers initiative of the Department of Education provides funding for school- and community-based after-school programs through a state-level competitive process. Funds can be used to promote physical activity through recreation programs.

Using Evidence-Based Curricula

Physical activity curricula should ensure that an after-school program is able to meet its outcome goals. Many after-school programs use physical activity curriculum packages marketed by outside organizations. Following are examples of after-school programs that use evidence-based curricula:

• The City of Las Vegas's Safekey After-school Program partners with the Southern Nevada Health District to bring the Coordinated Approach to Child Health (CATCH) Kids Club to children between the ages of 5 and 11 at its 68 after-school sites. The curriculum is marketed by FlagHouse, Inc., to schools and after-school programs. The after-school-specific version of the curriculum was piloted in 16 after-school sites and, based on the results, was subsequently adopted in hundreds of after-school sites around the nation. The program encourages healthy eating habits, physical activity, and parental involvement (CATCH n.d.).

• The 21st Century Community Learning Centers, Lincoln, Nebraska, use the Spark after-school physical activity program, which includes an after-school-specific curriculum featuring "cultural and aerobic games, dances from around the world, and enjoyable skill and sport activities written in scope and sequence," as well as activities such as jump rope, parachute play, jogging games, fitness circuits, and beanbag activities (Spark n.d.). This research-tested curriculum is supported by staff training, equipment, and follow-up support from the developers. Lincoln's use of the program is funded by a federal Carol M. White grant.

Additional Reading and Resources

The Healthy Out-of-School Time (HOST) Coalition recently finalized evidence-based, practical quality standards for providing children with healthy food, beverages, and physical activity in out-of-school time. The charge to this project, funded by the Robert Wood Johnson Foundation, was to recommend healthy eating and physical activity standards that foster the best possible nutrition and physical activity outcomes for children in grades K-12 attending programs outside of school hours.

Promoting Physical Activity and Healthy Nutrition in Afterschool Settings, published by the Department of Health and Human Services, is a useful resource that includes strategies for enacting health and nutrition guidelines and standards. It is available at www.centuray21me.org/staticme21/resources/fitness_nutrition.pdf.

The Quaker Chewy Get Active: Be Healthy Afterschool Toolkit, developed by the Afterschool Alliance and Quaker Oats, offers creative, easy-to-implement ideas for incorporating health and wellness into after-school programs, including lesson plans, activities, and games in addition to a comprehensive set of health-related resources that programs can access. It is available at http://afterschoolalliance.org/documents/QuakerGetActiveToolKit.pdf.

First Lady Michelle Obama's Let's Move campaign has recognized the value and importance of after-school programs, and many of the recommendations put forward in the White House Task Force on Childhood Obesity Report to the President echo the current efforts and initiatives of the after-school field. The Let's Move website includes a variety of action steps that after-school programs and families can use. It is available at www.letsmove.gov/.

The Alliance for a Healthier Generation (AFHG) website offers before-school and after-school providers an excellent page of tips, ideas, and success stories that address both physical activity and nutrition and snacks. The tips are available at www.healthiergeneration.org/take_action\out-of-school_time. Additionally, AFHG operates the no-cost Healthy Schools Program, which offers free resources, tips, and tools for promoting healthy lifestyles in after-school programs. Online registration for the program is available at https://host.healthiergeneration.org.

Action for Healthy Kids and the National Football League developed ReCharge! Energizing After-School, a fun-for-kids curriculum designed to teach students about good nutrition and engage them in physical activity. ReCharge! is a complete, easy-to-use kit with lesson plans, equipment ideas, and information for families. It is available at www.actionforhealthykids.org/what-we-do/534.

The Center for Collaborative Solutions' Healthy Behavior Initiative has recently released a free and comprehensive publication, Step-by-Step Guide to Developing Exemplary Practices in Healthy Eating, Physical Activity and Food Security in Afterschool Programs. It is available at www.ccscenter.org/afterschool/Step-By-Step%20Guide.

References

Afterschool Alliance. 2009. America after 3PM. www.afterschoolalliance.org/AA3PM.cfm.

Afterschool Investments Project. 2006. *Promoting physical activity and healthy nutrition in afterschool settings: Strategies for program leaders and policy makers*. Washington, DC: U.S. Department of Health and Human Services.

CANFit, Partnership for Public Health/Public Health Institute, Samuels & Associates. 2009. *Promoting Healthier Afterschool Environments: Opportunities and Challenges*. The California Endowment. Oakland. CA.

CATCH. n.d. www.catchinfo.org/catchmagalog.html.

Centers for Disease Control and Prevention. 2002. Physical activity levels among children aged 9-13 years. *MMWR: Morbid. Mortal. Wkly. Rep.* 52(33):785-8.

Centers for Disease Control and Prevention. 2012. Overweight and obesity. www.cdc.gov/obesity/stateprograms/index.html.

Fletcher, A. 2010. Changing lives, saving lives: A step-by-step guide to developing exemplary practices in healthy eating, physical activity and food security in afterschool programs. Healthy Behaviors Initiative. www.ccscenter.org/afterschool/Step-By-Step%20Guide.

Lee, S.M., C.R. Burgeson, J.E. Fulton, and C.G. Spain. 2007. Physical education and physical activity: Results from the School Health Policies and Programs Study 2006. *J. School Health* 77(8):435-68.

Mahoney, J.L. 2011. Adolescent summer care arrangements and risk for obesity the following school year. *J. Adolesc.* 34(4):737-49.

Mahoney, J.L. and L. Heather. 2005. Afterschool program participation and the development of child obesity and peer acceptance. *Appl. Dev. Sci.* 9(4):202-15.

Miller, K.E., D.F. Sabo, M.P. Farrell, G.M. Barnes, and M.J. Melnick. 1998. *The Women's Sports Foundation Report: Sport and Teen Pregnancy*. Women's Sports Foundation. New York, NY.

National AfterSchool Association Standards for Healthy Eating and Physical Activity in Out-of-School Time Programs. 2011. www.niost.org/pdf/host/Healthy_Eating_and_Physical_Activity_Standards.pdf.

Riley, R., T. Peterson, A. Kanter, G. Moreno, and W. Goode. 2000. *Afterschool Programs: Keeping Kids Safe and Smart*. Washington, DC: U.S. Department of Education.

Spark. n.d. www.sparkpe.org/after-school/.

U.S. Department of Education. n.d. Carol M. White physical education program. www2.ed.gov/programs/whitephysed/applicant.html.

Mass Media

Bess H. Marcus, PhD

Department of Family and Preventive Medicine, University of California San Diego

Mass media campaigns increasingly are being used as part of a public health approach to address physical inactivity. The best mass media campaigns have a clear focus, include paid and earned media placements, and reach a wide population. Connecting campaigns with national, state, or local partnerships and establishing clear links to community programs and policy and environmental change strategies appear to be promising approaches. All campaigns, regardless of their focus, need to include a clear and identifiable message or "brand" and sufficient media exposure. Effective campaigns typically include political support, sustained funding, and well-established partnerships that support the many settings in which physical activity can occur.

The chapters in this section describe communication strategies used in several mass media campaigns to promote physical activity: a community-wide social marketing campaign in West Virginia, a mass media campaign to promote physical activity in Hawai'i, a U.S. national campaign to promote activity in children, and national campaigns in Canada, Australia, and New Zealand. Each chapter tells a different story about the challenges and opportunities inherent in promoting physical activity via mass media.

Mass media campaigns must be included in public health approaches to promoting physical activity. These campaigns have the potential to create broad interest in physical activity, increase the potential for change, and influence social norms regarding active and sedentary lifestyles. Several examples in this section highlight the fact that government support can play an important role in successful mass media campaigns, because government can provide the sustained support needed to fund a dose of mass media sufficient to increase and sustain community awareness. Successful campaigns also need adequate planning, good formative message development, and sufficient media duration and intensity. Without these key components, it is unlikely that campaigns will produce change in the target population.

Finally, campaign planners must invest in quality evaluation at all stages of mass media campaign programming. First, they should ensure that rigorous formative research, which requires time and effort and should entail both qualitative and quantitative methods, is used to create optimal messages. Second, process evaluation of a campaign is important for understanding which audiences were reached by campaign activities and which ones were not. Third, outcome evaluations need to use the strongest research designs and measures so that campaign planners can determine what worked and can ensure that the next campaign is even more successful.

CHAPTER 6

VERB: It's What You Do! and VERB Scorecard
Bringing a National Campaign to Communities

Marian Huhman, PhD
University of Illinois at Urbana-Champaign

Judy Berkowitz, PhD
Battelle Institute

NPAP Tactics and Strategies Used in This Program

Mass Media Sector

STRATEGY 1: Encourage public health agencies to form partnerships with other agencies across the eight sectors to combine resources around common themes in promoting physical activity.

STRATEGY 2: Enact federal legislation to support a sustained physical activity mass media campaign.

STRATEGY 3: Develop consistent mass communication messages that promote physical activity, have a clear and standardized "brand," and are consistent with the Physical Activity Guidelines for Americans.

STRATEGY 4: Ensure that messages and physical activity plans developed by state and local public health agencies and key stakeholders from the eight sectors are consistent with national messages.

STRATEGY 5: Sequence, plan, and provide campaign activities in a prospective, coordinated manner. Support and link campaign messages to community-level programs, policies, and environmental supports.

STRATEGY 6: Encourage mass media professionals to become informed about the importance of physical activity and the potential role they can play in promoting physical activity.

The VERB: It's What You Do! social marketing campaign used mass media, school and community promotions, the Internet, and partnerships with national organizations and local communities to encourage children aged 9 to 13 years (tweens) to be physically active every day.

Program Description

Sponsored by the Centers for Disease Control and Prevention (CDC), VERB implemented mass media and promotions nationally from 2002 to 2006 in four phases that spanned roughly one year each. The first phase focused on building a strong brand and brand awareness among tweens. During phases 2 through 4, the campaign emphasized providing opportunities for tweens to experience the brand and to sample the product (physical activity) through experiential marketing—national promotional tours, community events, and school and community promotions. The specifics of the branding strategy (Asbury, Wong, Price, & Nolin 2008), the experiential marketing tactics (Heitzler, Asbury, & Kusner 2008), the description of the marketing activities for the four phases (including efforts that targeted the general market and specific ethnic groups) (Huhman et al., 2008), and an overview of the evaluation methods (Berkowitz et al., 2008) are summarized in a June 2008 supplement to the *American Journal of Preventive Medicine*. The remainder of this chapter focuses on the national and community partnership component of VERB, which was slower to develop than national VERB and, in many ways, was more complex.

VERB created a demand for physical activity, and communities supplied the opportunities for tweens to be physically active where they lived. As a public health effort, VERB was created to engage communities as campaign partners by helping them assess their needs, build capacity, and customize VERB-related activities to meet those needs. As willing and eager partners, communities wanted to own at least parts of the planning and implementation processes, which often was not practical or efficient in the fast-paced world of the private sector advertising and media groups. The creative agencies and media organizations were not used to community coalitions or task forces as partners, and they often could not accommodate the community's preferences for venues and times. Plus, the creative team from the Centers for Disease Control and Prevention (CDC) and the creative agencies were very concerned that all communications to the target audience be "on brand." They worried that loss of the cool factor of VERB by well-intentioned but adult-centric or unexciting community events would dilute the assets of the young VERB brand. Thus, for the first two years, VERB planners and communities grappled with the best ways to partner with each other. Communities were ready to partner, but VERB was cautious until the brand was firmly established and campaign products were developed that were appropriate for communities to use.

After the VERB brand was established and partners learned about the importance of brand protection, the strategy that evolved entailed communities' using the VERB brand guidelines to develop materials for their community that featured the VERB logo, bringing VERB's cachet to the community's efforts. VERB also provided activity toolkits with appealing premiums for schools and organizations to use with tweens. CDC's VERB Partnership Team consulted with community partners to ensure that their message was consistent with that of the national campaign by helping them (1) reframe their physical activity programs as fun and exciting and avoid a *should do, good for you* message,

(2) connect the VERB brand to the point-of-purchase, and (3) drive tweens to the opportunities, places, and programs where they could "purchase" the product of physical activity. The VERB brand created a desire to be physically active, and communities provided the places for tweens to be active.

One of the most comprehensive and successful community programs was VERB Summer Scorecard, later shortened to VERB Scorecard, which Lexington, Kentucky, implemented in the summer of 2004 and continued for several summers. A high-functioning coalition of more than 50 members from businesses, schools, health services, recreation centers, and the transportation system, as well as parents and coaches, decided to focus its efforts on youth physical activity. The centerpiece of VERB Summer Scorecard was the actual scorecard, a wallet-sized card with 24 squares on it; each square represented one hour of physical activity. Participating businesses and recreational outlets stamped the cards and gave tweens discounts on physical activities and events, such as free swimming at community pools and reduced admission prices to skating rinks and sports clinics (figure 6.1).

The coalition used a planning and implementation approach called "community-based prevention marketing," developed by the Florida Prevention Research Center (FPRC) (figure 6.2). Community-based prevention marketing uses the four Ps of marketing—product, price, place, and promotion—as an implementation framework. With assistance from the FPRC, the coalition quickly developed a marketing mindset and worked to develop the *places* for tweens to be active at the right *price* and even negotiated with the transportation system that a scorecard could be used as bus fare—thus removing an important barrier for tweens getting to their preferred places to be active.

CDC's VERB team helped keep program development costs low for the coalition by providing the extensive audience research about tweens and parents that had been conducted by CDC to develop the VERB brand and messages. This was possible because the Lexington staff recognized that many of the research findings for the same target audience were applicable regardless of geographic location. CDC's team

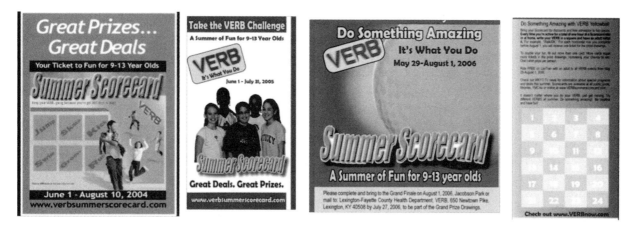

Figure 6.1 The VERB Summer Scorecards from Lexington's (left to right) 2004, 2005, and 2006 community-based campaigns listed the discounts and special events available for tweens. Tweens also tracked their physical activity hours on the VERB Scorecard (far right) and then redeemed completed cards for great prizes.

Reprinted, by permission, from Nutrition and Fitness Coalition.

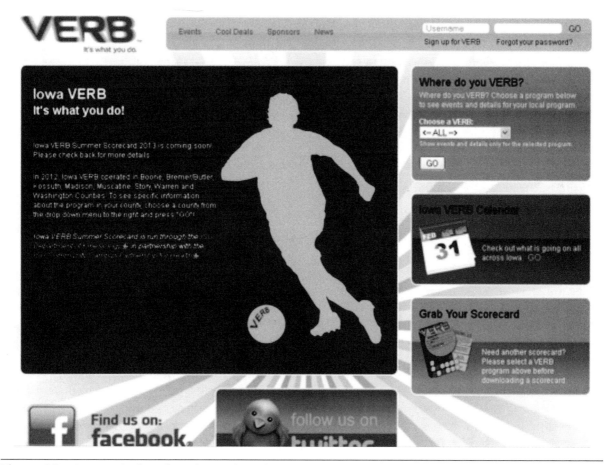

Figure 6.2 Community-based marketing from the VERB website.

Reprinted, by permission, from Iowa State University. Available: http://www.iowaverb.org

supported the Lexington coalition's efforts through consultation on the brand guidelines and local marketing strategies. CDC's evaluation team provided guidance on the coalition's plans for evaluation. By the end of 2006, 17 other communities in several states (e.g., Indiana, Iowa, and Florida) had adapted the Lexington VERB Scorecard program for their community.

VERB Summer Scorecard in Sarasota, Florida, closely modeled the Lexington program and was evaluated through a partnership with the FPRC. Some other U.S. communities have programs planned for 2011, five years after VERB's national funding ended.

Program Evaluation

National VERB was evaluated extensively. Process evaluation, which assesses how faithfully the campaign was implemented, included monitoring the reach and frequency of the advertising, conducting a national tracking survey to monitor the likeability of the VERB brand, and assessing the number of promotions and events, attendance at events, and receptiveness of tweens to the promotional events. VERB conducted an annual outcome evaluation through nationally representative telephone surveys. The evaluation surveyed tweens and parents regarding their attitudes and behaviors related to physical activity. The survey tool, the Youth Media Campaign Longitudinal Survey, was developed specifically for VERB and was found to be reliable and valid (Welk et al. 2007). The survey is available at www.cdc.gov/youthcampaign.

The outcome evaluation showed that after year one of the campaign, 74% of U.S. tweens were aware of VERB and 90% of those who were aware understood at least one of the key messages. Subgroups of tweens (e.g., girls, younger tweens) who were aware of the campaign did more physical activity than tweens who were not. After the second year, total population-level effects (no significant differences across gender, age, race, socioeconomic status) were found for six of the seven attitude and behavioral primary outcomes. After evaluators controlled for baseline levels of physical activity, tweens who were aware of VERB reported more physical activity sessions in their free time than did tweens who were not aware of the campaign. After four years of the campaign, the final outcome analysis showed continuing effects, and a dose response analysis found that increasing amounts of VERB exposure resulted in stronger attitude and behavioral effects. Some positive VERB effects were sustained as tweens aged into their later teen years.

VERB Summer Scorecard in Lexington was assessed with process and outcome measures. In 2004, tweens redeemed more than 350 completed VERB Scorecards that reported more than 8,400 hours of physical activity during the 13-week community campaign. Participants redeemed more than twice as many completed VERB Scorecards in 2005 and 2006. Scorecard participants were more likely to be physically active than were tweens who did not participate. In addition to affecting the individual-level variables, the efforts in Lexington led to changes in macro-level variables, affecting the local health department's relationship with local media, public transportation, and businesses.

The Sarasota County program evaluators used a post-only comparison group design to evaluate their 2005 Summer Scorecard program. They found that tweens who participated in the intervention were more likely to be physically active than tweens in the comparison group and more physically active than youth in the intervention community who did not participate in the scorecard program. Sarasota evaluators also used their scorecard program experiences to study community capacity to implement and sustain health interventions.

Linkage to National Physical Activity Plan

The campaign used six of the eight strategies included in the Mass Media Sector of the National Physical Activity Plan (NPAP).

Strategy 1: Encourage public health agencies to form partnerships with other agencies across the eight sectors to combine resources around common themes in promoting physical activity. VERB partnered with more than 50 county and local public health departments, coalitions, and task forces in 20 cities; national organizations (e.g., Girl Scouts); and marketing and media businesses that wanted to dedicate resources to a physical activity mission. VERB worked across sectors at the national level and supported community-level programs that partnered with health departments, local businesses, transportation systems, schools, and recreational facilities. These activities exemplify two of the three tactics described in Strategy 1 of the Mass Media Sector of the National Physical Activity Plan (NPAP). www.physicalactivityplan.org/media_st1.php.

Strategy 2: Enact federal legislation to support a sustained physical activity mass media campaign. A congressional appropriation funded the CDC to develop and implement a campaign that became VERB. The program was funded for five years for a total of $340 million. The VERB campaign exemplifies Strategy 2 for the Mass Media component of the NPAP (www.physicalactivityplan.org/media_st2.php).

Strategy 3: Develop consistent mass communication messages that promote physical activity, have a clear and standardized "brand," and are consistent with the Physical Activity Guidelines for Americans. The foundation of the campaign was the VERB brand, which was associated in the minds of tweens with the fun, cool, and social benefits of physical activity. Although the tween messages never mentioned getting the recommended 60 minutes of physical activity a day, VERB parent materials encouraged parents to help their children be physically active at recommended levels. These activities exemplify one of the tactics of Strategy 3 for the Mass Media Sector of the NPAP (www.physicalactivityplan.org/media_st3.php).

Strategy 4: Ensure that messages and physical activity plans developed by state and local public health agencies and key stakeholders from the eight sectors are consistent with national messages. CDC directed media partners, national organizations, and community partners to follow carefully the brand guidelines developed by CDC for using the national campaign VERB logo, including color, typeface, and context guidelines for using the logo, as recommended in Strategy 4 of the Mass Media Sector of the NPAP (www.physicalactivityplan.org/media_st4.php).

Strategy 5: Sequence, plan, and provide campaign activities in a prospective, coordinated manner. Support and link campaign messages to community-level programs, policies, and environmental supports. VERB's initial attempts to coordinate national promotions in nine local communities during year one had mixed results. VERB administrators learned that communities needed time to develop events, programs, and activities that matched their interests and resources. VERB also needed to provide tangibles (e.g., promotional items) to support communities, but CDC was still developing and refining those resources. The most comprehensive, and some of the most successful, community VERB programs used the systematic planning approach of community-based prevention marketing. Coordinating mass media efforts with community planning is recommended as a tactic of Strategy 5 of the Mass Media Sector of the NPAP (www.physicalactivityplan.org/media_st5.php).

Strategy 6: Encourage mass media professionals to become informed about the importance of physical activity and the potential role they can play in promoting physical activity. When VERB purchased media placement, media companies (e.g., Disney, Nickelodeon) offered the campaign added-value opportunities such as producing VERB ads with their talent (i.e., TV stars, cartoon characters) and placing the ads on their channels and in their national print media (e.g., *Sports Illustrated Kids*). VERB found that youth physical activity and obesity prevention appealed to everyone, including high-profile media companies such as Black Entertainment Television (BET), AOL (originally known as America Online), and Warner Bros (WB). Media companies wanted to go the extra mile and help to ensure VERB's success. These activities exemplify two of the four tactics recommended for Strategy 6 of the Mass Media Sector of the NPAP (www.physicalactivityplan.org/media_st6.php).

Evidence Base Used During Program Development

Between 2001 and 2005, the CDC's Guide to Community Preventive Services issued recommendations regarding evidence-based, community-level interventions to promote physical activity. The guide strongly recommended community-wide campaigns but could not recommend mass media interventions because insufficient evidence exists regarding their effectiveness. These two approaches share some characteristics with VERB, but VERB is not a typical example of either approach. Community-wide campaigns generally are tailored to a community, balance marketing and nonmarketing approaches, and mobilize substantial local partnerships (e.g., the adult-focused Wheeling Walks). VERB built a strong brand as a foundation for messages, emphasized social marketing, and involved national-local partnerships. VERB was also more than a mass media intervention (e.g., it included school and community promotions). Research indicates that social marketing is effective when done correctly, with examples including the "truth" campaign for prevention of tobacco use in adolescents, campaigns to promote low-fat milk (1% Milk campaign), campaigns to promote use of seat belts, and non-health-related campaigns such as promotion of recycling. Although no large campaigns have focused on physical activity in children, there is increasing evidence that social marketing approaches can be effective in promoting physical activity (Gordon, McDermott, Stead, & Angus. 2006).

The success of VERB substantially adds to the evidence that social marketing campaigns to promote physical activity can be effective in general and can be effective specifically in children.

Populations Best Served by the Program

The VERB national campaign targeted all U.S. tweens. This age group was chosen because group members are beginning to make their own lifestyle choices but still are strongly influenced by their parents.

VERB's national and community partners also targeted the tween age group but in some cases further segmented the audience. For example, some of the communities using the scorecard program specified that they were targeting moderately active tweens or "passives," which they defined as tweens who participated in no physical activity.

Lessons Learned

CDC's VERB team recommends the following:

If the physical activity promotion strategy is built around a brand, and the brand is meant to provide an identity that communities can leverage, build the brand presence first. Develop marketing materials for communities that they can adapt while the national campaign is being established. Examples include turnkey kits for physical activities in the classroom or an after-school program, press releases, tip sheets for engaging community partners, and guidelines for parents. These types of materials provide communities with something on which they can build.

Consider a system of categories to determine the right match for partner involvement. CDC's VERB team used a tiered model in which the tier 1 or ideal community or national partner had four characteristics:

1. An existing coalition or community network that facilitated access to the supply of physical activity opportunities in the community

2. A champion within the network who provided leadership and ensured follow-through

3. Its own funding (including donated media time and space) to support community-wide campaigns or promotional events

4. A firm understanding of the social marketing model and "a marketing mindset"

Partners at the tier 2 level had contact with the national campaign planners, some funding resources, and some understanding of a marketing mindset and ability to protect the brand. VERB helped these partners conduct on-brand events and promotions with their own resources.

Tier 3 partners included schools, recreational centers, and similar organizations that had none of the previously described characteristics and no funding resources. VERB provided these partners with a turnkey kit that they could implement in a classroom or an after-school

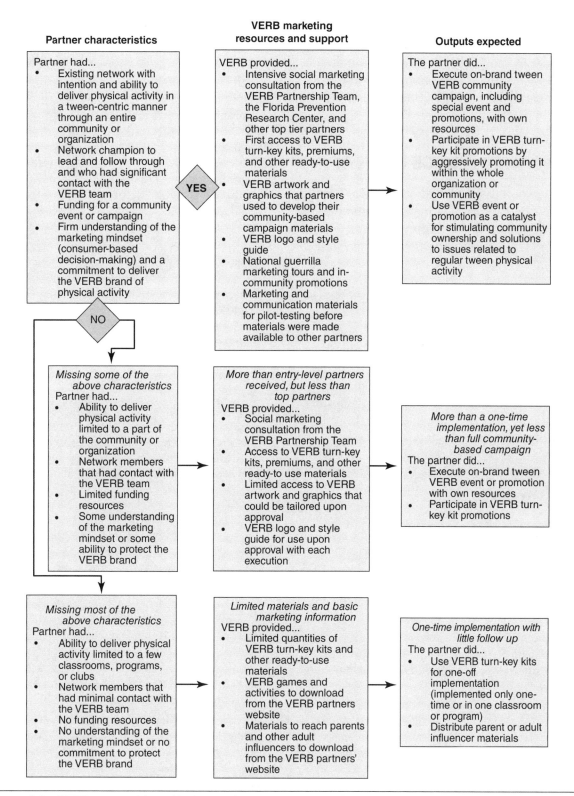

Figure 6.3 VERB partnerships: aligning marketing resources with partner characteristics.

Reprinted from *American Journal of Preventative Medicine,* Vol. 34 (6S), R. Bretthauer-Mueller et al., "Catalyzing community action within a national campaign: VERB™ community and national partnerships," pgs. S210-S221, copyright 2008, with permission of Elsevier.

program. Using this tiered approach based on the community partner's level of readiness allowed CDC to target its limited partnership and staffing resources to communities that were able to create sustainable efforts (figure 6.3)

Tips for Working Across Sectors

It is important to negotiate a process for timely clearance and approval of marketing and media materials, a step that often is needed when working with public health agencies. VERB negotiated an expedited clearance process that was essential for the timelines needed across several sectors, especially media organizations and businesses.

Another important strategy is to build in expectations with the creative team members that communities and national partners will carry the mass media messages to their constituents and communities, thereby sustaining the behavior in the target audience. Establish strong brand protection guidelines and provide careful oversight of partners' implementation to ensure that partners' efforts are consistent with the brand specifications.

Additional Reading and Resources

VERB legacy products and tools and data for the outcome evaluation are available at www.cdc.gov/youthcampaign.

Articles in the June 2008 Supplement to the *American Journal of Preventive Medicine* are available at www.cdc.gov/youthcampaign. The following are especially relevant:

Bretthauer-Mueller, R., J.M. Berkowitz, M. Thomas, et al. (2008). Catalyzing community action within a national campaign: VERB community and national partnerships. *American Journal of Preventive Medicine, 34*(6S).S210-1.

Wong, F.L., M. Greenwell, S. Gates, and J.M. Berkowitz. (2008). It's what you do! Reflections on the VERB™ campaign *American Journal of Preventive Medicine, 34*(6S),S175-82.

Materials related to the Lexington and Sarasota County VERB Summer Scorecard programs:

Alfonso, M.L., J.E. Nickelson, D.L. Hogeboom, J. French, C.A. Bryant, R.J. McDermott, and J.A. Baldwin.(2008). Assessing local capacity for health intervention. *Evaluation and Program Planning, 31,*145-59.

Bryant, C.A., A.H. Courtney, R.J. McDermott, M.L. Alfonso, J.A. Baldwin, J. Nickelson, K.R. McCormack Brown, R.D. Debate, L.M. Phillips, Z. Thompson, and Y. Zhu. (2010). Promoting physical activity among youth through community-based prevention marketing. *Journal of School Health,* 80(5), 214-24.

Bryant, C.A., K. McCormack Brown, R.J. McDermott, R.D. Debate, M.A. Alfonso, J.L. Baldwin, P. Monaghan, and L.M. Phillips. 2009. Community-based prevention marketing: A new planning framework for designing and tailoring health promotion interventions. In: *Emerging Theories in Health Promotion Practice and Research: Strategies for Improving Public Health.* 2nd ed. R. DiClemente, R.A. Crosby, and M.C. Kegler, Eds. San Francisco: Jossey-Bass.

DeBate, R.D., J. Baldwin, Z. Thompson, J.E. Nickelson, M. Alfonso, C.A. Bryant, L.M. Phillips, and R.J. McDermott. (2009). VERB Summer Scorecard: Findings from a multi-level community-based physical activity intervention for tweens. *American Journal of Community Psychology.* 44, 363-73.

References

Asbury, L.D, F.L Wong, S.M. Price, and M.J. Nolin. 2008. The VERBcampaign: Applying a branding strategy in public health. *American Journal of Preventive Medicine, 34* (6S), S183-S187.

Berkowitz, J.M., M. Huhman, C.D. Heitzler, L.D. Potter M.J. Nolin, and S.W. Banspach. 2008. Overview of formative, process, and outcome evaluation methods used in the VERB™ campaign. *American Journal of Preventive Medicine, 34* (6S), S222-S229.

Gordon, R., L., M. McDermott, M. Stead, and K. Angus. 2006. The effectiveness of social marketing to improve health: What's the evidence? *Public Health, 120,* (12):1133-9.

Heitzler, C.D., L.D. Asbury, and S.L. Kusner. 2008. Bringing "play" to life: The use of experiential marketing in the VERBcampaign. *American Journal of Preventive Medicine, 34* (6S), S188-S193.

Huhman, M., J.M. Berkowitz, F.L. Wong, E. Prosper, M. Gray, D. Prince, and J. Yuen. 2008. The VERB-campaign's strategy for reaching African-American, Hispanic, Asian, and American Indian children and parents. *American Journal of Preventive Medicine, 34* (6S), S194-S209.

Welk, G.J., E. Wickel, M. Peterson, C.D. Heitzler, J.E. Fulton, and L.D. Potter. 2007. Reliability and validity of physical activity questions on the Youth Media Campaign Longitudinal Survey. *Medicine & Science in Sports & Exercise, 39* (4), 612-21.

CHAPTER 7

Start.Living.Healthy
Using Mass Media to Increase Physical Activity in Hawai`i

Jay Maddock, PhD
University of Hawai`i at Mānoa

Alice Silbanuz, BA
Hawai`i Department of Health

Lola Irvin, MED
Hawai`i Department of Health

Bill Reger-Nash, EdD
West Virginia University

NPAP Tactics and Strategies Used in This Program

Mass Media Sector

STRATEGY 1: Encourage public health agencies to form partnerships with other agencies across the eight sectors to combine resources around common themes in promoting physical activity.

STRATEGY 3: Develop consistent mass communication messages that promote physical activity, have a clear and standardized "brand," and are consistent with the most current Physical Activity Guidelines for Americans.

STRATEGY 5: Sequence, plan, and provide campaign messages in a prospective coordinated manner. Support and link campaign messages to community-level programs, policies, and environmental supports.

Start.Living.Healthy uses paid and earned media to encourage adults ages 35 to 55 to walk at least 30 minutes a day. Based on the Theory of Planned Behavior, the campaign titled Step It Up, Hawai`i presents common decision points to allow people to decide to become active.

Program Description

Start.Living.Healthy is a social marketing umbrella campaign designed as part of the Healthy Hawai`i Initiative (HHI) (Maddock et al. 2006), an ongoing, multilevel, statewide, mass media-led intervention in Hawaii. HHI, which is funded by the tobacco settlement, addresses tobacco control, physical activity, and nutrition in Hawaii. Start.Living.Healthy is the state's umbrella brand for all physical activity and nutrition messages. It has been used since 2002 and is widely known in Hawai`i. The HHI is housed in the Hawai`i State Department of Health and includes a steering committee of community stakeholders.

Campaign Foundations

The walking campaign was the third phase of the overall social marketing campaign. In phase I of the overall campaign, messages were developed for individuals in the precontemplation stage of change for physical activity and nutrition. Results of the campaign showed high awareness and increased knowledge about government recommendations for physical activity and nutrition (Maddock and Johnson 2006). In phase II, a research-tested mass media campaign to encourage individuals to switch to low-fat milk was adapted and culturally tailored to the population. This campaign was very successful, with more than 10 percent of high-fat milk drinkers switching to low-fat milk (Maddock et al. 2006).

To plan for phase III, the management team of the HHI conducted extensive formative research (Maddock et al. 2008b), using the data from its psychosocial surveillance system (Maddock et al. 2003). Data showed that (1) a large percentage of adults were in the contemplation and preparation stages (Marcus et al. 1992) for physical activity, and (2) the percentage of adults meeting physical activity guidelines decreased significantly with increasing age: 58.4 percent of 25- to 34-year-olds, 49.2 percent of 35- to 44-year-olds, and 48.2 percent of 55- to 64-year-olds (Centers for Disease Control and Prevention 2007). The management team decided to promote regular walking among 35- to 55-year-olds for this campaign as a means of helping Hawai`i residents meet the national recommendations (Pate et al. 1995).

Identifying Target Behaviors

Next, program planners identified the target behavior for the campaigns. The national guidelines for physical activity at the time were 30 minutes or more of moderate physical activity a day, on most days of the week, or 20 minutes or more of vigorous physical activity on three or more days per week (Pate et al. 1995). These recommendations were seen as too complex to convey in a cluttered world of mass media sound bites. In addition, recommending vigorous exercise to 35- to 55-year-olds who are not sufficiently active seemed impractical. National surveillance data showed that walking was the activity most frequently reported by adults who met the guidelines (Simpson et al. 2003), and moderate-intensity walking is consistent with the Physical Activity Guidelines for Americans (Physical Activity Guidelines Advisory Committee 2008). Therefore, the program planners chose moderate-intensity walking as the target behavior.

Preproduction Research

Preproduction research was carried out in two phases. In the first phase, program staff conducted open-ended elicitation surveys to generate key beliefs about exercising 30 minutes a day. They asked 32 clerical, skilled, and trade workers, ages 35 to 55 years, to generate key beliefs on social norms, attitudes, and perceived behavioral control for physical activity. The responses yielded unique Theory of Planned Behavior belief statements. Staff then created a quantitative survey to measure these key beliefs and assess self-reported behaviors related to regular walking. Snowballing sampling methods were used, and the survey was sent to all county health offices in the state of Hawaii. Health department staff used their contacts in the local communities to recruit 35- to 55-year-old adults to complete the survey. Respondents were classified into those who performed the behavior at the recommended level (i.e., at least 30 minutes of physical activity, five days a week; $N = 85$), and those who did not ($N = 300$). A discriminant functional analysis was conducted to assess which beliefs differed between the groups. Program staff then used the beliefs most different between the groups as the basis for developing the media messages. The significantly different variables were (1) "I don't have enough time," (2) "I think I should exercise 30 minutes a day most days of the week," and (3) "It is hard staying motivated."

Production Testing

The program hired a creative team to develop message concepts based on the key beliefs identified in the preproduction phase. The team presented three concepts to the steering committee, which rejected one message that did not clearly articulate the core concepts. The remaining two messages were titled All in the Family and Decision Point. The All in the Family message was based on Wheeling Walks, a research-tested mass media program (Reger et al. 2002). In the All in the Family approach, participants were introduced to someone who successfully improved his or her health through the motivation and support of a family member.

The Decision Point message focused on making choices and taking small steps to follow a more healthy lifestyle. The actors were presented with a decision point between a sedentary activity (e.g., watching television) and a more active activity (e.g., walking with friends during their planned time together). Another spot posed a choice between taking the elevator or the stairs. These two approaches were then tested with two separate focus groups of males and females.

Focus group participants were adults ages 35 to 55 who were active less than 150 minutes per week. During the groups, facilitators presented the two concepts (i.e., All in the Family and Decision Point). Participants discussed what they liked and did not like about the two approaches and whether the approaches influenced their core beliefs regarding these behaviors. The order in which the campaigns were introduced was switched for the two groups to control for order effects. Participants marked their responses on paper during the focus group so that statistics could be calculated after the group.

The All in the Family approach was not well received. Only three participants (15.8 percent) found it believable, and few (10.5 percent) thought that the advertisements would get them to start walking. The general feeling was that the family approach was overdone and that the spots were not exciting or motivating enough to maintain behavior change. The Decision Point approach fared much better. Most participants (89.5 percent) found it believable, and almost all thought it would motivate them to become active (94.7 percent). Participants liked the tone of the advertisements, found them empowering, and were more accepting of the advice offered to improve their health. Based on this feedback, program planners selected the Decision Point advertisements for development.

Campaign Launch

HHI used results from the formative research to develop three 30-second television commercials, four 30-second radio commercials, mall advertisements, and posters for the walking campaign. The campaign method was patterned after the Wheeling Walks campaign, which is also presented in this book. Staff made other decisions about the campaign logistics based on HHI's previous evaluation data. Decisions on media channels were based on evaluation data from the successful 1% or Less campaign (Maddock et al. 2007). The intensive walking campaign lasted 10 weeks, similar to Wheeling Walks (Reger et al. 2002). The overall campaign brand was Start.Living.Healthy, which has been used by HHI since 2002 and is well recognized in the community. The specific campaign slogan was Step It Up, Hawai`i!

The campaign was launched on April 4, 2007, with a press conference led by the lieutenant governor. Program staff began writing a weekly column on walking, which appeared in the state's largest newspaper. All 65,000 government employees received a pay stub message encouraging walking. Media relations events resulted in earned mass media campaign message communication worth approximately $51,000. Gross rating points were 2,205 for television and 3,443 for radio. Campaign posters were placed in 300 locations, including malls and doctors' offices, across the state. The campaign website received more than 2,000 visits during the campaign.

Program Evaluation

The data for this study were collected as part of an ongoing statewide surveillance survey for physical activity and nutrition (Maddock et al. 2003). A stratified, random-digit dialing system was used to reach a random sample of 3,600 of Hawaii's noninstitutionalized adult population on all major inhabited islands: 1,800 from the island of Oahu, 600 from Hawaii, 600 from Kauai, 500 from Maui, 75 from Molokai, and 25 from Lanai. The disproportionate design was randomized across counties and included both listed and unlisted telephone numbers. The sample size was selected to give statewide precision estimates of ±2 percent.

This analysis used only the results from the 2007 cross-sectional survey, which was conducted immediately following the conclusion of the campaign and included variables that provided data on the potential knowledge gap.

Overall, 54 percent of respondents said that they had heard (via prompted recall) of the Start.Living.Healthy campaign in the prior six months, and 70.3 percent of respondents recalled seeing or hearing the message "people should walk 30 minutes a day for at least 5 days a week." Sixty-four percent of all respondents recalled hearing that "walking gives you energy." About 50 percent recalled the messages that "there is benefit in walking only 10 minutes" (52.7 percent) and that "walking gives you time, because you have more energy to do things" (49.0 percent). Overall, half (51.7 percent) of respondents recalled seeing Start. Living.Healthy advertisements on television, including 12.2 percent who said that they had seen "a lot" of such commercials. Recall of radio commercials was much lower—only 20 percent of all respondents recalled having heard Start. Living.Healthy radio ads. Fewer than half of all respondents (42.9 percent) recalled seeing news stories about the campaign. A complete analysis of campaign awareness by subgroups has been reported by Buchthal and colleagues (2011). Smaller pre- and postcampaign surveys of 400 people examined attitudes and behavior. No significant differences were seen for the Theory of Planned Behavior variables or behavior, indicating little or no effect of the campaign on changing the underlying theoretical variables or walking behavior (Maddock et al. 2008a).

Linkage to the National Physical Activity Plan

The Start.Living.Healthy walking campaign was consistent with three strategies of the Mass Media Sector of the National Physical Activity Plan.

Strategy 1: Encourage public health agencies to form partnerships with other agencies across the eight sectors to combine resources around common themes in promoting physical activity. Public and private partnerships were essential to increasing the penetration of the campaign. The Hawai`i Department of Health and the University of Hawai`i already had a long-standing partnership and formed the core of the campaign. In addition, the lieutenant governor served as the spokesperson for the campaign. The state Office of Human Resources allowed campaign messages to be placed on the paystubs of all state employees. In the private sector, the *Honolulu Advertiser*, the state's largest newspaper, provided a free weekly column for the entire campaign.

Strategy 3: Develop consistent mass communication messages that promote physical activity, have a clear and standardized "brand," and are consistent with the most current Physical Activity Guidelines for Americans. The campaign used the well-tested brand called Start. Living.Healthy. This is the state's umbrella brand for all physical activity and nutrition messages. It has been used since 2002 and is widely known in Hawai`i. All of the messages encouraged 30 minutes of physical activity a day, consistent with national recommendations.

Strategy 5: Sequence, plan, and provide campaign messages in a prospective coordinated manner. Support and link campaign messages to community-level programs, policies, and environmental supports. This campaign was phase III of an overall campaign. It built directly on an earlier campaign geared toward people in the precontemplation stage of change; that program was titled You've Got to Start Somewhere. The campaign is part of the broader HHI, which uses a social ecological approach to create change in communities and schools and promote policy for physical activity.

Evidence Base Used During Program Development

This program was developed using the Theory of Planned Behavior (Montano and Kasprzyk 2002), which has been tested in numerous research studies and found to be applicable to many behaviors, including physical activity (Nigg et al. 2009). The campaign used the principles of other research-tested campaigns, including Wheeling Walks, Active Australia, and the earlier Start.Living.Healthy campaigns (figure 7.1). The entire campaign was based on the six steps proposed by Noar (2006) for effective mass media campaigns.

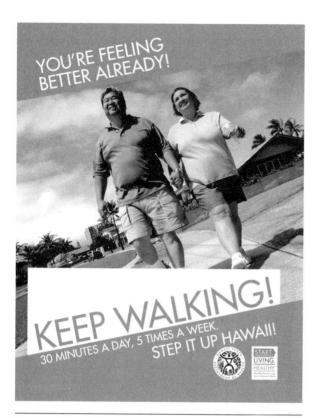

Figure 7.1   Flier used to promote Start.Living. Healthy's walking program.

©Jay Maddock, Lola Irvin, Alice Silbanuz, and Bill Reger-Nash.

Populations Best Served by the Program

This program was designed for 35- to 55-year-olds in multiethnic Hawai`i. Women and all ethnic groups, including Native Hawaiians and Filipinos, had a high recall of the campaign and a positive response to the advertisements. However, recall of the campaign was lower among those at 130 percent or less of the federal poverty line and those with less than a high school education, indicating that the campaign did not reach some at-risk populations (Buchthal et al. 2011).

Lessons Learned

Start planning early. To develop an effective theory-based campaign, allow at least six months prior to the kickoff event. Political and funding realities often make it difficult to secure this preparation time, but it is necessary to ensure that all of the steps are taken and that theory is truly integrated into the campaign.

Recognize that what worked in another community may not work in your community. We were surprised that the Wheeling Walks–style commercials called All in the Family did not test well in the target population. Taking campaigns that worked in one location and implementing them in a new location, instead of looking at the underlying deep structure around cultural norms and expectations, often does not work well.

Use public figures cautiously. The lieutenant governor appeared in one of the campaign spots and also hosted the kickoff events. During this time, he was considering a run for governor. This caused statewide controversy. Several news stories questioned whether it was appropriate for him to appear in the spots. Now that a new governor of a different political party has been elected, the program cannot use any of the campaign materials that feature the lieutenant governor.

Tips for Working Across Sectors

This program is part of the larger HHI. The HHI seeks to increase physical activity using the social ecological approach and partners with several groups throughout the state, including the state departments of transportation, parks and recreation, and land and natural resources; community coalitions; county governments; and nongovernmental agencies. Partnership is an ongoing iterative process that is never complete. In areas in which the program has been successful, key factors have included articulating an enticing vision of the future, understanding the goals of partners, developing roles for all partners, sharing credit, and celebrating successes.

Additional Reading and Resources

Campaign Advertisements are available at www.healthyhawaii.com/about/about_start_

living_healthy/step_it_up_hawaii_media_campaign.htm.

References

Buchthal, O.V., A.L. Doff, L.A. Hsu, A. Silbanuz, K.M. Heinrich, and J.E. Maddock. 2011. Avoiding a knowledge gap in a multiethnic statewide social marketing campaign—Is cultural tailoring sufficient? *J Health Commun*. 16:314-27.

Centers for Disease Control and Prevention. 2007. *Behavioral Risk Factor Surveillance System Survey Data*. Atlanta, GA: U.S. Department of Health and Human Services, Centers for Disease Control and Prevention.

Maddock, J.E., and C. Johnson. 2006. Effects of a social marketing campaign on chronic disease related behaviors in a multi-ethnic community. *Int. J. Behav. Med*. 13:S141.

Maddock, J.E., C.A. Maglione, J.D. Barnett, C. Cabot, J. Jackson, and B. Reger-Nash. 2007. Statewide implementation of the 1 Percent or Less campaign. *Health Educ. Behav*. 34:953-63.

Maddock, J.E., C. Marshall, C.R. Nigg, and J.D. Barnett. 2003. Development and first year results of a psychosocial surveillance system for chronic disease related health behaviors. *Calif. J. Health Promot*. 1(5):54-64.

Maddock, J.E., L. Takeuchi, B. Nett, C. Tanaka, L. Irvin, C. Matsuoka, and B. Wood. 2006. Evaluation of a statewide program to reduce chronic disease: The Healthy Hawai`i Initiative, 2000-2004. *Eval. Prog. Plann*. 29:293-300.

Maddock, J.E., A. Silbanuz, L. Irvin, and B. Reger-Nash. 2008. Using social marketing to increase physical activity and improve nutrition in Hawaii. *Ann. Behav. Med*. 35:s95.

Maddock, J.E., A. Silbanuz, and B. Reger-Nash. 2008. Formative research to develop a mass media campaign to increase physical activity and nutrition in a multiethnic state. *J. Health Commun*. 13:208-15.

Marcus, B.H., V.C. Selby, R.S. Niaura, and J.S. Rossi. 1992. Self-efficacy and the stages of exercise behavior change. *Res. Q. Exerc. Sport* 63:60-6.

Nigg, C.R., S. Lippke, and J.E. Maddock. 2009. Factorial invariance of the Theory of Planned Behavior applied to physical activity across gender, age and ethnic groups. *Psychol. Sport Exerc*. 10:219-25.

Montano, D.E. and D. Kasprzyk. 2002. The theory of reasoned action and the theory of planned behavior. In: *Health Education and Behavior*. 3rd ed. K. Glanz, B. Rimer, and F. Lewis, Eds. San Francisco: Jossey-Bass.

Noar, S.M. 2006. A 10-year retrospective of research in health mass media campaigns: Where do we go from here? *J. Health Commun*. 11:1-22.

Pate, R.R., M. Pratt, S.N. Blair, W.L. Haskell, C.A. Macera, et al. 1995. Physical activity and public health—A recommendation from the Centers for Disease Control and Prevention and the American College of Sports Medicine. *JAMA*. 273:402-7.

Physical Activity Guidelines Advisory Committee. 2008. *Physical Activity Guidelines Advisory Committee Report*. Washington, DC: USDHHS.

Reger, B., L. Cooper, S. Booth, H. Smith, A. Bauman, M. Wootan, S. Middlestat, B. Marcus, and F. Greer. 2002. Wheeling Walks: A community campaign using paid media to encourage walking among sedentary older adults. *Prev. Med*. 353:285-92.

Simpson, M.E., M. Serdula, D.A. Galuska, C. Gillespie, R. Donehoo, C. Mecera, and K. Mack. 2003. Walking trends among US adults: The Behavioral Risk Factor Surveillance System, 1987-2000. *Am. J. Prev. Med*. 25:95-100.

CHAPTER 8

ParticipACTION
The National Voice of Physical Activity and Sport Participation in Canada

Amy E. Latimer-Cheung, PhD
Queen's University

Kelly Murumets
ParticipACTION

Guy Faulkner, PhD
University of Toronto

NPAP Tactics and Strategies Used in This Program

Mass Media Sector

STRATEGY 1: Encourage public health agencies to form partnerships with other agencies across the eight sectors to combine resources around common themes in promoting physical activity.

STRATEGY 2: Enact federal legislation to support a sustained physical activity mass media campaign.

STRATEGY 3: Develop consistent mass communication messages that promote physical activity, have a clear and standardized "brand," and are consistent with the most current physical activity guidelines.

STRATEGY 4: Ensure that messages and physical activity plans developed by state and local public health agencies and key stakeholders from the eight sectors are consistent with national messages.

STRATEGY 5: Sequence, plan, and provide campaign activities in a prospective, coordinated manner.

Support and link campaign messages to community-level programs, policies, and environmental supports.

STRATEGY 6: Encourage mass media professionals to become informed about the importance of physical activity and the potential role they can play in promoting physical activity.

STRATEGY 7: Encourage local, state, and federal public health agencies and key stakeholders from the eight sectors to integrate into their physical activity plans and programs Web- and new media-based physical activity interventions that are supported by evidence.

STRATEGY 8: Expand the definition of media for mediated interventions to include new and emerging technologies such as global positioning systems, video gaming, and other technologies. Identify funding for research to develop evidence that supports or opposes the use of existing and emerging technologies for increasing physical activity.

ParticipACTION is a national not-for-profit organization solely dedicated to inspiring and supporting active living and sport participation for Canadians. Established in 1971, ParticipACTION operated for nearly 30 years and was a leading catalyst to encourage healthy, active living for all Canadians. The organization and its message became a Canadian source of influence, recognition, and pride (figure 8.1). In December 2000, ParticipACTION closed its doors because of insufficient resources. With the looming physical inactivity crisis, however,

ParticipACTION received a renewed commitment from the Canadian government and was revitalized in February 2007; its 3-year vision, mission, and strategic goals for 2009-2012, the period immediately after its revitalization, are discussed in this chapter. Since this chapter was written, ParticipACTION has renewed its vision, mission, and strategic plan for 2012-2015. Details of recent strategic initiatives are available on the ParticipACTION website.

Program Description

Within a year of its revitalization, ParticipACTION undertook a comprehensive strategic planning process (figure 8.2). The ParticipACTION board of directors and advisory committees and experts from across Canada who work in relevant areas (i.e., research, health promotion, government) provided input into the process. The resulting three-year strategic plan for 2009 to 2012 is presented in figure 8.2. This plan has been critical in guiding decision making. It has helped to streamline organizational activities, ensuring that ParticipACTION continually moves in a direction consistent with its mission and vision.

Strategic Plan

The plan identified three strategic focus areas: communications, capacity building, and knowledge exchange. These areas were selected because they leverage the strengths of the organization and provide value to the physical activity sector in Canada (i.e., all organizations with an interest in promoting physical activity and sport participation). ParticipACTION also recognized that a single organization cannot address the inactivity crisis on its own. Reflecting the need for a unified approach to tackling inactivity, these focus areas emphasize providing resources and support to empower partner organizations within and across the physical activity sector. The objectives associated with each area of focus are described next.

ParticipACTION's communications objectives include (1) delivering messages through multimedia for the purpose of raising awareness, educating, inspiring, and supporting behavior change and (2) coordinating communications

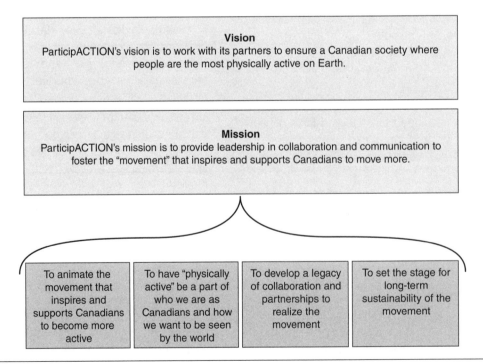

Figure 8.1 ParticipACTION's vision and mission statement for 2009-2012.

Reprinted, by permission, from ParticipACTION.

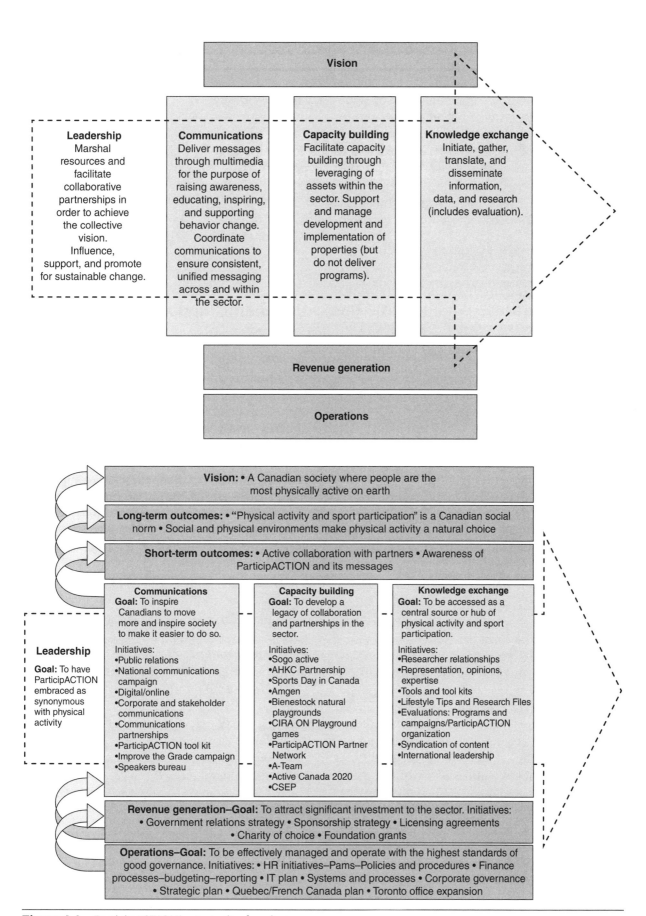

Figure 8.2 ParticipACTION's strategic planning process.

Reprinted, by permission, from ParticipACTION.

to ensure consistent, unified messaging across and within the physical activity sector. Since its renewal in 2007, ParticipACTION has undertaken three multifaceted mass media campaigns as one of its approaches to meeting these communications objectives. The target audience, time frame, and timing for each campaign were determined by identifying the needs of the physical activity sector and conducting extensive evaluation. The campaigns are archived on ParticipACTION's website (www.participaction.com).

ParticipACTION's capacity building objectives include (1) leveraging strengths within the physical activity sector by forging partnerships with and between organizations committed to promoting physical activity and sport participation in Canada and (2) supporting and managing the development and implementation of physical activity and sport participation initiatives (but not delivering programs). As a strategy for meeting the first objective, ParticipACTION created the ParticipACTION Partnership Network (PPN). The PPN is a robust network of organizations dedicated to physical activity and sport participation. Through the PPN, members expand their awareness of and access to resources, initiatives, and expertise within the physical activity sector while minimizing the duplication of efforts. In addition, the PPN coordinates and builds on existing infrastructure and communication channels to provide a mechanism for disseminating consistent messaging about physical activity and sport participation broadly across Canada.

ParticipACTION's objective for knowledge exchange is to position itself as a hub of information, data, and research related to physical activity and sport participation. ParticipACTION aims to make the latest research findings accessible to policy makers and practitioners in an effort to encourage evidence-informed decision making. In turn, ParticipACTION works to raise awareness among researchers regarding the gaps in the physical activity and sport participation evidence base that policy makers and practitioners have identified. To facilitate these knowledge exchange processes, ParticipACTION established three advisory groups: a research advisory group, a policy advisory group, and a marketing and communications advisory group. Group members have extensive expertise and are able to keep ParticipACTION informed of the latest research evidence and practice issues. ParticipACTION also is committed to creating new knowledge by publishing findings from its ongoing evaluation activities.

All of the activities ParticipACTION undertakes to meet its strategic objectives are listed in figure 8.2. To further demonstrate how ParticipACTION is accomplishing its strategic objectives, several exemplary activities for each focus area are presented in the following.

Communications Activities

The Think Again campaign, launched in January 2011, exemplifies how ParticipACTION meets its communication objectives. The campaign focused strategically on promoting awareness of the Canadian Physical Activity Guidelines for children and youth by targeting mothers, who exert a key influence on children's physical activity (Gustafson and Rhodes 2006), and youth. Using a comprehensive, integrated approach, the campaign disseminated information via national media (television advertisements, print and magazine advertisements and advertorials, and digital displays), social media (blog posts, Facebook posts, and tweets), the ParticipACTION website, and public relations outreach activities (press releases, direct media contact). A preliminary campaign evaluation indicated that, consistent with ParticipACTION's goal of raising awareness, a greater proportion of mothers, compared with the general population, recalled (without prompting) seeing an ad about children's physical activity (41 percent versus 35 percent). Forty percent of mothers who saw the ad accurately recalled the key campaign message without prompting. Although the remaining mothers could not recall the key message exactly, the majority did recall a message consistent with children's physical activity.

The Think Again campaign met the second objective, coordinating a consistent message across the physical activity sector, in several ways. The campaign's specific focus on mothers and youth allowed ParticipACTION to marshal its resources to support national and government initiatives that launched new physical activity guidelines and aimed to get children and youth more active. ParticipACTION provided organizations in its PPN with co-branding opportunities on its television and print media materials. As a result, PPN organizations could adopt ParticipACTION materials as their own, thus saving the organizations thousands of dollars on campaign production costs and ensuring a consistent national physical activity promotion message. Ten partner organizations took advantage of this opportunity, including national organizations (e.g., the YMCA), provincial organizations (e.g., the Nova Scotia Provincial Government), and municipal organizations (e.g., the Chatham-Kent Public Health Unit).

Capacity-Building Activities

Sogo Active, now known as the ParticipACTION Teen Challenge, illustrates the types of activities it undertakes to meet its objective related to building capacity in program development. Sogo Active is a youth-focused physical activity movement that encourages youth to find fun reasons and new opportunities to incorporate physical activity into their daily lives. Coordinated primarily through an online portal, the program encourages youth to sign up for and participate in Sogo Challenges. Youth themselves and community organizations (e.g., community centers, sport leagues, yoga studios) put forth the challenges. ParticipACTION supports the challenges by maintaining the online portal and providing small grants for community groups to host challenge events. In this way, ParticipACTION does not replicate services provided by organizations that offer physical activity programs for youth. Rather, ParticipACTION provides these organizations with resources to support their programs and empowers youth to become active agents in tackling the physical inactivity crisis.

Knowledge Exchange Activities

As an example of its knowledge exchange activities, ParticipACTION collaborates with the Canadian Fitness and Lifestyle Research Institute, a national not-for-profit research agency, to produce The Research File and the Lifestyle Tips series. The Research File includes monthly reports summarizing research findings on various topics related to physical activity. The Lifestyle Tips series, also published monthly, offers practical suggestions for daily physical activity. These reports are available on the ParticipACTION website.

Program Evaluation

ParticipACTION conducts regular and ongoing evaluations of all its activities. This section discusses why ParticipACTION places an emphasis on evaluation, what it evaluates, and how it conducts its evaluations. It also describe the baseline evaluation that was conducted immediately before ParticipACTION's relaunch. The data collected at that time serve as a benchmark for all subsequent evaluations, and they position ParticipACTION as a natural experiment that allows researchers to study the effectiveness of national strategies for promoting physical activity and sport participation.

Why?

The data gathered from ongoing evaluations provide evidence that ParticipACTION is accomplishing its strategic goals and moving toward its vision. This evidence is used to demonstrate accountability to funders and to build a strong case when they are seeking new funding opportunities. In line with its commitment to evidence-based practice, ParticipACTION relies heavily on the outcomes of its evaluations to inform the development of new initiatives. For example, data from previous campaign evaluations were integral in shaping decisions about modes of dissemination for the campaign released in January 2011. The availability of data from specific initiatives and campaigns also puts ParticipACTION in a position to generate new research knowledge about the effectiveness of physical activity and sport participation initiatives—an objective within the organization's knowledge exchange strategy.

What?

Using the strategic framework (figure 8.2) as a starting point, ParticipACTION has developed a logic model to guide its evaluation approach. The logic model outlines the organization's long- and short-term goals as well as the activities it will undertake to achieve these goals. Metrics have been assigned to evaluate each goal and activity. These metrics are diverse and include outcomes related to awareness (e.g., unaided recall of the ParticipACTION brand), usage (e.g., the number of website visits), exposure (e.g., the number of media impressions), behavior (e.g., the number of mothers who have looked for more information about physical activity for their children since viewing a campaign ad), uptake (e.g., the number of community organizations that have hosted a Sogo Challenge), and satisfaction (e.g., the satisfaction of members within the PPN). From 2010 to 2011, ParticipACTION conducted 17 individual evaluations, including evaluations of its campaigns and activities such as Sogo Active. It surveyed the general public, members of the PPN, the advisory groups, the staff, and the board of directors in order to provide input on ParticipACTION's activities.

How?

Because ParticipACTION is constantly involved in evaluation, it has been essential for the organization to establish streamlined, cost-effective procedures for data collection. Thus, it uses a professional research agency to conduct surveys of the general population. Survey participants are drawn from existing community panels, allowing ParticipACTION to survey specific segments of the population quickly and easily. The surveys are developed by ParticipACTION, with input from the research agency and the advisory groups. Surveys of partners and staff have been conducted online using a commercially available online survey interface. Many of the metrics related to usage are generated from online tracking tools monitoring outcomes, such as website visits and downloads. ParticipACTION monitors its media impact through a partnership with a communications firm with established protocols for measuring media impressions and uptake.

Baseline Evaluation: A Natural Experiment

With support from a strategic funding opportunity from the Canadian Institutes of Health Research, an independent research team collected extensive baseline data before the official relaunch of ParticipACTION in 2007. This was an important research opportunity, because limitations in the evaluation of the original ParticipACTION weakened the organization's ability to understand its real impact on physical activity. At the time of ParticipACTION's initial launch in 1971 (Bauman et al. 2004), formal evaluation techniques designed to assess the effectiveness of public health programs were limited. The relaunch of ParticipACTION presented a unique opportunity to address this gap by collecting baseline data as a basis for future, ongoing evaluation in the form of a natural experiment.

Two primary projects were embedded within the baseline data collection. First, the evaluation team assessed baseline awareness and understanding of ParticipACTION at an individual level using a population-based survey of 4,650 Canadians conducted over six months, from August 2007 to February 2008 (see Spence et al. 2009). Approximately 8 percent of Canadians were aware of ParticipACTION unprompted, and 82 percent were aware when prompted. Both education and income were significant correlates of awareness. Notably, higher education and income were associated with greater odds of ParticipACTION awareness. Second, the team collected baseline data concerning organizational capacity for physical activity promotion in Canada using an Internet-based survey instrument and interviews with key informants across Canada. Key informants painted a generally positive picture of current organizational capacity to promote physical activity messages, programs, and services in Canada (e.g., Faulkner et al. 2009). Overall, these studies provide the basis for assessing the short-, mid-, and long-term impact of ParticipACTION at the individual level (in terms of awareness, attitudes, and behavior) and the organizational level (in terms of organizational capacity, readiness, and advocacy regarding physical activity).

In 2012, five years after baseline data collection, additional research funding from the Canadian Institutes of Health Research was received to conduct a follow-up evaluation. The baseline data collection will be replicated and extended to determine the impact of ParticipACTION's activities since its revitalization in 2007.

Linkage to the National Physical Activity Plan

ParticipACTION's activities are relevant to multiple sectors identified in the National Physical Activity Plan (NPAP). For example, its activities incorporate the NPAP sectors Volunteer and Nonprofit; Public Health; Parks, Recreation, Fitness, and Sports; and, most of all, Mass Media. This section relates ParticipACTION's activities to each of the NPAP mass media strategies. Like the NPAP, ParticipACTION recognizes the importance of consistent and coordinated messages that promote participation in physical activity and sport. The implementation of the PPN and the development of detailed brand, government, media, and public relations strategies are central activities that contribute to ParticipACTION's success in accomplishing this goal.

Strategy 1: Encourage public health agencies to form partnerships with other agencies across the eight sectors to combine resources around common themes in promoting physical activity. The PPN includes members from all sectors and encourages cross-sector dialogue and resource sharing.

Strategy 2: Enact federal legislation to support a sustained physical activity mass media campaign. ParticipACTION has developed a government relations strategy (available on request) to ensure that physical activity and sport participation have a prominent place on the government's funding and policy agenda. The Canadian government does not have its own physical activity mass media campaign but rather relies on ParticipACTION to be the national voice on this issue.

Strategy 3: Develop consistent mass communication messages that promote physical activity, have a clear and standardized "brand," and are consistent with the most current physical activity guidelines. In accordance with standard marketing practices, ParticipACTION has a brand strategy with a brand pyramid (available on request). Up to 94 percent of Canadian adults are familiar with the ParticipACTION brand. ParticipACTION's messages are aligned entirely with the most current Canadian Physical Activity Guidelines (refer to the 2011 Think Again campaign). ParticipACTION was a principal partner in the release of the new Canadian Physical Activity Guidelines.

Strategy 4: Ensure that messages and physical activity plans developed by state and local public health agencies and key stakeholders from the eight sectors are consistent with national messages. ParticipACTION participates in the Federal, Provincial, and Territorial Social Marketing Working Group and has initiated the PPN to encourage consistent messaging across the sector.

Strategy 5: Sequence, plan, and provide campaign activities in a prospective, coordinated manner. Support and link campaign messages to community-level programs, policies, and environmental supports. When launching a campaign, ParticipACTION undertakes an extensive planning process, setting short-, medium-, and long-term objectives. Campaigns are linked to the sector through the PPN.

Strategy 6: Encourage mass media professionals to become informed about the importance of physical activity and the potential role they can play in promoting physical activity. Using strategic objectives for knowledge exchange, ParticipACTION has established a media and public relations strategy to educate and advocate for heightened awareness of physical activity and sport participation issues among media personnel. This strategy also involves promoting the PPN so that messages can be deployed by local organizations.

Strategy 7: Encourage local, state, and federal public health agencies and key stakeholders from the eight sectors to integrate into their physical activity plans and programs Web- and new media-based physical activity interventions that are supported by evidence. To facilitate this process, ParticipACTION has initiated the development of a national Canadian physical activity plan, Active Canada 20/20. The plan aims to provide an integrated multisectoral platform to tackle the physical inactivity crisis.

Strategy 8: Expand the definition of media for mediated interventions to include new and emerging technologies such as global positioning systems, video gaming, and other technologies. Identify funding for research to develop evidence that supports or opposes the use of existing and emerging technologies for increasing physical activity. ParticipACTION's Think Again campaign exemplifies the use of emerging technology to communicate physical activity and sport participation messages. The campaign uses traditional media (print, television) as well as social media and public relations to disseminate key messages.

Evidence Base Used During Program Development

ParticipACTION strives to model evidence-based practice. When developing its strategic plan, ParticipACTION conducted an extensive market analysis, drawing on evidence from large epidemiological studies that documented Canadians' physical activity patterns (e.g., Bryan and Katzmarzyk 2009; Iannotti et al. 2009). Current evidence from research and practice serves as the foundation of each ParticipACTION mass media campaign (e.g., Colley et al. 2011; Latimer et al. 2010; Tremblay et al. 2011a, 2011b). For example, the concept for the 2011 Think Again campaign emerged from a national report that documented parents' lack of awareness of their children's levels of inactivity (Active Healthy Kids Canada 2009). The content of the campaign was determined through extensive focus group testing with the target audience. Decisions related to modes of dissemination were based on evaluations of ParticipACTION's previous campaigns.

ParticipACTION's partnerships with researchers and practitioners and its commitment to evaluation and knowledge exchange are key components of its success in developing and implementing evidence-based practice. Partnerships with researchers and research agencies facilitate access to and interpretation of the most current research evidence. Regular interaction with practitioners ensures that ParticipACTION's activities align with current trends in the field. Having its own extensive database that documents the effectiveness of its practices ensures that ParticipACTION directs its resources to initiatives that will continue to move the organization forward. Moreover, having a strategic goal of knowledge exchange ensures that the organization is abreast of emerging evidence and that the use of evidence is at the forefront of all decision-making processes.

Populations Best Served by the Program

ParticipACTION's long-term goal is to get all Canadians moving more. However, in alignment with the priorities of the physical activity sector, many of ParticipACTION's recent initiatives emphasize promoting physical activity and sport participation among children and youth. Each activity ParticipACTION undertakes has a specific target group, including (but not limited to) mothers of young children, policy makers, researchers, practitioners, media personnel, and government officials.

Lessons Learned

Since its revitalization in 2007, ParticipACTION has learned some key lessons.

Have a Plan . . . for Everything

ParticipACTION has an extensive strategic plan as well as plans for brand development, communication, evaluation, and government, media, and public relations. By developing and implementing these plans, ParticipACTION can ensure that all of its activities are aligned with the organization's vision, that actions are evidence informed, and that metrics of evaluation are matched appropriately to the outcomes of the plan.

Use Advisory Groups

One of ParticipACTION's organizational strengths is its willingness to listen to and learn from the physical activity sector in Canada. Being receptive to feedback from its two advisory groups has allowed ParticipACTION to shape and strengthen many of its initiatives to reflect cutting-edge research and to respond to the needs of the sector.

Keep the Organization's Message Simple and Targeted

Nationwide initiatives promoting physical activity and sport participation often require a substantial investment of time and financial resources. As a consequence, organizations often try to ensure value for their investment by covering multiple issues at once and targeting broad segments of the population. However, ParticipACTION has learned that simple, targeted messages are quite valuable. The target audience can more easily comprehend, internalize, and implement a simple message than a complex one. As a result, physical activity organizations must adjust and align their own initiatives with simple messages.

Work in Partnership With the Physical Activity Sector

ParticipACTION has carefully aligned its efforts with the physical activity sector's needs and activities. This alignment ensures that the sector presents a coordinated and consistent message to the public and policy makers, while also optimizing resources.

Tips for Working Across Sectors

Although working across sectors (e.g., health, education, physical activity) can be challenging at times, its value is immeasurable. The inactivity crisis cannot be overcome by a single organization or a single sector for that matter. Rather, all sectors with an interest in enhancing the health of the population must work together to tackle the issue of inactivity. A coordinated effort across sectors capitalizes on, leverages resources for, and strengthens initiatives to promote physical activity and sport participation. ParticipACTION has been especially successful in facilitating cross-sectoral activities through its PPN. The PPN has created channels of communication between sectors, and it provides a mechanism for sharing resources. The PPN builds capacity at the grass roots community level.

Summary

ParticipACTION is a national not-for-profit organization committed to getting Canadians moving. The activities it undertakes to accomplish this goal are guided by detailed strategic plans for communication, capacity building, and knowledge exchange. Central to ParticipACTION's success has been its efforts to work in partnership with and across sectors. This collaborative approach capitalizes on the strengths of organizations within the physical activity sector and optimizes resources. Consistent with the fundamental principles underlying the National Physical Activity Plan, the philosophy of ParticipACTION is that the only way to tackle the inactivity crisis is through unified and comprehensive initiatives across all sectors including, but not limited to, the industry, education, health care, and public sectors.

Additional Reading and Resources

Visit the ParticipACTION website at www.participaction.com. The website includes detailed descriptions of current initiatives underway and an archive of all previous mass media campaigns.

ParticipACTION and its activities have been featured in two special issues of academic journals: The *Canadian Journal of Public Health*, available for free download from http://journal.cpha.ca/index.php/cjph/issue/view/248; and the *International Journal of Behavioral Nutrition and Physical Activity*, available for free download from www.ijbnpa.org/series/participaction.

References

Active Healthy Kids Canada. 2009. The 2009 report card on physical activity for children and youth. www.activehealthykids.ca/ReportCard/ArchivedReportCards.aspx.

Bauman, A., J. Madill, C.L .Craig, and A. Salmon. 2004. ParticipAction: This mouse roared, but did it get the cheese? *Can. J. Public Health* 95(Suppl. 2):S14-19.

Bryan, S.N., and P.T. Katzmarzyk. 2009. Are Canadians meeting the guidelines for moderate and vigorous leisure-time physical activity? *Appl. Physiol. Nutr. Metab.* 34(4):707-5.

Colley, R.C., D. Garriguet, I. Janssen, C.L. Craig, J. Clarke, and M.S. Tremblay. 2011. Physical activity of Canadian children and youth: accelerometer results from the 2007 to 2009 Canadian Health Measures Survey. *Health Rep.* 22(1):15-23.

Faulkner, G., C. McCloy, R.C. Plotnikoff, A. Bauman, L.R. Brawley, K. Chad, L. Gauvin, J.C. Spence, and M.S. Tremblay. 2009. ParticipAction: Baseline assessment of the capacity available to the "new ParticipAction": A qualitative study of Canadian organizations. *Int. J. Behav. Nutr. Phys. Act.* 6:87.

Gustafson, S.L., and R.E. Rhodes. 2006. Parental correlates of physical activity in children and early adolescents. *Sports Med.* 36(1):79-97.

Iannotti, R.J., M.D. Kogan, I. Janssen, and W.F. Boyce. 2009. Patterns of adolescent physical activity, screen-based media use, and positive and negative health indicators in the U.S. and Canada. *J. Adolesc. Health* 44(5):493-9.

Latimer, A.E., L.R. Brawley, and R.L. Bassett. 2010. A systematic review of three approaches for constructing physical activity messages: What messages work and what improvements are needed? *Int. J. Behav. Nutr. Phys. Act.* 7(1):36.

Spence, J.C., L.R. Brawley, C.L. Craig, R.C. Plotnikoff, M.S. Tremblay, A. Bauman, G.E.J. Faulkner, K. Chad, and M.I. Clark. 2009. ParticipAction: Awareness of the ParticipAction campaign among Canadian Adults—Testing the knowledge gap hypothesis and a hierarchy-of-effects model. *Int. J. Behav. Nutr. Phys. Act.* 6:85.

Tremblay, M.S., A.G. Leblanc, I. Janssen, M.E. Kho, A. Hicks, K. Murumets, et al. 2011a. Canadian sedentary behavior guidelines for children and youth. *Appl. Physiol. Nutr. Metab.* 36(1):59-71.

Tremblay, M.S., D.E. Warburton, I. Janssen, D.H. Paterson, A.E. Latimer, R.E. Rhodes, et al. 2011b. New Canadian physical activity guidelines. *Appl. Physiol. Nutr. Metab.* 36(1):36-58.

CHAPTER 9

Wheeling Walks

A Targeted Mass Media–Led Physical Activity Campaign

Bill Reger-Nash, EdD
West Virginia University

Keith Zullig, PhD
West Virginia University

Adrian Bauman, PhD, FAFPHM
Sydney University

Lesley Cottrell, PhD
West Virginia University

Christiaan G. Abildso, PhD, MPH
West Virginia University

Matthew Gurka, PhD
West Virginia University

NPAP Tactics and Strategies Used in This Program

Mass Media Sector

STRATEGY 1: Encourage public health agencies to form partnerships with other agencies across the eight sectors to combine resources around common themes to promote physical activity.

STRATEGY 3: Develop consistent mass communication messages that promote physical activity, have a clear and standardized "brand," and are consistent with the most current Physical Activity Guidelines for Americans.

STRATEGY 4: Ensure that messages and physical activity plans developed by state and local public health agencies and key stakeholders from the eight sectors are consistent with national messages.

STRATEGY 5: Sequence, plan, and provide campaign activities in a prospective, coordinated manner. Support and link campaign messages to community-level programs, policies, and environmental supports.

STRATEGY 6: Encourage mass media professionals to become informed about the importance of physical activity and the potential role they can play in promoting physical activity.

Physical inactivity contributes significantly to morbidity and mortality in the United States (U.S. Department of Health and Human Services 2008; Lee et al. 2012). Therefore, establishing the effectiveness of whole-community interventions to promote physical activity is an important component of health promotion and disease prevention. The Wheeling Walks campaign used a community-wide social marketing campaign to promote 30 minutes or more of daily moderate-intensity walking among insufficiently active 50- to 65-year-old residents of Wheeling, West Virginia (Reger et al. 2002). The project garnered policy support from multiple agencies, with a focus on changing individual behavior, the community, and the environment in support of physical activity. Mass media–led social marketing is a cost-effective method for influencing defined population groups within a targeted geographic region.

Program Description

The Wheeling Walks intervention was conducted between June 1999 and June 2002 in Wheeling, West Virginia. To build on the strengths of the community, a participatory planning process (Green and Kreuter 2005; Minkler and Wallerstein 2003) was initiated in August 1999. The process involved 37 community members from local and state health agencies; business; industry; labor unions; hospitals; health clinics serving low-income residents; the National Association for the Advancement of Colored People; regional voluntary associations such as the American Heart Association, the American Cancer Society, and Diabetes Associations; civic groups such as Kiwanis and Rotary; local parks and recreation agencies; public and private schools; colleges; faith-based groups; and government offices (García et al. 2009). The participatory planning group met for one hour per week for 12 consecutive weeks to better understand the public health challenge of physical inactivity and to work collaboratively toward a solution. From this group, task forces were established to identify the potential target behavior (walking); an at-risk population (residents 50-65 years of age); campaign components (paid media, media relations to generate earned media, public health activities, policy, environment, and evaluation); potential funding sources; infrastructure challenges; and potential intersectoral partners. Twenty months of planning preceded the 12-month social marketing intervention, which included an initial intensive eight-week paid mass media–led campaign, an earned media–led booster with extensive media relations and no paid ads during the fifth month, and a final paid mass media–led booster campaign during month 11. The participatory planning process successfully brought together community representatives to own the public health problem of physical inactivity. The majority of the participatory planning members volunteered to become the Wheeling Walks Community Advisory Board and to work collaboratively in campaign planning, fund-raising, implementation, and evaluation.

Characteristics of Wheeling

- Located in northern West Virginia (Ohio and Marshall Counties)
- Population 31,420 (in 2000)
- 92.7 percent of population Caucasian
- 21.6 percent of population 65 years or older
- 18.0 percent of population below poverty
- West Virginia per capita income 75 percent of the national average (in 2001).
- Two daily newspapers
- Two television stations
- 12 radio stations

www.census.gov

Mass Media

Mass-reach media has the potential to communicate to large segments of the population and set the agenda for community-wide change (Bauman and Chau 2009). The initial mass media–led campaign began April 17, 2001, and ran for eight weeks, with paid print, television, and radio messages (produced by Zimmerman and Markman of Santa Monica, California). Formative research determined that lack of time and perceived lack of energy were the two most common barriers to regular physical activity that the target audience reported. Therefore, the advertisements focused on helping the target audience overcome these specific barriers to regular walking. (See www.wheelingwalks.org/WW_TrainingManual/TM_index.asp.)

People live in a media-cluttered world and are bombarded with myriad messages to support their unhealthy behaviors. The Wheeling Walks campaign communicated a single overarching tagline, "Walk at least 30 minutes daily," to more than 85 percent of the target population during the first eight-week campaign. The prime-time television and radio advertising purchase included 683 prime-time 30-second television ads and 1,988 prime-time 60-second radio ads, which represented more than 5,100 television and 3,400 radio gross rating points (Reger et al. 2002). Each gross rating point represents a theoretical campaign exposure to

1 percent of the market. Thus, accumulation of 100 television and radio gross rating points suggests that up to 100 percent of the market would be exposed to the television and radio ads. The campaign also ran 28 one-eighth-page ads (see figure 9.1) in the local daily newspaper and aired 1,164 thirty-second cable television ads.

Media relations events communicated campaign messages without purchasing advertisements, a process known as "earned media." Public health campaign organizers cannot present information alone to news gatekeepers (Abroms and Maibach 2008). Rather, campaign messages must be linked to newsworthy events. Therefore, the initial phase of the campaign included five media relations events, spaced approximately two weeks apart.

The campaign kickoff, for example, was held in the brightly decorated foyer of the Wheeling Civic Center. Approximately 200 people attended this event, which included a dais of local dignitaries, such as the mayor, the medical director of the local health department, and representatives of the participating organizations. The campaign kickoff message was disseminated by television, radio, and newspaper to more than 100,000 consumers in the media catchment area through coverage of this event. A weekly column on walking was included in the Sunday edition of the largest daily newspaper (figure 9.2).

The eight-week campaign included public health education activities designed to facilitate walking-related social networking and social support. These included a speakers' bureau and worksite wellness walking campaigns. Physicians volunteered to write prescriptions for walking, as appropriate to their patients' health status and needs. A professional engineer from West Virginia University conducted a workshop titled Walkable Wheeling to help community leaders appreciate the role that public policy and

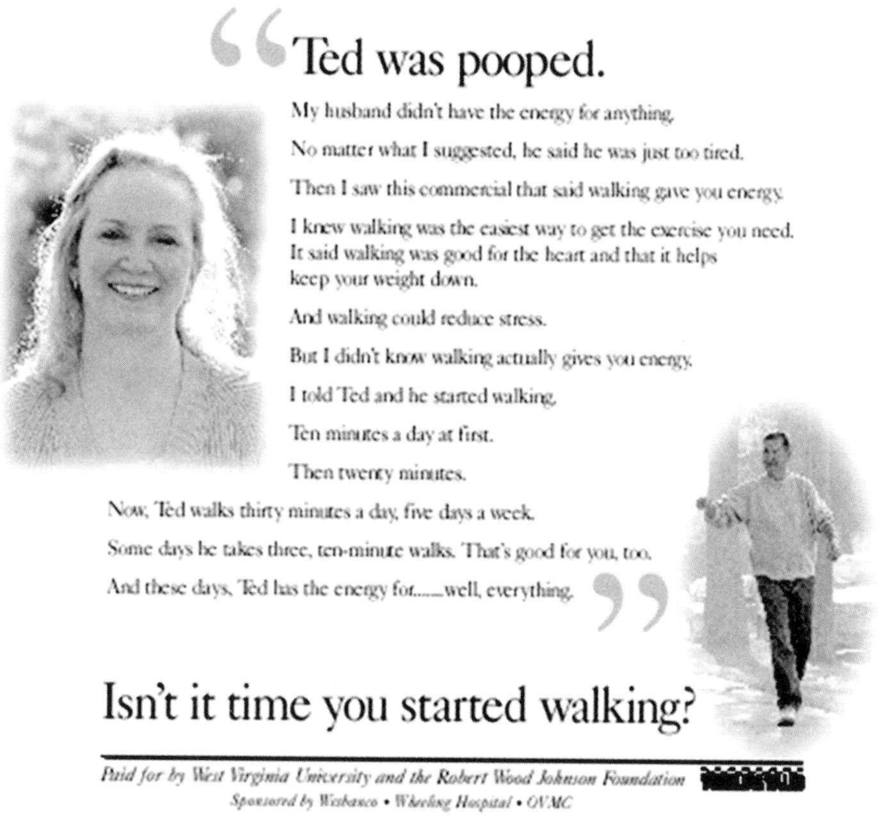

Figure 9.1   Print newspaper advertisement, which featured the same actors as in the TV commercials.
Reprinted, by permission, from Zimmerman and Markman, Inc.

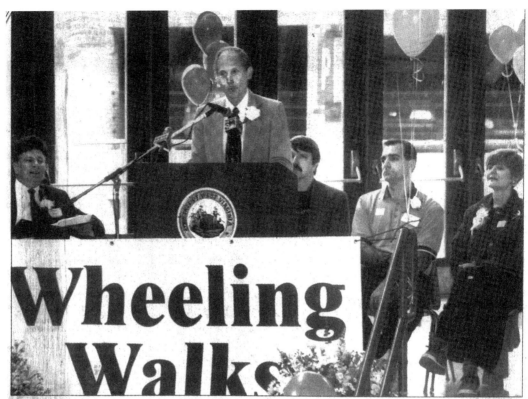

Photo by Scott McCloskey

The kick-off of "Wheeling Walks" was held this morning at the Wheeling Civic Center before a large and enthusiastic crowd. Bill Reger, of West Virginia University, at the podium is the project director. From left, Wheeling Mayor Nick Sparachane, Dr. William Mercer, director of the Ohio County Health Department, Joe Slavik, manager of the Howard Long Wellness Center and Kristine Molnar, president-Upper Ohio Valley Region of WesBanco.

Figure 9.2 Newspaper column from the Wheeling News-Register that highlighted the Wheeling Walks campaign kickoff.

Reprinted, by permission, from J. Michael Myer, 2001, *Wheeling News-Register.*

the physical environment can play in enabling and reinforcing or discouraging walking. The mayor of Wheeling established the Walkable Wheeling Task Force, which has met every two months since May 2001 to promote programs, policy, and environmental change.

A four-week media relations booster campaign was planned to generate earned media during September 2001. The catastrophic terrorist events of September 11, 2001, resulted in the cancellation of this phase of campaign actions. The campaign conducted booster activities during month 11, March 2002, which included 521 and 370 local network television and radio gross rating points, respectively. The campaign also purchased four 1/8th-page newspaper ads and orchestrated four media relations events. A multiweek walking clinic, which attracted

more than 300 participants, was cosponsored with Ogden Newspapers, which also sponsored the United States National 20K running championship in Wheeling. Because of the Wheeling Walks campaign, a walking category was added to the running event.

Funding

In 1999, the West Virginia Bureau for Public Health provided a $20,000 participatory planning grant to address the growing problem of obesity in Wheeling, and the Benedum Foundation provided a $30,000 grant for the development of the campaign message and materials. In 2001, the Robert Wood Johnson Foundation provided a $354,000 grant for the design, implementation, and evaluation of the targeted physical activity intervention. Additional funding was provided by Wesbanco ($15,000), a Wheeling-based bank; the West Virginia Tobacco settlement fund ($20,000 to examine the impact of walking on tobacco use); and two local hospitals ($17,500).

Program Evaluation

Process evaluation data comprised the number of community events, number of participants, ads purchased, earned media hits, and self-reported campaign awareness. In addition, the campaign monitored task force commitment and engagement with Wheeling Walks over time. Impact evaluation used a quasi-experimental design with a demographically matched comparison community. Data were collected from cohort samples through four waves (baseline, 3 months, 6 months, and 12 months after baseline) of random-digit-dial telephone surveys in Wheeling and Parkersburg, West Virginia, a comparison community on the Ohio River (Reger-Nash et al. 2005a). Impact data included assessment of awareness, behavioral intention, and walking behaviors from baseline to 3 and 12 months after baseline.

The participatory planning process served as a springboard for process and impact changes, which have resulted in the long-term sustainability of the intervention. The 37 participatory planning members represented more than 10 sectors of the community. Some members of the original Walkable Wheeling Task Force (now called the Ohio Valley Trail Partners) continue to lead the efforts to effect policy and environmental changes 10 years later. Changes observed over time among the task force members included increased commitment, shared purpose, and interagency trust across the planning process (Reger-Nash et al. 2006a). Impact evaluation surveys showed high community campaign awareness in Wheeling, with 92 percent and 89 percent awareness reported by wave 2 and wave 4 respondents (3 and 12 months after baseline), respectively (Reger-Nash et al. 2005a). The television ads specifically were recalled by 77 percent of wave 2 and 93 per-

cent of wave 4 Wheeling respondents. Eighty-one and 83 percent of telephone respondents reported an awareness of the campaign in the news (earned media) for wave 2 and wave 4, respectively. Overall, Wheeling, the intervention community, showed a 14 percent increase in the likelihood of walking (attained at least 30 minutes, five days per week) compared with the matched control community. This change among the most inactive at baseline was observed immediately after the most intense social marketing campaign and was still in place 12 months later. The mass media campaign was integrated with other strategies, including health professional advice programs and environmental and policy change initiatives. The latter involved developing and maintaining partnerships across sectors, and these elements have been maintained for more than a decade. As a result, rail-trail mileage in the Wheeling area has more than doubled since 2002, and a regional trail plan is now complete (see www.wheelingheritage.org/pdf_docs/WHTX.pdf). This community program shows the effects of mass media as an initial catalyst to community awareness, promotion of interagency engagement, and development of sustainable structures to carry forward the process of building environments that support physical activity.

Linkage to the National Physical Activity Plan

Wheeling Walks was an exemplary community-wide program that optimizes the principles outlined in the Mass Media Sector of the National Physical Activity Plan. The campaign had a clear message and a local "brand," and it consisted of a planned sequence of messages, public relations, and community programming. The most important principle was that paid mass media was required as an initial focus of Wheeling Walks, but this was integrated into a comprehensive set of community activities that were broader than the mass communications component alone. The maintenance of the local task forces epitomized partnership formation, which led to the sustained environmental and policy work to build infrastructure to support physical activity in the community. This best-practice approach requires local leadership to take over and sustain community programs after formal funding has ceased.

The efforts of the Wheeling Walks intervention model support the strategies in the Mass Media Sector of the National Physical Activity Plan:

Strategy 1: Encourage public health agencies to form partnerships with other agencies across the eight sectors to combine resources around common themes to promote physical activity. From the inception of the intervention, the transdisciplinary campaign team worked diligently to partner with key community groups. For example, the participatory planning task forces of Wheeling Walks formed partnerships with the local hospitals, which have a vested interest in addressing health problems related to physical activity. Hospital representatives served on the task forces and advisory board, and the hospitals contributed $17,500 to deliver the campaign's targeted message. Educational programs, such as the 20 Weeks to the 20K walking workshop, were held in the community facilities of our intervention partners. The West Virginia Bureau for Public Health contributed $20,000 to the campaign's mass media purchases to help address the comorbidities of inactivity and tobacco use.

Strategy 3: Develop consistent mass communication messages that promote physical activity, have a clear and standardized "brand," and are consistent with the most current Physical Activity Guidelines for Americans. The local Wheeling Walks message was clearly "branded" and showed high population reach, with recognition by 90 percent of the target population. The campaign promoted a single unequivocal message, "Walk at least 30 minutes daily," which was developed in accordance with the 1996 Surgeon General's Report on Physical Activity and Health and remains consistent with the 2008 Physical Activity Guidelines for Americans.

Strategy 4: Ensure that messages and physical activity plans developed by state and local public health agencies and key stakeholders from the eight sectors are consistent with national messages. Some of the early community work suggested that the campaign should be titled One Mile or More, For Sure! However, formative research indicated that "Walk at least 30 minutes daily" was a more effective message and consistent with the 1996 Surgeon General guidelines. In addition, Wheeling Walks procedures were consistent with the second tactic identified in Strategy 4: "Develop a . . . training manual on the use of the mass media messages . . . for use by state and local campaigns and key stakeholders. Involve users in creation of these tools." Campaign leaders and community stakeholders developed an implementation guide that is generalizable to other settings and communities. This manual is freely available at www.wheelingwalks.org/WW_Training-Manual/TM_index.asp.

Strategy 5: Sequence, plan, and provide campaign activities in a prospective, coordinated manner. Support and link campaign messages to community-level programs, policies, and environmental supports. The Wheeling Walks intervention approach called for broad-based community capacity building, which led to policy-related changes. This was conducted at the local city level. The Wheeling Walks model supports the National Physical Activity Plan and the West Virginia State Physical Activity Plan.

Strategy 6: Encourage mass media professionals to become informed about the importance of physical activity and the potential role they can play in promoting physical activity. Over time, the Wheeling model has been refined. During the initial campaign, the mass media gatekeepers were clearly supportive of the efforts. In Morgantown, West Virginia, the same mass media community intervention model was used from 2003 to 2005. In that city, the local newspaper became a major proponent of improvements in pedestrian infrastructure. When the Morgantown Municipal Pedestrian Safety Board developed a tax schedule to fund changes to better support walking in the city, the local newspaper, *The Dominion Post*, hosted a public forum to further promote the idea. The newspaper has been willing to cover news events related to walking and bicycling, almost regardless of the content.

Evidence Base Used During Program Development

Promoting small changes across a large number of people in a community is more of a public health approach than are intensive interventions that focus on large changes among a few individuals (Rodgers et al. 2004). The 1996 Surgeon General's Report on Physical Activity and Health recommended engaging in at least 30 minutes of daily moderate intensity physical activity and stated that walking is an excellent way of attaining the recommended amount of physical activity.

Following the guidance provided by the Ottawa Charter for Health Promotion (1986), Wheeling Walks used a participatory planning process (Reger et al. 2002) to mobilize the community to address physical inactivity among the target population (Green and Kreuter 2005). The goals were to better appreciate the epidemiological, behavioral, environmental, and policy aspects of the problem and to work with the community to develop sustainable solutions to them.

Research has shown that mass media can be used effectively to communicate targeted messages to select populations (Snyder and Hamilton 2002). By following the CDC Prevention Guide (www.thecommunityguide.org/index.html) recommendations, programmers can effectively integrate mass media into a multicomponent campaign (Kahn et al. 2002). In Wheeling, the campaign messages were designed using the Theory of Planned Behavior (Ajzen 2002) and the Communications Hierarchy of Effects Theory (McGuire 1984).

Populations Best Served by the Program

Often the segments of the population most in need are those least likely to become involved in health promotion programs. The needs assessment for Wheeling Walks demonstrated that nearly 80 percent of those ages 55 to 64 years were insufficiently active (West Virginia Department of Health and Human Resources

2001). Paid mass media offers the possibility of directing communications specifically to audience segments or subpopulations. For example, Nielsen television ratings specify which subpopulations are watching individual television programs. Similar targeting is possible when purchasing newspaper and radio advertising.

The most powerful single source of information in the United States is television (Nielsen Company 2009). Wheeling Walks identified a segment of the Wheeling-Steubenville television broadcast mass media market, insufficiently active 50- to 65-year-old residents of Wheeling, as its target population. There are 215 network television and 210 cable television mass media markets within the United States. Most of these markets are served by at least one daily newspaper and several dominant radio stations. These avenues enable providers to bombard the population segment to communicate a message.

Specific replication efforts explored the potential implications of generalizing the Wheeling Walks program to other settings and age groups. In Welch Walks (Reger-Nash et al. 2005b), the age group was expanded to include those ages 35 to 65 years. BC Walks (Reger-Nash et al. 2006b) and WV Walks (Reger-Nash et al. 2008) focused on residents ages 40 to 65 years. The results of these campaigns (briefly described later in the chapter) were not as robust as those for Wheeling Walks.

Lessons Learned

A single unambiguous message (campaign theme, brand, or tagline) is critical for effective public communication (Snyder and Hamilton 2002). Problems in public health are so numerous that practitioners and researchers often attempt to do and communicate too much. To attempt to do everything is to do nothing. Adequate planning with formative research can help to avoid pitfalls in the implementation of a program into a community.

Available funding will determine the amount of time needed for planning. Wheeling Walks (Reger et al. 2002) and the subsequent WV Walks program (Reger-Nash et al. 2008) had little money when planning began, and each community intervention required 18 months to plan. By contrast, BC Walks had significant funding through the New York State Health Department (Reger-Nash et al. 2006b) at the start of the program. In this case, the planning period was shorter, with a six-month time frame from initial planning to social marketing campaign implementation. Developing a "logic model" of the expected impacts and outcomes of the program at each stage can be a useful planning tool (Huhman et al. 2004; Reger-Nash et al. 2011).

Paid mass media facilitates effective targeting of subpopulations within a community. By purchasing newspaper and prime-time television and radio advertisements, campaign planners are able to focus specifically on certain populations within defined geographic boundaries.

Mass media markets are not always as they appear. First, program planners need to verify that the television, radio, and newspaper media markets cover the targeted region. The experience of the WV Walks campaign in Morgantown, West Virginia, was illustrative. Although most Morgantown residents receive their local network television from West Virginia affiliates, program planners learned late that approximately one fourth of the region was covered by the Pittsburgh television market, which was too expensive to purchase for the small number of targeted residents. Media coverage was also an issue in the quasi-experimental design for evaluation, as planners tried to ensure that comparison communities were uncontaminated by the media campaign messaging in the intervention region.

The community model described here can be scaled up or down. Welch, West Virginia, used another version of this community intervention model in a much smaller community, with a total budget of $10,000. That program created change in knowledge, but not behavior, in the low-income community of 5,000 (Reger-Nash et al. 2005b). BC Walks represented a more rigorous, scaled-up implementation of the model in Broome County, New York, a community in excess of 200,000. That campaign resulted in a statistically significant increase in campaign awareness and walking (Reger-Nash et al. 2006b). WV Walks, which targeted the 15-county area of north-central West Virginia,

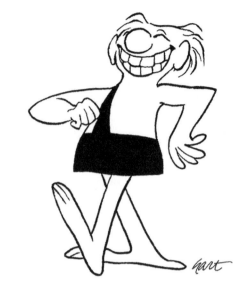

"B.C. Walks" logo appears with permission of John L. Hart FLP.

resulted in a significant 12 percent increase in the likelihood of walking in the intervention community compared with the control community (Reger-Nash et al. 2008). These replication studies, which adapted the original Wheeling Walks campaign, produced smaller but consistently reliable results.

By making slight modifications to professionally prepared mass media materials, programmers can adapt advertising packages and generic messages to fit different communities. Media relations provide an opportunity to tailor campaign materials to the local community, as live local personalities and talents are incorporated into staged media events. The Wheeling experience showed that the mass media can catalyze and synergize targeted intervention efforts at the community level to influence change. Social marketing activities done correctly, with initial extensive and paid mass media, can serve as high-energy, high-profile initial intervention elements, which a community can then embrace as a significant value-added component.

Tips for Working Across Sectors

The effectiveness of a community-wide effort is predicated on involving a broad spectrum of community sectors in the intervention. Promoting physical activity requires involving much more than the health sector, as education, urban planning, recreation, and other sectors all play key roles in developing sustainable policy and environmental infrastructure for physical activity. Many of these groups will be in competition with one another for local government resources and may be reluctant to support an initiative that is perceived to be "owned" by only one agency. For Wheeling Walks, a steering committee linked the campaign to West Virginia University and the County Health Department, both perceived to be politically neutral. Invitations were also extended to labor unions, low-income advocacy groups, public and private schools, all local colleges, voluntary associations, faith and minority-based groups, civic organizations, and health-related professional organizations. By initially working together for the 12 weeks of the participatory planning process, the planning group developed better collaboration and a shared agenda. Campaign news updates were sent to groups that were unwilling or unable to attend the participatory planning sessions, in order to keep them involved. The Walkable Wheeling Task Force continues to serve the policy and environmental needs of the community, as is illustrated at www.wheelingheritage.org/pdf_docs/WHTX.pdf.

A key feature of the Wheeling Walks model was that it used mass media to initiate community actions. The models used in communities elsewhere in West Virginia and New York State (Welch Walks, WV Walks, and BC Walks) were derived from the initial Wheeling program and reported smaller but still clear community effects on walking. A public health program should be tested, replicated, and, if deemed effective, generalized (disseminated) across a state or larger region (Bauman and Nutbeam 2013). This up-scaling appears warranted based on the results of this set of community-level mass media campaigns. These campaigns also support the potential for mass media as an initial step in increasing physical activity at the population level.

Additional Reading and Resource

Canadian Public Health Association, Health and Welfare Canada, and World Health Organization.

1986. Ottawa charter for health promotion. Paper presented at the First International Conference on Health Promotion, Ottawa, Canada.

References

Abroms, L.C., and E.W. Maibach. 2008. The effectiveness of mass communication to change public behavior. *Ann. Rev. Public Health* 29:219-34.

Ajzen, I. 2002. Perceived behavioral control, self-efficacy, locus of control, and the theory of planned behavior. *J. Appl. Soc. Psychol.* 32(4):665-83.

Bauman, A., and J. Chau. 2009. The role of media in promoting physical activity. *Journal of Physical Activity and Health* 6(Suppl 2):S196-210.

Bauman, A. and D. Nutbeam. 2013. *Evaluation in a Nutshell: A Practical Guide to the Evaluation of Health Promotion Programs* 2nd Ed. Sydney, Australia: McGraw-Hill.

García, R., A. Bracho, P. Cantero, and B.A. Glenn. 2009. "Pushing" physical activity, and justice. *Prev. Med.* 49(4):330-3.

Green, L.W., and M.W. Kreuter. 2005. *Health Program Planning: An Educational and Ecological Approach.* 4th ed. New York: McGraw-Hill.

Huhman, M., C. Heitzler, and F. Wong. 2004. The VERB™ campaign logic model: A tool for planning and evaluation. *Prev. Chronic Dis.* 1(3). www.cdc.gov/pcd/issues/2004/jul/04_0033.htm.

Kahn, E.B., L.T. Ramsey, R.C. Brownson, G.W. Heath, E.H. Howze, K.E. Powell, et al. 2002. The effectiveness of interventions to increase physical activity: A systematic review. *Am. J. Prev. Med.* 22(Suppl 4):73-107.

Lee, I.M., E.J. Shiroma, F. Lobelo, P. Puska, S.N. Blair, and P.T. Katzmarzyk. 2012. Effect of physical inactivity on major non-communicable diseases worldwide: an analysis of burden of disease and life expectancy. *The Lancet,* 380(9838), 9-19.

McGuire, W.J. 1984. Public communication as a strategy for inducing health-promoting behavioral change. *Prev. Med.* 13(3):299-313.

Minkler, M.E., and N.E. Wallerstein. 2003. *Community Based Participatory Research for Health.* San Francisco: Jossey-Bass.

The Nielsen Company. 2009. A2/M2 Three screen report: 1st quarter 2009. http://blog.nielsen.com/nielsenwire/wp-content/uploads/2009/05/nielsen_threescreenreport_q109.pdf.

Reger, B., L. Cooper, S. Booth-Butterfield, H. Smith, A. Bauman, M. Wootan, et al. 2002. Wheeling walks: A community campaign using paid media to encourage walking among sedentary older adults. *Prev. Med.* 35(3):285-92.

Reger-Nash, B., A. Bauman, S. Booth-Butterfield, L. Cooper, H. Smith, T. Chey, et al. 2005a. Wheeling walks: Evaluation of a media-based community intervention. *Family and Community Health* 28(1):64-78.

Reger-Nash, B., A. Bauman, L. Cooper, T. Chey, and K. Simon. 2006a. Evaluating communitywide walking interventions. *Eval. Program Plann.* 29:251-9.

Reger-Nash, B., A. Bauman, L. Cooper, T. Chey, K.J. Simon, M. Brann, et al. 2008. WV walks: Replication with expanded reach. *Journal of Physical Activity and Health* 5(1):19-27.

Reger-Nash, B., A. Bauman, B. Smith, C. Craig, C.G. Abildso, and K.M. Leyden. 2011. Organizing an effective communitywide physical activity campaign: A step-by-step guide. *ACSM's Health Fit. J.* 15(5):21-7.

Reger-Nash, B., L. Cooper, J. Orren, and D. Cook. 2005b. Marketing used to promote walking in McDowell County. *WV Med. J.* 101(3):106.

Reger-Nash, B., P. Fell, D. Spicer, B.D. Fisher, L. Cooper, T. Chey, et al. 2006b. BC walks: Replication of a communitywide physical activity campaign, *Prev.*

Chronic Dis. 3:A90. www.cdc.gov/pcd/issues/2006/jul/05_0138.htm.

Rodgers, A., M. Ezzati, S. Vander Hoorn, A.D. Lopez, R.-B. Lin, C.J.L. Murray, et al. 2004. Distribution of major health risks: Findings from the global burden of disease study. *PLoS Med.* 1(1):e27.

Snyder, L.B., and M.A. Hamilton. 2002. A meta-analysis of us health campaign effects on behavior: Emphasize enforcement, exposure, and new information, and beware the secular trend. In: *Public Health Communication: Evidence for Behavior Change* (pp. 357-83). R. Hornik, Ed. Mahwah, NJ: Lawrence Erlbaum.

U.S. Department of Health and Human Services. 1996. *Physical Activity and Health: a Report of the Surgeon General.* Atlanta, GA: National Center for Chronic Disease Prevention and Health Promotion.

U.S. Department of Health and Human Services. 2008. *2008 Physical Activity Guidelines for Americans* (p. 61). Atlanta, GA: Office of Disease Prevention and Health Promotion.

West Virginia Department of Health and Human Resources, Bureau for Public Health, Office of Epidemiology and Health Promotion. 2001. *West Virginia 1999 Behavioral Risk Factor Survey.* Charleston, WV.

CHAPTER 10

Mass Media Campaigns to Promote Physical Activity
Australia and New Zealand as Case Studies

Adrian Bauman, PhD, FAFPHM
Sydney University

Grant McLean, BA (hons)
Sport and Recreation New Zealand (SPARC)

Sue Walker, PhD
Sport and Recreation New Zealand (SPARC)

Trevor Shilton, MSc
Heart Foundation and University of Western Australia

Bill Bellew, MPH, DPH
Sydney University

Mass media campaigns increasingly are being used as part of a public health approach to addressing physical inactivity. They are purposive and usually include paid media placements that have a wide population reach. In this chapter, we provide three examples of mass reach campaigns that used paid communications through the media to promote moderate-intensity, regular physical activity (PA) to adult populations in Australia and New Zealand.

The first was a national campaign in New Zealand, Push Play, led by the national sport and recreation agency, between 1999 and 2009. The next example is the Active Australia campaign, conducted initially in New South Wales and subsequently in other states. It emanated from Active Australia, a federal partnership of health departments and sport and recreation departments, and lasted from 1998 to 2001. The last example is from the state of Western Australia, where the Find Thirty campaign has been conducted for almost a decade; here we report findings from the first phase of this initiative, 2002 to 2006.

One feature of the campaigns is worth noting. All three were strongly grounded in intersectoral national or state partnerships or task forces and had clear links to community programs and policy and environmental change strategies, in addition to the mass reach communications. These features, plus a focus on defining a clear brand for physical activity, use of marketing strategies, and sufficient media exposure, made the three campaigns more typical of social marketing than simple mass media campaigns (Maibach et al. 2002). The three campaigns are described separately and then compared with each other and with the mass media strategies recommended in the U.S. National Physical Activity Plan.

New Zealand: Push Play

Mass media campaigns are often developed by government to highlight health issues, promote awareness, and increase community engagement. In New Zealand, the comprehensive program, Push Play, was facilitated by the national sport agency initially named the Hillary Commission and later called SPARC, Sport and Recreation New Zealand, which managed and delivered the Push Play mass media and social marketing campaign.

Program Description

Push Play (phase 1: 1999-2002; phases 2 and 3: 2003-2009) was a national mass media campaign to promote physical activity. The campaign built gradually over several years, with the initial focus (phase 1) to raise awareness of the 30-minutes-a-day physical activity message among New Zealand adults. Push Play later focused on defining and targeting priority subpopulations through an audience segmentation analysis (phase 2). Phase 3 included a specific focus on young people. The campaign emanated from New Zealand's response to the U.S. Surgeon General's Report on Physical Activity and Health; a National Health Committee report, *Active for Life: A Call for Action* (1998); and the Hillary Commission's (now SPARC) *Physical Activity Taskforce Report: More People, More Active, More Often* (1998). The latter recommended a comprehensive multisectoral approach to promoting physical activity for health, starting with a national mass media campaign. The strategy initiated a joint policy statement on physical activity signed by both the Hillary Commission and the Ministry of Health.

Details of the Push Play campaign are shown in table 10.1, left column. Phase 1 promoted 30 minutes of daily, moderate-intensity physical activity as a fun and easy-to-achieve goal that New Zealand adults could integrate into community life. The objectives were to increase awareness of the benefits of physical activity and to encourage people to think about becoming more physically active. The campaign was supported by community-level and health care programs and events. The latter included a physician's written advice and referral for patients to become more physically active, using a Green Prescription (Elley 2003). The Green prescription was an evidence-based tool for primary care doctors to prescribe physical activity, and these were disseminated, and physicians trained, through the Push Play initiative. The Push Play campaign was launched in 1999 with two 15-second silent commercials that showed a person in a sedentary pose with signal distortion lines across the screen and a written message "Do not adjust your set, adjust your life." These

were followed by a longer message showing a variety of New Zealanders making choices to include physical activity in their lives. The campaign logo for Push Play looked like a green "play" button on a video recorder, suggesting that people make a start to become more active. Push Play was built as a social marketing brand to reflect the positive values of being upbeat, fresh and clean, fun, Kiwi, family-based, and physically active.

In addition to paid major media, extensive resources and merchandising supported the campaign. Other national initiatives were implemented under the umbrella of Push Play, including the well-evaluated Green Prescription Scheme for General Practitioners (family physicians) (Elley et al. 2003) and He Oranga Poutama (since 1997), a program encouraging healthy lifestyles for Maori (the indigenous New Zealand population). Regional sports trusts, which are independent nongovernment sports agencies, worked with local public health agencies to develop and promote local events, including local celebrations of the national Push Play Day.

Phase 2 of the Push Play campaign moved from focusing on raising awareness among the general population to targeting less active population subgroups. A national survey of physical activity barriers and motivators called Obstacles to Action (SPARC 2003) provided audience segmentation research for this phase. From 2003 through the end of the campaign, Push Play media focused on inactive population groups. New Push Play mass media, resource development, and on-the-ground initiatives (e.g., the Activator, Push Play Nation, Push Play Family Challenge) were aimed at providing specific information and resources for these groups.

Phase 3 of Push Play (2006-2009) targeted children and young people and coincided with SPARC's issuing PA guidelines for youth, which recommended that youth participate in 60 minutes of physical activity on most days and limit time spent watching television (SPARC 2007). SPARC and the Ministries of Health and Education developed this phase jointly. It included mass media and used the school setting for resource and program marketing and distribution.

Table 10.1 Elements of the Australian and New Zealand Mass Media Campaigns

Characteristic	Push Play NZ 1999-2009	Active Australia 1998-2000	Find Thirty, Western Australia 2002-2006
Demography, setting	NZ, population 4.3 million, mix urban and rural; 1 in 7 indigenous (Maori).	State of NSW, Australia; highly multicultural mix, population 7 million; >85% in coastal communities; 2% indigenous.	Western Australia; growing population , currently 2.3 million; most in urban Perth; 3% indigenous.
Phases of campaign and target population	Phase 1: 1999-2002; middle-aged adults. Phase 2: target segments. Phase 3: youth campaign.	Phase 1: adults 25-60 years old. Phase 2: seniors 55-75 years old. Both carried out in NSW state only.	Phase 1: 2002-2006 of annual Find Thirty campaigns; targeted middle-aged adults in state of Western Australia.
Formative evaluation	Use of population surveillance data; focus groups and consultations in 1999; identified generic approach, message, logo.	Extensive use of population PA data and qualitative focus group to develop messages for phases 1 and 2.	Use of population data and formative research (TNS Social Research 2006).
Implementation: cost, reach, TARPs and GRPs	Phase 1: $3 million (NZD)* TARPs: every adult had seen each Push Play message 5-8 times.	Phase 1: $700,000 (AUD)* funding; 800 TARPs reaching 65% of the target audience in prime time.	$700,000 funding; average 800 TARPs in three media waves per year. Lower TARPs in maintenance periods.
Research design	Serial cross-sectional surveys 1999-2002; smaller tracking surveys thereafter.	Phase 1: independent population samples in NSW; comparison in rest of Australia; and cohort pre-post only in NSW.**	Up to 14 small sample serial cross-sectional tracking surveys from 2002 (year 1) to 2006.
Initial or baseline awareness	Specific PP message 29.8% at year 1, recognized logo 13.5%.	Pre-campaign exact message recall 2.1%, prompted recall 12.9%.*** *Phase 2: 3.9%*	Spontaneous recall in year 1 was 43%, subsequent median 45%; prompted recall 84%, subsequent median 77%; spontaneous slogan recall 22% at end of year 1; subsequent median 17%.
Peak awareness	Specific PP message 57.2% at year 3; recognized logo 52.0%.	Phase 1: Post-campaign exact recall 20.9%, prompted recall 50.7%. *Phase 2: 48.5%*	
Other impact reported	In phase 1, no sustained changes in PA levels, although in other population surveys, 3% increase in PA was noted among adults between 1997 and 2001.	In phase 1, knowledge items and efficacy about PA increased in NSW; no change elsewhere; PA showed a small increase in NSW, decreased elsewhere.	Understand how much PA is needed for health baseline 44%, subsequent median 57%. Sufficient PA 51% at year 1, subsequent median estimate 65.5%.

GRP = gross rating points; NZ = New Zealand; NSW = New South Wales; PA = physical activity; PP = Push Play; TARPs = target audience rating points. TARPs are similar to GRPs in North America.

*Dollar values are Australian dollars (AUD) and New Zealand dollars (NZD) and at the times of these campaigns were typically 70 to 80 cents US (AUD) and around 60 cents US (NZD).

**For details of this research design see (Bauman et al. 2001).

***Note that these are "ghost" (spurious baseline) values, because they were measured before the campaign had ever been shown.

Program Evaluation

Phase 1 of Push Play was evaluated with annual cross-sectional population surveys (1999-2002) that monitored the impact of the campaign on message awareness, recognition of the Push Play logo, intention to be active, and recent activity (table 10.1). Process evaluation data suggested sufficient media purchased to reach almost all adults at least once and for them to have seen a Push Play message approximately five to eight times. Phase 1 of the Push Play media campaign was successful in reaching the general adult population and increasing awareness in this broad population group (see table 10.1; also Bauman et al. 2003). A key element in its success was the supportive role played by community programs, primary care programs, and regional events.

Cross-sectional tracking surveys of the Push Play campaign were continued for phases 2 and 3 between 2004 and 2009. This monitoring indicated a continuation of strong recognition of the Push Play message (averaging 50 percent unprompted and 80 percent prompted among the target group). There was a trend toward stronger message recognition and intention to change behavior and even some increase in reported physical activity among the broad target groups. Parents also were surveyed to assess their awareness of the Push Play guidelines for young people and allied initiatives targeting young people. Levels of awareness tended to be lower than in phase 1, possibly reflecting the addition of new messages and some confusion around the messages for 30-minute (adult) and 60-minute (children) recommendations. Independent national physical activity prevalence surveys conducted by SPARC (2007-2008) and the Ministry of Health (2002-2003 and 2006-2007) found that physical activity levels (48-52 percent meeting the 30-minute guideline) among adults remained stable during the period of the Push Play campaign's implementation (both the mass media and allied community initiatives).

Lessons Learned

The Push Play mass media campaigns demonstrated good reach into the general popula-tion and in targeted messages to particular subgroups. Collaborative local messaging and associated activities contributed to the campaign's success. The long-term sustainability of the Push Play campaign was noteworthy, and even since its formal suspension in 2009, local regions and areas continue to market events under the Push Play brand.

The key features that made this campaign successful included the development and sustained use of a strong recognizable brand with repeated use of paid television mass media throughout the campaign. Further, the overarching tagline was a simple, consistent core message for all marketing (with consistent messaging referring to 30 minutes or half an hour of physical activity daily). The Push Play campaign had strong links to community-based initiatives across settings—sport and recreation, primary care, community events, and schools—and capitalized on cross-government agency policy and program support, including national and regional strategies and national physical activity guidelines (adults and young people). To increase the longevity of the initiative, it was supported by an interdisciplinary advisory group (consisting of practitioners, marketing experts, social science professionals, and researchers) and was subject to ongoing monitoring, evaluation, and review of the impact and relevance of the campaign.

Active Australia Campaign Phases 1 and 2

The Active Australia partnership between the health sector and the sport and recreation sector was an important national initiative to promote physical activity in the late 1990s. A first step in Active Australia was to pilot a mass media campaign in one state that focused on the new moderate intensity physical activity recommendation.

Program Description

The Active Australia mass media program phases 1 and 2 were conducted in the State of New South Wales (NSW) Australia in March

1998 and March 1999. Focusing primarily on people who were insufficiently active, phase 1 targeted people aged 25 to 60 years, and phase 2 targeted people aged 55 years and older. A complementary program activity in phases 1 and 2 targeted general practitioners (family physicians), other health professionals, and sport, recreation, and fitness professionals. Both phases of the program featured the slogan "Exercise. You only have to take it regularly, not seriously."

The communication objectives of phases 1 and 2 were to increase the target population's awareness of the benefits of regular, moderate physical activity (in particular of importance of 30 minutes of accumulated, moderate intensity exercise) and to maintain motivation among people who were already sufficiently active. Details of the campaigns are shown in the middle column in table 10.1.

The campaign was managed by the NSW State Health Department, in collaboration with state and national health and sport and recreation departments, as part of an overall Active Australia initiative. Media components consisted of paid television advertising (two 15-second television commercials), paid advertisements in metropolitan and rural print media, a multilingual component for minority communities, community-level support from Health Service and Sport and Recreation regional staff (including a toll-free telephone line), and marketing of program merchandise to optimize media exposure. The total media costs were $700,000. The television component of the program had a weighting of 800 target audience rating points from some 200 showings of the message across New South Wales, reaching 65 percent of the target audience during prime viewing time. In addition, six weeks of paid media inserts (portraying local and domestic environments for moderate activity) were run in the weekend editions (Saturday and Sunday) of lifestyle magazines and daily newspapers. A mail-out was used to inform primary care physicians about the new moderate-intensity physical activity message. Information packs were sent to all public health professionals two months before the campaign launch, and physical activity counseling kits were mailed to all

6,500 family physicians across the state. Local and regional initiatives included community-based walking and physical activity events, promotions organized by health sector staff in some areas, and the use of regional and community-level media (Bauman et al. 2001); these were part of a statewide physical activity plan (Simply Active Every Day 2004).

Phase 2 targeted older adults and intentionally coincided with the United Nations International Year of Older Persons. The NSW State Health Department again coordinated the program, this time targeting people aged 55 years and older. The total budget was smaller than that of phase 1, less than $500,000 for communications in NSW. Paid media messages coincided with Seniors Week. The television commercial depicted a "tin man" who becomes aware that being physically active is healthy, fun, and involves only moderate levels of physical activity. Planning was integrated across agencies, including the Department of Sport and Recreation and Health. In addition, the Department of Veterans Affairs sent 30,000 resource kits to veteran health professionals across Australia (Commonwealth Department of Health and Ageing 2000).

Program Evaluation

Before launch, the program partners conducted extensive formative research, both quantitative and qualitative, to inform message and program development. Qualitative research was used to determine the communication concepts most likely to resonate with target audiences. For phase 1, a quasi-experimental research design was used, with independent population samples surveyed before and after the March 1998 program in NSW and independent samples surveyed at the same times in the rest of Australia. A NSW cohort sample of 1,185, representing a response rate of 87.2 percent (Bauman et al. 2001), was also surveyed. The surveys showed high rates of exact program theme and specific tagline recall, which increased significantly in the NSW cohort and independent samples but not in the comparison sample from the rest of Australia (see table 10.1). For phase 2, a NSW cohort of 1,102 older adults was assessed before and after the campaign. Prompted recall of the tin man message increased from 3.9 percent to 48.5 percent following the campaign, and recognition of the overarching Active Australia slogan "Exercise. You only have to take it regularly, not seriously" increased from 33 percent before to 64.1 percent after the program. Intention to be more active improved marginally, and self-efficacy increased significantly between pre- and postprogram surveys, but there was no change in reported actual physical activity (Australian Sports Commission 2000). In summary, evaluation was reasonably comprehensive for a mass media campaign and provided good evidence that observed effects on awareness and understanding of the physical activity message could be attributed specifically to the campaign.

Lessons Learned

The main findings of the evaluation of the NSW Active Australia campaign are discussed subsequently. The findings suggest that mass media campaigns have an important role in increasing awareness of physical activity but that this communication takes place in a socio-cultural milieu that reinforces sedentary lifestyles. This suggests that campaigns alone may not result in a measurable population-level effect on behavior; an integrated set of multi-sectoral population health strategies and services are needed to support, maintain, and extend the reach of the mass media component. Active Australia was informed by quantitative and qualitative formative research that established baseline levels of the problem, identified target audience segments, set specific communication objectives, and pretested communications concepts and advertising materials.

Western Australia's Find Thirty— It's Not a Big Exercise

In Australia, some campaigns are developed by government but are sustained by not-for-profit (nongovernment) organizations; as an example, the Find Thirty initiative was maintained by the Heart Foundation in Western Australia for several years as a serial set of reinforcing social marketing campaigns.

Program Description

Find Thirty was a community-wide social marketing program undertaken by the West Australian Department of Health (2002-2006). Find Thirty targeted Western Australian adults aged 20 to 54 years (see table 10.1, right column). Later, the state Department of Health contracted the National Heart Foundation in Western Australia to conduct another Find Thirty campaign (2008-2011). This section describes the 2002-2006 program and its development and evaluation.

The initial Find Thirty campaign objectives were to increase awareness of the type and frequency of physical activity necessary for good health; demonstrate how moderate-intensity physical activity could be incorporated into everyday life (modeling active living); and cognitively reframe the daily recommended 30 minutes of PA as relatively easy to achieve. The Find Thirty campaign was based on social cognitive theory, with the tag line "It's not a big exercise" conveying the message that physical activity could be incorporated easily into the day and the fact that it's easy to find the 30 minutes needed for good health.

Find Thirty featured three television advertisements in its first campaign wave in April and May 2002. A wide range of additional strategies supported the television campaign. These included information for the general public; targeted communications to primary care physicians and other health professionals; public relations and regional activities; publications and merchandise carrying the campaign message; signage on taxi tops, billboards and bus shelters; and the website www.findthirty.com. Added media included purchased weather segments that featured celebrity endorsement in news bulletins. The campaign's television budget across 2002-2006 was approximately $600,000 per annum. To put this in context, the State of Western Australia has just three commercial television stations, which serve a total population of two million people, with three-quarters living in the capital city of Perth. In 2004, new materials were developed that showed how physical activity can be accumulated in bouts of 10 minutes or more. The television messages showed people being active while on hold on the phone, while waiting for an appointment, and while waiting for a download on a computer. These added the dimension that physical activity can be incidental, accumulated in short bouts, and easily fit into everyday life.

Program Evaluation

Continuous formative research was used to inform the development of sequential phases of the Find Thirty 2002-2011 campaign. Enablers and barriers to being active were examined by segments of interest, with a particular focus on people who are not sufficiently active, low socioeconomic status groups, rural residents, and indigenous people. For the 2002 campaign, program planners conducted research to determine the suitability of creative concepts, advertising executions, enjoyment, and perceived salience of the proposed communications. Impact evaluation of the Find Thirty 2002-2006 campaign used a campaign tracking survey, with weekly computer-assisted telephone interviews of random samples of adults. The objectives of this evaluation were to assess the impact of television messages in the campaign on awareness, understanding of the 30-minute physical activity message, beliefs, attitudes, intentions. and behavior (see table 10.1).

Lessons Learned

The West Australian campaign identified the importance of ongoing formative research to reduce the chance of delivery failure; mass media production is an expensive undertaking, and program promoters may have only one chance to convey their message and select appropriate communication (creative concepts, channel selection). For mass-reach strategies, it is essential to obtain appropriate government agency support and funding for specific campaigns. The duration of the Find Thirty campaign was contingent on sustained government support and state physical activity

task force imprimatur. As with the other two campaigns, a critical element of success was the link to other sectors (especially transport) and to community programs to extend the reach of the campaign and create important policy synergies. Finally, the West Australian campaign was a multiyear serial campaign under an overarching theme and tagline. This allowed for a sequenced approach, building from messages about physical activity to more action-focused messages providing examples of active living and information about accumulating PA across the day.

Linkage to the National Physical Activity Plan

The U.S. National Physical Activity Plan Mass Media Sector includes eight recommended strategies. Table 10.2 demonstrates that the three Australasian campaigns were concordant with these strategies even though the campaigns were initiated a decade before the National Physical Activity Plan.

The U.S. NPAP describes the need for partnerships, interagency policy congruence, and sustained messaging (Strategies 1-3 of the Mass Media Sector). In particular, the Push Play and Find Thirty campaigns in New Zealand and Australia had long durations, and all three campaigns were initiated and overseen by state or federal task forces and agencies. All three campaigns were responsive to the need for message and brand consistency (Strategies 3 and 4), even when themes or target groups changed. Campaign planning identified a sequence of campaign elements over several years, using a strategic framework to create and sustain community awareness and interest in physical activity (Strategy 5) (see table 10.2). All three campaigns worked with the media industry and engaged in media advocacy to add value to the PA messages (Strategy 6). Finally, although these three campaigns incorporated some web and Internet engagement, they partly preceded the recent surge in web 2.0 approaches, which could be included in contemporary mass reach campaigns, especially those targeting youth (Bauman and Chau 2009).

Table 10.2 Mass Media Recommendations of the U.S. National Physical Activity Plan: How Well Did the Australian and New Zealand Campaigns Do?

Characteristics and Strategy*	Push Play NZ 1999-2009	Active Australia 1998-2000	Find Thirty, Western Australia 2002-2007
Form partnerships with other agencies; PA task forces (1)	Developed from national sport agency (Hillary Commission, later Sport and Recreation New Zealand, SPARC). Links to education and health sectors throughout. Push Play was supported by a national physical activity and strategy (Healthy Eating—Healthy Action), led by the Ministry of Health in partnership with government agencies including SPARC (NZ Ministry of Health 2008).	Developed and closely collaborated with state inter-sectoral NSW Physical Activity Task Force work program; multiple agencies and sectors contributed to campaign components.	Started by state health department and then taken over by Heart Foundation to continue delivery. Linked to 10-year strategy of cross-governmental PA task force; embedded in statewide policy for PA and walking. Good links to walking and cycling messages with transport sector.
Obtain funding for sustained mass media campaign (2)	Sustained 9-year campaign from same lead agency with Push Play brand, with different populations targeted.	Funding for 3-year Active Australia campaign provided; campaign adopted by other states in years 2 and 3.	4-year funding for phase 1. Find Thirty has been adopted by two other state jurisdictions in Australia.
Develop consistent message local to national, brand, logo (3, 4)	Push Play with logo of a fast-forward button on a VCR, indicating activation or getting movement; logo sustained across campaign years and target groups.	Clear brand and message. "Exercise. You only have to take it regularly, not seriously."	"Find Thirty—It's not a big exercise" as tagline and theme through all messages and communication channels.
Sequence campaign elements, link to policy, programs (5)	Phase 1: 1999-2002 targeted middle-aged adults; phase 2: defined and targeted inactive population segments; phase 3: 2006-2009 targeted young people.	Clear campaign plan, starting phase 1 with motivated but inactive middle-aged adults, and year 2, seniors aged 55-75 years.	Phase 1 targeted PA dose, i.e., 30 minutes. Phase 2 indicated that 30 minutes can be accumulated in doses of 10 minutes or more. After 2006, the focus was on sessions, i.e., "Find thirty every day."
Educate the media, engage media channels (6)	Worked with media locally and nationally in NZ.	Worked with media to generate publicity. Separate PR agency: "unpaid media"; value of unpaid coverage generated estimated at $300,000.	Strong focus on ongoing public relations media. Collaboration with added value ideas such as buying space in weather bulletins.

Characteristics and Strategy*	Push Play NZ 1999-2009	Active Australia 1998-2000	Find Thirty, Western Australia 2002-2007
Use web, new media as supportive new technologies (7, 8)	Online components, PA "activators," interactive website. Especially in phase 3, added new media.	Toll-free telephone line supported phase 1 and 2: provided a consumer link to regional sport and recreational services	Campaign website developed. Consumer input regarding ways to Find Thirty. Otherwise limited (preceded new media).
Additional information: *written manual *documentation * policy and environmental support *most innovative features	Resources and information on Push Play available at www.sparc.org.nz/en-nz/communities-and-clubs/Push-Play/. Innovation included community connection to local sport and recreation delivery network and local messaging; cultural adaptation and local flexibility; sustainability and duration.	Campaign support manual developed for local health and sport/recreation sectors; PA counseling kits mailed to family physicians. Phase 1: Community activities supported the campaign (local walking events; flyers attached to pay slips). Phase 2: community grants scheme. School and municipality funding to networks to support PA. Innovation: was the first large media campaign linked to a large interagency PA task force.	A manual and materials developed to assist regional and rural uptake. Innovation included consistency of the Find Thirty brand/slogan; link of this slogan to the PA guideline about 30 minutes; thorough and ongoing formative research to "get the message right"; strong engagement of walking and transport messages; linked to a cross-governmental task force; thorough and ongoing impact evaluation.

PA = physical activity.

*Strategy numbers from the National Physical Activity Plan, Mass Media Sector are in parentheses.

Summary

Campaigns led by mass-reach media should be included in public health approaches to promoting physical activity. The examples from Australasia described in this chapter indicate that such campaigns have the potential to create interest in physical activity, catalyze the potential for change, and influence social norms regarding inactive lifestyles. Important elements of effective campaigns include political support, sustained funding, and well-established interagency partnerships that support the myriad settings and sectors in which physical activity can be promoted.

Overarching government support was a consistent feature of these three campaigns, providing the sustained support to fund a sufficient dose of mass media to increase and sustain community awareness. This is the *sine qua non* of media campaigns, and without adequate planning, good formative message development, and sufficient media duration and intensity, little can be expected from these initiatives. Further, embedding campaigns in large-scale national or state-level planning for physical activity and having the policy support from a task force are essential features illustrated here. Having met these conditions, the three Australasian campaigns achieved substantial reach into their respective target communities. The populations targeted were mostly middle-aged adults, with the exception of phase 3 of Push Play, which targeted young people.

Finally, investing in quality evaluation at all stages of mass media campaign programming (Bauman et al 2006) is important. Formative research to optimize message development requires time and effort and needs to be rigorous and comprehensive, usually using a mix of qualitative and quantitative research. Process evaluation of the reach of campaign activities includes an assessment of audience reached (target audience rating points or gross rating points). These measures indicate that media placement occurred as intended and exposure was likely to be sufficient to achieve mass reach. In addition, tracking the population reach of other campaign resources, use of ancillary community programs, and participation in related mass events are crucial. Impact evaluation needs to be rigorous, using the best research designs and measures that the program can afford; such evaluation indicates to program developers what works, in turn leading to better subsequent campaigns. All three of these campaigns, especially Push Play and Find Thirty, emphasized evaluation and used the results to improve subsequent programs. We have much to learn from these efforts at promoting physical activity in Australia and New Zealand and from the comprehensive way in which campaigns were nested in broader policy frameworks and linked to good evaluation.

References

Bauman, A., Bellew, B., Vita, P., Brown, W., Owen, N. March 2002. Getting Australia active: towards better practice for the promotion of physical activity. National Public Health Partnership. Melbourne, Australia, (pp. 80-81). ISBN: 0-9580326-2-9. Accessible from archive at: fulltext.ausport.gov.au/fulltext/2002/nphp/gaa.asp.

Bauman, A., B. Bellew, N. Owen, and P. Vita. 2001. Impact of an Australian mass media campaign targeting physical activity in 1998. *Am. J. Prev. Med.* 21(1):41-7.

Bauman, A., B.J. Smith, E.W. Maibach, and B. Reger-Nash. 2006. Evaluation of mass media campaigns for physical activity. *Eval. Prog. Plann.* 29:3:312-22.

Bauman, A., G. McLean, D. Hurdle, S. Walker, J. Boyd, I. van Aalst, and H. Carr. 2003. Evaluation of the national "Push Play" campaign in New Zealand: Creating population awareness of physical activity. *NZ Med. J.* 116(1179):U535.

Bauman, A., and J. Chau. 2009. The role of media in promoting physical activity. *Journal of Physical Activity and Health.* 6(Suppl 2):S196-210.

Bull, F., R. Milligan, M. Rosenberg, and H. McGowan. 2000. *Physical Activity Levels of Western Austra-lian Adults 1999.* Perth, Western Australia: Health Department of Western Australia and Sport and Recreation.

Commonwealth Department of Health and Ageing. 2000. Annual Report 1999/2000. Canberra, Australia: Author. www.health.gov.au/internet/main/publishing.nsf/.../outcome8.pdf

Elley, R., N. Kerse, B. Arroll, and E. Robinson. 2003. Effectiveness of counselling patients on physical activity in general practice: Cluster randomised controlled trial. *Br. Med. J.* 326:793.

Hillary Commission (Department of Sport, now Sport New Zealand), Wellington. 1998. *Physical Activity Task Force Report: More People, More Active, More Often.*

Maibach, E., M.L. Rothschild, and W.D. Novelli. 2002. Social marketing. In: *Health Behavior and Health Education* (pp. 437-461). 3rd ed. K. Glanz and B.K. Rimer, Eds. San Francisco, CA: Jossey-Bass.

Milligan, R., G.R. McCormack, and M. Rosenburg. 2007. *Physical Activity Levels of Western Austra-lian Adults 2006. Results from the Adult Physical Activity Survey.* Perth, Western Australia: Western Australian Government.

National Health Committee, New Zealand. 1998. Active for life: A call for action. http://nhc.health.govt.nz/publications/nhc-publications-pre-2011/active-life-call-action.

New Zealand Ministry of Health. 2008. Healthy Eating—Healthy Action, Oranga Kai—Oranga Pumau. Progress on Implementing the HEHA strategy 2008. www.moh.govt.nz/moh.nsf/indexmh/heha-progress-dec08.

Simply Active Every Day. 2004. NSW Physical Activity Task Force. A plan to promote physical activity in NSW 1998-2002. Evaluation report, NSW health department. www.health.nsw.gov.au/pubs/2004/pdf/simplyactive.pdf.

SPARC. 2003. *Obstacles to Action: Overview Report. A Study of New Zealanders Physical Activity and Nutrition.* A report produced by AC Nielsen for SPARC. Wellington, South Australia: SPARC.

SPARC. 2007. Physical activity guidelines for children and young people (5-18 years old). *Obstacles to Action: Overview Report. A Study of New Zea-landers Physical Activity and Nutrition.* A report produced by AC Nielsen for SPARC. Wellington, South Australia: SPARC. www.sparc.org.nz/en-nz/young-people/Activity-Guidelines-5-18-Years/.

TNS Social Research. 2006. Physical activity campaign track, October 2002–December 2005. TNS Social Research and Department of Health WA.

CHAPTER 11

Communication Strategies to Promote the 2008 Physical Activity Guidelines for Americans

Katrina L. Piercy, PhD, RD
U.S. Department of Health and Human Services, Office of Disease Prevention and Health Promotion

Kay Loughrey, MPH, MSM, RD, LDN
Whole Mind Wellness, LLC, Gaithersburg, Maryland

Jane D. Wargo, MA
Presidential Youth Fitness Program

NPAP Tactics and Strategies Used in This Program

Mass Media Sector

STRATEGY 3: Develop consistent mass communication messages that promote physical activity, have a clear and standardized "brand," and are consistent with the most current *Physical Activity Guidelines for Americans*.

Public Health Sector

STRATEGY 4: Disseminate tools and resources important to promoting physical activity, including resources that address the burden of disease due to inactivity, the implementation of evidence-based interventions, and funding opportunities for physical activity initiatives.

The *Physical Activity Guidelines for Americans,* issued on October 7, 2008, provide science-based guidance to help Americans ages 6 years and older improve their health through regular physical activity. Before 2008, the U.S. federal government had never issued comprehensive physical activity guidelines for the nation, although the guidelines were preceded by government-sponsored recommendations. For example, in 1995 the Centers for Disease Control and Prevention (CDC) and the American College of Sports Medicine (ACSM) published physical activity recommendations for public health; the report stated that adults should accumulate at least 30 minutes per day of moderate-intensity physical activity on most, preferably all, days per week. In 1996, *Physical Activity and Health: A Report of the Surgeon General* supported this same recommendation. This chapter provides background on the development of the Physical Activity Guidelines for Americans (PAG) and identifies communications activities and ongoing efforts to promote the guidelines.

Maintaining a healthy lifestyle includes a balance of both good nutrition and regular physical activity. Therefore, the PAG and the *Dietary Guidelines for Americans (DGA,* www.health.gov/dietaryguidelines) provide complementary and consistent advice for physical activity.

Acknowledgments: The authors thank Richard P. Troiano, PhD, federal coordinator for the development of the 2008 Physical Activity Guidelines for Americans and executive secretary of the Physical Activity Guidelines Advisory Committee; and Suzanne Hurley Zarus, Centers for Disease Control and Prevention, for their contributions to this chapter. The authors also acknowledge Rachel Polon, MPH, RD; Holly McPeak, MS; and Richard Olson, MD, MPH, from the HHS Office of Disease Prevention and Health Promotion for their contributions and assistance in editing.

The DGA were first released in 1980 and are federally mandated to be updated on a five-year cycle. The most recent release of the DGA in 2010 incorporates the recommendations from the PAG to provide guidance on the importance of being physically active and eating a healthy diet to promote good health and reduce the risk of chronic disease.

In October 2006, the U.S. Department of Health and Human Services (HHS) sponsored, and the Institute of Medicine planned, a workshop titled Adequacy of Evidence for Physical Activity Guidelines Development. On October 27, 2006, HHS Secretary Michael Leavitt announced plans for the development of federal Physical Activity Guidelines for Americans to be issued in 2008. HHS decided that the PAG would serve as a benchmark and a single, authoritative voice for providing science-based guidance on physical activity for health promotion. The department solicited expert advisory committee members through the *Federal Register* and simultaneously outlined a communications campaign to promote the messages of the PAG. In February 2007, Secretary Leavitt appointed 13 members to the PAG advisory committee and charged the committee to review existing scientific literature to identify whether sufficient evidence existed to develop a comprehensive set of physical activity recommendations and identify areas where further scientific research was needed.

Nine subcommittees of the advisory committee focused on specific topics: all-cause mortality, cardiorespiratory health, metabolic health, energy balance, musculoskeletal health, functional health, cancer, mental health, adverse events, and youth and understudied populations. The PAG advisory committee submitted its findings and recommendations to Secretary Leavitt in spring 2008. HHS staff used the PAG advisory committee report to develop the Physical Activity Guidelines for Americans.

Description of the Physical Activity Guidelines

The PAG affirm that it is acceptable for adults ages 18 and older to follow the CDC-ACSM recommendation and similar recommendations. However, the scientific evidence does not allow researchers to say, for example, whether the health benefits of 30 minutes of activity on five days a week differ from the health benefits of 50 minutes on three days a week. As a result, the guidelines allow for adults to accumulate two hours and 30 minutes a week in various ways. People can choose from many activities and can accumulate activities in bouts of 10 minutes throughout the week. In addition, adults can do moderate-intensity activity, vigorous-intensity activity, or a combination of the two. Muscle-strengthening activity is advised on two or more days per week. Unlike previous recommendations, the PAG provide more direct guidance for older adults, women who are pregnant or in the postpartum period, persons with chronic conditions, and persons with disabilities. Additionally, recommendations for children and adolescents ages 6 to 17 are included—60 minutes of activity each day plus muscle-strengthening and bone-strengthening activities at least three days a week.

The PAG include several key messages:

- Regular physical activity reduces the risk of many adverse health outcomes.

- Some physical activity is better than none.

- For most health outcomes, additional benefits occur as the amount of physical activity increases through higher intensity, greater frequency, or longer duration.

- Most health benefits occur with at least two hours and 30 minutes (150 minutes) per week of moderate-intensity physical activity, such as brisk walking. Additional benefits occur with more physical activity.

- Both aerobic (endurance) and muscle-strengthening (resistance) physical activities are beneficial.

- Health benefits occur for children and adolescents, young and middle-aged adults, older adults, and those in every racial and ethnic group, as well as for people with disabilities.

- The benefits of physical activity far outweigh the possibility of adverse outcomes.

Development of Communication Materials

HHS relied on user-centered methods (www. usability.gov) and evidence-based health literacy principles (Health literacy 2013) to ensure that communication surrounding the PAG was relevant and included steps people could take to incorporate more physical activity into their lives. User-centered methods were incorporated to ensure that the content of the materials was engaging, relevant, and appropriate to the audience. Health literacy principles played a critical role in guiding the development of consumer materials that were appropriate for people of different ages, genders, and cultural backgrounds. Materials, written at the fifth-grade level, were conversational and friendly and used the active voice. The materials used limited scientific jargon, explained new terms in several ways, and used interactive techniques. The material developers paid careful attention to the visual appearance of the materials, limiting line length and depth, using subheadings to break up text, and using photographs to amplify text.

The agency conducted two rounds of focus groups to help shape the messages. Its research was primarily on the U.S. adult population with low health literacy, most with less than a high school education, but the ability to read simple text. HHS wanted to ensure that the messages used to promote the PAG were relevant to the daily lives of U.S. adults, including the 77 million Americans with limited health literacy.

Focus Group Tagline and Icon Testing

Prior to the release of the PAG, the CDC conducted communications research related to individuals' understanding of physical activity and the PAG as well as message development and testing. It conducted two sets of focus groups in 2008; the first set included adults with limited health literacy and was conducted in Houston, Texas; Memphis, Tennessee; and Baltimore, Maryland. The second set, which included inactive adults who were contemplating becoming more physically active, was conducted in Richmond, Virginia, and Catons-

ville, Maryland. The goal of this research was to learn how to encourage understanding, awareness, and acceptance of the PAG among this segment of the U.S. population. The focus groups also provided information that served as the foundation for developing messages that were relevant, clear, and easy for the general public to understand. Focus group participants evaluated taglines and icons that might be used to promote the PAG; participants characterized the tagline "Be active. Be healthy. Be happy" as motivating, meaningful, and appealing.

Tagline and Concept Testing

In May 2008, the HHS Office of Disease Prevention and Health Promotion (ODPHP) contracted with the American Institutes for Research (AIR) to conduct six focus groups to examine consumer reactions to concepts and taglines for the PAG and to design a consumer booklet. AIR tested materials with consumers ages 25 to 64, in groups separated by gender and level of physical activity, in Chicago, Illinois; Jackson, Mississippi; and Bethesda, Maryland. The locations selected included large and small urban and suburban areas, different racial and ethnic populations, and different climates. Participants reacted to four creative concepts developed by AIR and five additional taglines. They also shared their perceptions of physical activity and their understanding of the word *guidelines*.

Concepts Tested

- Join the Movement
- Active Life
- Making it Easier
- Role Model

Taglines Tested

- Physical activity. Every move counts.
- Physical activity. Just what the doctor ordered.
- Be active. Be healthy. Be happy.
- Physical activity is for everyone. One step at a time.
- Physical activity is for everyone. Step it up!
- Physical activity. For your body, mind, and spirit.

Feedback from these focus groups showed a preference for the Role Model concept, which had a headline of "If I can do it, you can do it." Many mentioned that the concept made them feel motivated and, in some cases, reminded them of personal experiences in which they had been inspired to start being active by someone else who was more active than they were. The tagline "Be active. Be healthy. Be happy" was well received, and many people noted the connection between physical activity and a person's health and happiness. This research was consistent with the focus groups conducted on behalf of the CDC. Focus group participants also favored the use of success stories and quotes from "real people," as well as using images to depict "regular" people (e.g., family, friends, and neighbors) incorporating physical activity into their everyday lives. Additionally, the focus groups reinforced previous findings that self-efficacy and social support are important when promoting physical activity.

Field Testing of Consumer Booklet

Following focus group testing, ODPHP developed and field tested a booklet designed to have broad appeal for American adults, with an emphasis on persons with low literacy or limited time. The goal of the booklet was to inform people about how much activity they need, to convince them that being active at recommended levels is possible for them, and to suggest ways to add more activity into their busy lives. The format of the booklet was different from a typical linear approach to organizing content. Because most people are inactive and the concepts are complex, the biggest challenge was to help people think about how to start engaging in physical activity and learn how to build up gradually. Therefore, the booklet was designed to focus on various audience segments, mirroring progress through the Transtheoretical Stages of Change Model (precontemplation, contemplation, preparation, action, and maintenance). For example, the first chapter targeted people who are not currently active but are thinking about becoming more active (precontemplation or contemplation stage). The second chapter targeted people in the preparation phase, those who are doing

some activity and are planning to do more. Field testing demonstrated that the booklet was well matched to the experience, logic, and language of respondents and was well received as attractive, informative, understandable, and motivational.

Resources for the Key Message: Be Active Your Way

As a result of the focus groups, Be Active Your Way was selected as a key communication message. This message emphasized the importance of finding and doing the physical activities that a person enjoys. Several consumer guides, including a fact sheet and a booklet for adults, were developed using this message and following rigorous health literacy standards. These resources were part of a larger toolkit that HHS developed for the launch and shared with partner organizations. The PAG toolkit, accessible online (www.health.gov/paguidelines/adultguide/default.aspx), contains the following print resources (along with a CD of all materials):

Physical Activity Guidelines for Americans Toolkit Components

- 2008 Physical Activity Guidelines for Americans
- Be Active Your Way: A Guide for Adults (booklet)
- Be Active Your Way: A Fact Sheet for Adults
- Physical Activity Guidelines for Americans Toolkit User's Guide
- Posters (4)
- Event flyers (4)
- At-a-Glance: A Fact Sheet for Professionals
- Frequently Asked Questions
- Federal Resources
- PowerPoint presentation (available on CD–ROM only)

In 2011, HHS released Spanish versions of two resources from the PAG: *Be Active Your Way: A Guide for Adults* (booklet) and *Be Active Your Way: A Fact Sheet for Adults*. These documents were first translated into Spanish and then tested with a Hispanic audience to ensure that key messages were conveyed.

Be Active Your Way:
A Fact Sheet for Adults

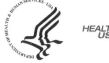 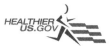

Finding out what kind and how much physical activity you need

How do I do it?
It's your choice. Pick an activity that's easy to fit into your life. Do at least 10 minutes of physical activity at a time. Choose **aerobic** activities that work for you. These make your heart beat faster and can make your heart, lungs, and blood vessels stronger and more fit. Also, do **strengthening** activities which make your muscles do more work than usual.

Why should I be physically active?
Physical activity can make you feel stronger and more alive. It is a fun way to be with your family or friends. It also helps you improve your health.

How many times a week should I be physically active?
It is up to you, but it is better to spread your activity throughout the week and to be active at least 3 days a week.

How do I build up more physical activity?
Do a little more each time. Once you feel comfortable, do it more often. Then you can trade activities at a moderate level for vigorous ones that take more effort. You can do moderate and vigorous activities in the same week.

How much physical activity do I need to do?

This chart tells you about the activities that are important for you to do. Do **both** aerobic activities and strengthening activities. Each offers important health benefits. And remember, some physical activity is better than none!

Aerobic Activities

If you choose activities at a **moderate** level, do at least **2 hours and 30 minutes** a week.	If you choose **vigorous** activities, do at least **1 hour and 15 minutes** a week.

- Slowly build up the amount of time you do physical activities. The more time you spend, the more health benefits you gain. Aim for twice the amount of activity in the box above.
- Do at least 10 minutes at a time.
- You can combine moderate and vigorous activities.

Muscle Strengthening Activities

Do these at least **2 days** a week.

- Include all the major muscle groups such as legs, hips, back, chest, stomach, shoulders, and arms.
- Exercises for each muscle group should be repeated 8 to 12 times per session.

Be Active, Healthy, and Happy!

Reprinted from Health and Human Services.

How can I tell an activity at a moderate level from a vigorous one?

Vigorous activities take more effort than moderate ones. Here are just a few moderate and vigorous aerobic physical activities. Do these for **10 minutes or more** at a time.

Moderate Activities	Vigorous Activities
(I can talk while I do them, but I can't sing.)	(I can only say a few words without stopping to catch my breath.)

Moderate Activities	Vigorous Activities
• Ballroom and line dancing	• Aerobic dance
• Biking on level ground or with few hills	• Biking faster than 10 miles per hour
• Canoeing	• Fast dancing
• General gardening (raking, trimming shrubs)	• Heavy gardening (digging, hoeing)
• Sports where you catch and throw (baseball, softball, volleyball)	• Hiking uphill
• Tennis (doubles)	• Jumping rope
• Using your manual wheelchair	• Martial arts (such as karate)
• Using hand cyclers—also called ergometers	• Race walking, jogging, or running
• Walking briskly	• Sports with a lot of running (basketball, hockey, soccer)
• Water aerobics	• Swimming fast or swimming laps
	• Tennis (singles)

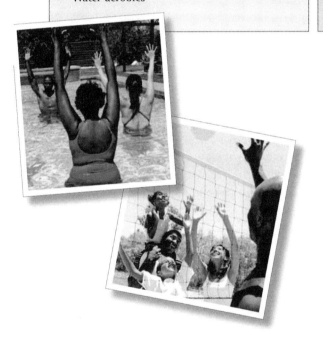

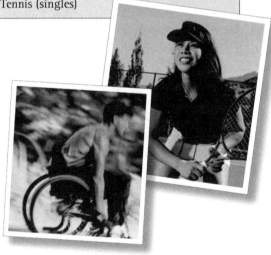

For more information, visit www.healthfinder.gov/getactive

Be active your way by choosing activities you enjoy!

ODPHP Publication No. U0038   October 2008

CDC Youth Physical Activity Guidelines Toolkit for Schools, Families, and Communities

Although many of the toolkit components focused on promoting the PAG for adults, the CDC Division of Adolescent and School Health developed a toolkit to promote the guidelines for youth. The Youth Physical Activity Guidelines Toolkit highlighted strategies that schools, families, and communities can use to support youth physical activity and targeted community leaders; physical education and health education teachers; physical activity coordinators at the school, district, and state levels; and physical activity practitioners working in health or community-based organizations. The toolkit is available at www.cdc.gov/HealthyYouth/physicalactivity/guidelines.htm.

Youth Physical Activity Guidelines Toolkit Components

- User guide (step-by-step guidance, customizable resources, fundamental strategies, and key examples of use pertaining to toolkit contents)
- Fact sheets
  - Youth Physical Activity: The Role of Schools
  - Youth Physical Activity: The Role of Communities
  - Youth Physical Activity: The Role of Families
- PowerPoint presentations
  - The Role of Schools in Promoting Youth Physical Activity
  - The Role of Communities in Promoting Youth Physical Activity
  - The Role of Families in Promoting Youth Physical Activity
  - The Role of Schools, Families, and Communities in Promoting Youth Physical Activity
- Poster: Be Active and Play, 60 Minutes Every Day!
- Video: Active Children and Adolescents: The Physical Activity Guidelines in Action

Communications Strategy

HHS used a three-fold communication strategy to promote the PAG: the launch, media outreach, and partnerships. The communications strategy was designed to raise awareness of the guidelines among professionals and consumers, develop partners, increase people's confidence in their ability to meet the guidelines, and ensure that Americans received consistent and accurate messages about the PAG from all sources. The following three sections detail the components of the strategy.

Launch

The Physical Activity Guidelines for Americans were launched on October 7, 2008. President Bush announced the guidelines at a White House event followed by an official launch by Secretary Leavitt at HHS. ODPHP and the President's Council on Fitness Sports and Nutrition (PCFSN) hosted a partnership forum immediately following the launch. Representatives from lead partner groups, including ACSM, the International Health, Racquet and Sportsclub Association (IHRSA), the National Association for Sport and Physical Education (NASPE), the National Coalition for Promoting Physical Activity (NCPPA), the YMCA, and the American Heart Association shared their plans to promote and disseminate the PAG.

Media Outreach

An extensive media outreach campaign followed the launch of the PAG. A majority of the media coverage was online, comprising 48% of the visibility, followed by print with 27% and television with 25%. Coverage of the PAG generated more than 15 million message contacts during October, November, and December 2008. Stories on msn.com, MSNBC, and CNN provided an especially strong online presence. Coverage also appeared on regional affiliates of major broadcast networks, including ABC, NBC, FOX, and CW. Articles in *USA Today*, the *New York Times*, the *Chicago Tribune*, the *Washington Post*, and other major newspapers helped the PAG to reach a broad, national audience.

News Release

For Immediate Release
Tuesday, October 7, 2008

Contact: HHS Press Office

HHS Announces Physical Activity Guidelines for Americans

Adults gain substantial health benefits from two and a half hours a week of moderate aerobic physical activity, and children benefit from an hour or more of physical activity a day, according to the new Physical Activity Guidelines for Americans. The comprehensive set of recommendations for people of all ages and physical conditions was released today by the U.S. Department of Health and Human Services.

The guidelines are designed so people can easily fit physical activity into their daily plan and incorporate activities they enjoy.

Physical activity benefits children and adolescents, young and middle-aged adults, older adults, and those in every studied racial and ethnic group, the report said.

"It's important for all Americans to be active, and the guidelines are a roadmap to include physical activity in their daily routine," HHS Secretary Mike Leavitt said. "The evidence is clear—regular physical activity over months and years produces long-term health benefits and reduces the risk of many diseases. The more physically active you are, the more health benefits you gain."

Regular physical activity reduces the risk in adults of early death; coronary heart disease, stroke, high blood pressure, type 2 diabetes, colon and breast cancer, and depression. It can improve thinking ability in older adults and the ability to engage in activities needed for daily living. The recommended amount of physical activity in children and adolescents improves cardiorespiratory and muscular fitness as well as bone health and contributes to favorable body composition.

The Physical Activity Guidelines for Americans are the most comprehensive of their kind. They are based on the first thorough review of scientific research about physical activity and health in more than a decade. A 13-member advisory committee appointed in April 2007 by Secretary Leavitt reviewed research and produced an extensive report.

Key guidelines by group:

Children and adolescents—One hour or more of moderate or vigorous aerobic physical activity a day, including vigorous intensity physical activity at least three days a week. Examples of moderate intensity aerobic activities include hiking, skateboarding, bicycle riding, and brisk walking. Vigorous intensity aerobic activities include bicycle riding, jumping rope, running and sports such as soccer, basketball, and ice or field hockey. Children and adolescents should incorporate muscle-strengthening activities, such as rope climbing, sit-ups, and tug-of war, three days a week. Bone-strengthening activities, such as jumping rope, running, and skipping, are recommended three days a week.

Adults—Adults gain substantial health benefits from two and one half hours a week of moderate-intensity aerobic physical activity, or one hour and 15 minutes of vigorous physical activity. Walking briskly, water aerobics, ballroom dancing, and general gardening are examples of moderate intensity aerobic activities. Vigorous-intensity aerobic activities include racewalking, jogging or running, swimming laps, jumping rope, and hiking uphill or with a heavy backpack. Aerobic activity should be performed in episodes of at least 10 minutes. For more extensive health benefits, adults should increase their aerobic physical activity to five hours a week moderate-intensity or two and one half hours a week of vigorous-intensity aerobic physical activity. Adults should incorporate muscle strengthening activities, such as weight training, push-ups, sit-ups, and carrying heavy loads or heavy gardening, at least two days a week.

Older adults—Older adults should follow the guidelines for other adults when it is within their physical capacity. If a chronic condition prohibits their ability to follow those guidelines, they should be as physically active as their abilities and conditions allow. If they are at risk of falling, they should also do exercises that maintain or improve balance.

Women during pregnancy—Healthy women should get at least two and one half hours of moderate-intensity aerobic activity a week during pregnancy and the time after delivery, preferably spread through the week. Pregnant women who habitually engage in vigorous aerobic activity or who are highly active can continue during pregnancy and the time after delivery, provided they remain healthy and discuss with their health care provider how and when activity should be adjusted over time.

Adults with disabilities—Those who are able should get at least two and one half hours of moderate aerobic activity a week, or one hour and 15 minutes of vigorous aerobic activity a week. They should incorporate muscle-strengthening activities involving all major muscle groups two or more days a week. When they are not able to meet the guidelines, they should engage in regular physical activity according to their abilities and should avoid inactivity.

People with chronic medical conditions—Adults with chronic conditions get important health benefits from regular physical activity. They should do so with the guidance of a health care provider.

For more information about the Physical Activity Guidelines for Americans, visit www.hhs.gov or www.health.gov/paguidelines.

Reprinted from Health and Human Services.

Radio Media Tour

Following the launch, the Surgeon General, Steven Galson, MD, promoted the PAG through a variety of outlets that were coordinated through a contractor with CDC. A media campaign reached more than 60 cities during the live on-air portion and many additional locations through replays. A podcast was created for the HHS Health Beat, and the Surgeon General was interviewed for a National Institutes of Health (NIH) Vodcast Radio episode that aired in February 2009. A three-part series about the PAG also aired on NIH radio during February and March 2009.

E-Marketing and Web

HHS used a variety of e-marketing and web techniques to reach the public in a cost-effective manner, including blogs and podcasts, e-newsletter articles, and announcements sent to listservs, external partners, advocates, professionals, educators, and policy makers. Consistent messages and resources related to the PAG were posted on a variety of websites, including those of ODPHP, PCFSN, and CDC. A Wikipedia article provided an overview of the health benefits of physical activity and the key PAG recommendations for adults and youth: http://en.wikipedia.org/wiki/Physical_Activity_Guidelines_for_Americans.

The agency also used Healthfinder.gov to deliver messages about the PAG and provide resources, tips and links for additional information. It conducted extensive focus group testing and research with more than 750 people to inform the content of the Healthfinder material. Healthfinder.gov distributed seasonal e-cards that could be personalized and sent to family and friends to encourage them to be active. The Be Active Your Way quiz, found on the PAG website, is linked to physical activity information found on Healthfinder.gov. The quiz widget can be copied and used on other sites to promote the PAG.

CDC Exercise Videos

CDC created a series of videos that help explain the physical activity guidelines, provide tips on how to meet them, and demonstrate proper techniques for muscle strengthening exercises. These videos were based on usability testing conducted in fall 2008. The testing showed that the general public prefers simple explanations, simple visuals, icons, and personal testimonies of meeting the PAG. The videos can be accessed at www.cdc.gov/physicalactivity/everyone/videos/index.html.

Partnerships

Partnerships have been a critical component of the PAG communications strategy, and partners continue to disseminate key physical activity messages within their communities. PAG leaders created the Physical Activity Guidelines for Americans Supporter Network prior to the release of the guidelines, and key partners were invited to attend the launch and share their ideas for dissemination. By October 2009, the supporter network included more than 3,400 organizations; by 2011, it included more than 5,100. The PAG gained support from a variety of sectors, including government, education, and nonprofit and community-based organizations. Organizations interested in becoming a part of the supporter network can sign up through the PAG website, www.health.gov/paguidelines/.

Members of the supporter network attended webinars on the guidelines between January 2009 and January 2011. Hosted by ODPHP in collaboration with PCFSN and CDC, the webinars covered a range of topics, including CDC's Guide to Community Preventive Services, evidence-based strategies on physical activity, and the National Physical Activity Plan. During the webinars, supporters updated participants on implementation of the PAG in their communities.

Be Active Your Way Blog

The Be Active Your Way blog was created to stimulate a virtual dialog among professionals interested in helping Americans be more active. Launched on November 4, 2009, the blog provides a forum where professionals can learn from and connect with each other through content that is updated weekly and comments in response to the content. Additionally, the blog highlights a number of community-based programs that participating organizations are using to increase physical activity in their communities.

Lessons Learned

There were several challenges in communicating the PAG to the public. Given the tight timeline and limited funding, a strong effort was made to communicate the messages of the PAG to the public in a variety of ways, as described in this chapter. For future iterations of the PAG, it will be necessary to have a strong communications plan in place, with sufficient time to fully develop and test messages.

Timeline

One challenge in developing and releasing the PAG was the tight timeline to complete the project prior to the end of the Bush administration. Secretary Leavitt announced plans for the PAG in 2006 and, in just under 2 years, the guidelines were released. The condensed timeline made it challenging to fully develop a large and comprehensive communications plan to be released concurrently with the PAG. Unlike the DGA, the PAG are not federally mandated; however, it may be helpful to have a timeline for subsequent iterations of the PAG so that funding, time, and staff can be allocated for the advisory committee report, policy document, and supporting consumer materials. This would provide an opportunity for the department to highlight the importance of physical activity in a regular manner, similar to the nutrition messages delivered in the DGA.

Communications

Experts in communication assisted with writing the PAG to help address some of the key communication challenges, including appropriately targeting the intended audience, clarifying target amounts of activity, defining levels of intensity, and supporting dissemination and maintaining public awareness (Troiano and Buchner 2011). Although focus groups were conducted to test the tagline and concepts, it would also be helpful to have the language of key messages tested to identify messages that resonate with the key target audience. The goal would be to develop messages that promote action, not simply awareness of the recommendations.

Partners

Partners played a key role in disseminating the PAG, and several lessons can be learned from partner relationships. Solid commitments with actionable items and clear roles for each partner can help target messages to specific audiences. This will ensure that messages reach a variety of sectors, including youth, who are targeted through schools, coaches, and parents. The message needs to be consistent across partners, including health care providers, from whom many consumers get their health information. Changing people's behaviors to increase physical activity will require a significant change in the culture of our country. This culture shift would benefit from engaging partners across a wide variety of sectors, such as CEOs of large corporations and educational leaders, who could provide opportunities for physical activity throughout the work and school day.

Tips for Working Across Sectors

The PAG were a successful collaborative effort across many sectors of HHS. The PAG steering committee consisted of representatives within the ODPHP, PCFSN, and the Physical Activity and Health Branch of CDC. The primary coordinating office was ODPHP, whereas CDC managed the literature review and scientific management. The advisory committee consisted of experts in academia across the United States. In addition, the Food and Nutrition Board and the Board on Population Health and Public Health Practice, both of the Institute of Medicine, were integral in planning the workshop Adequacy of Evidence for Physical Activity Guidelines Development. Additional names and titles of individuals who assisted with the PAG process are outlined in the report of the PAG advisory committee, representing the teamwork required to complete the PAG.

Summary

As this chapter highlights, participating agencies communicated key messages of the PAG with minimal resources. ODPHP, PCFSN, and CDC, along with partner agencies and the supporter network, continue to promote the PAG

and the importance of regular physical activity. These agencies recommend that a scientific advisory committee review the science and make recommendations to update the guidelines every 10 years. Revised guidelines should be accompanied by a robust communication campaign that highlights the new recommendations and reiterates the core messages of the Physical Activity Guidelines for Americans.

Additional Reading and Resources

Physical Activity Guidelines for Americans policy document: www.health.gov/paguidelines/pdf/paguide.pdf

Physical Activity Guidelines Advisory Committee Report: www.health.gov/paguidelines/Report/Default.aspx

Partnership Toolkit: /www.health.gov/paguidelines/adultguide/default.aspx

CDC Toolkit for Youth: www.cdc.gov/HealthyYouth/physicalactivity/guidelines.htm

List of federal websites that promote physical activity: www.health.gov/paguidelines/federalresources.aspx E-cards to promote physical activity: http://healthfinder.gov/ecards/cards.aspx?jscript = 1

Recorded radio media tour, HHS HealthBeat: www.hhs.gov/news/healthbeat/2009/04/20090414a.html.

The Surgeon General interview, National Institutes of Health (NIH) Vodcast Radio episode (February 23, 2009): www.nih.gov/news/radio/feb2009/20090220PAG.htm (transcript)

www.youtube.com/watch?v = bn5gr4Jc3to (video)

NIH radio three-part series; www.nih.gov/news/radio/podcast/2009/e0077.htm;

www.nih.gov/news/radio/podcast/2009/e0078.htm

www.nih.gov/news/radio/podcast/2009/e0079.htm

References

Health literacy. 2013. http://health.gov/communication/literacy/.

Troiano, R.P., and D.M. Buchner. 2011. National Guidelines for Physical Activity. In: *Physical Activity and Public Health Practice* (pp. 196-209). B.E. Ainsworth and C.A. Macera, Eds. CRC Press, Boca Raton, FL.

Health Care

Robert Sallis, MD, FAAFP, FASCM

Kaiser Permanente Medical Center

The association between physical activity and good health has been well established. In fact, research has shown there is a dose-response relationship between a person's activity level and his or her health status. That is, those who are active and fit tend to live longer and healthier lives, whereas those who are sedentary and unfit are more likely to suffer from chronic disease and to die at a younger age. Research also has shown that the connection between physical activity and health exists in every subgroup of the population. The research across race and ethnic groups, age groups, and genders is clear—people who are physically active are healthier and live longer than those who are sedentary. Exercise really is a powerful medicine that can be used to prevent and treat myriad conditions.

Unfortunately, health care systems generally have ignored this research and have not integrated it into standard disease prevention and treatment paradigms, thereby failing to harness the power of exercise to prevent and treat disease. This is troubling, given that our society is experiencing an explosion of noncommunicable diseases that result in large part from sedentary lifestyles. Can you imagine if a pill or medical procedure provided even a fraction of the proven health benefits of exercise? Surely it would be the most widely prescribed therapy known to humankind, and patients would demand access to it! Thus, it is time for health care providers to begin advising patients, particularly those at risk for or diagnosed with chronic diseases such as diabetes, heart disease, and high blood pressure, to engage in regular physical activity.

Health care is America's largest industry, and its costs threaten to become unsustainable if we don't change the way we practice medicine. Most experts agree, and studies suggest, that a focus on preventing disease will achieve better results at lower cost than our current system's emphasis on pills and procedures. Increasing physical activity among patients is a key health care strategy that has the potential to prevent and treat disease at a low cost.

This section of the book presents five programs that are working to make the connection between exercise and health. The starting point for making this connection is to assess and prescribe exercise at every patient encounter by looking at physical activity as a "vital sign"; chapters 13 (Sallis) and 15 (Joy et al.) describe initiatives that have successfully adopted this approach. Another important strategy is to develop a health care systems approach to promoting physical activity as a treatment for disease, and chapter 16 by Ballard describes how this can be done. A final key strategy is to improve education for physicians about physical activity and health, not just for patients but for themselves as well. The chapters by Kennedy and Phillips and Bilodeau provide excellent examples of how to do this. These chapters provide both motivation and a blueprint that other health care systems can use to harness the power of physical activity to improve the health and longevity of the patients they serve.

CHAPTER 12

Institute of Lifestyle Medicine

Mary A. Kennedy, MS
Institute of Lifestyle Medicine,
Joslin Diabetes Center, Boston MA
Harvard Medical School

Edward M. Phillips, MD
Institute of Lifestyle Medicine,
Joslin Diabetes Center, Boston MA
Harvard Medical School

NPAP Tactics and Strategies Used in This Program

Health Care Sector

STRATEGY 5: Include physical activity education in the training of all health care professionals.

The Institute of Lifestyle Medicine (ILM) is a nonprofit professional education, research, and advocacy organization that is leading a comprehensive effort to reduce lifestyle-related death and disease in society through clinician-directed interventions with patients. Edward M. Phillips, MD, founded the ILM at Harvard Medical School (HMS) and Spaulding Rehabilitation Hospital (SRH) in 2007. In 2013 the institute transitioned from SRH to the Joslin Diabetes Center, a Harvard teaching affiliate. The ILM offers concrete tools and training to health care professionals, conducts research to demonstrate the efficacy of lifestyle medicine education, and advocates for national adoption of lifestyle medicine and reform of medical education to include lifestyle medicine. It also promotes health improvement by empowering clinicians to adopt healthier habits, facilitate behavior change, and stimulate a culture of health and wellness for their patients.

Program Description

The ILM as it exists today took several years to evolve. It began as an effort to educate physicians about a new way to effectively and efficiently address weight management in their patients by incorporating health coaching techniques into clinical encounters. Although government agencies, private employers, and insurance companies have developed programs to address obesity and promote wellness, the medical profession is lagging in its efforts to educate physicians about physical inactivity and other lifestyle behaviors and train them to address these issues. The ILM seeks to fill the void of wellness education for physicians and other health care professionals.

Introducing the Concept of Lifestyle Medicine

In 2004, Dr. Phillips collaborated with Margaret Moore, MBA, founder and CEO of Wellcoaches, to write and publish an online continuing medical education (CME) program offered through the HMS Department of Continuing Education. This course, Lifestyle Medicine for Weight Management, was supported by a small grant from the HMS Department of Physical Medicine and Rehabilitation, where Dr. Phillips is an assistant professor. This unique online education module used the term *lifestyle medicine* to describe the skills physicians need to deal effectively with the obesity crisis. Many of the competencies needed to address obesity—including health coaching—are not taught in medical school. This course was one of the first to provide a template for clinical interventions using rudimentary coaching techniques to help patients with weight management. Since its release in 2005, more than 2,000 clinicians from over 100 countries have completed this course (www.harvardlifestylemedicine.org).

Gaining an International Reach

Leaders of a wellness program at Apollo Hospitals in Hyderabad, India, learned about the online weight management course and requested in-depth, onsite training in lifestyle medicine for their clinicians. A second small grant from HMS allowed Dr. Phillips to expand the material taught in the online course and create a two-day interactive training curriculum that covered exercise prescription, stress management, nutrition, smoking, physician health, obesity, and behavior change theory. The course included a personal health assessment and coaching demonstration and provided CME credits from HMS. Harvard clinicians taught the course in four Indian cities in March 2006, which proved timely, considering the recent epidemic of lifestyle illnesses that the country was experiencing. At end of two weeks in India, there was a clear need to establish a formalized institute to serve as a resource for clinicians worldwide seeking to learn the skills to effectively counsel patients about lifestyle interventions.

Forming the Right Partnerships

Drawing on their experiences in India, the course facilitators agreed that the time was right to establish an institute that would serve as a resource for clinicians who wanted to counsel their patients about lifestyle interventions. Dr. Phillips agreed to lead the effort to form the ILM. His home institution, SRH, and academic home, HMS, agreed to host the institute, and key national organizations such as the American College of Sports Medicine supported it. The ILM was launched on October 1, 2007.

Building on Established Expertise

The ILM was structured with education at its core, and, for that reason, its leaders focused on that agenda first. Following completion of the courses in India, momentum had been building to establish similar courses in the United States. As a first step toward achieving that goal, ILM created a one-day CME course titled Introduction to Lifestyle Medicine. This course, developed to provide a general introduction to lifestyle medicine, drew 125 attendees when it was first held in Boston in fall 2008. The feedback from the course was very positive; however, participants made it clear that they needed concrete tools to make changes to their practices. ILM leaders used this feedback to update the course. The name was changed to Lifestyle Medicine: Tools for Promoting Healthy Change, and the format was updated to provide more resources that the attendees could readily use in their work. This updated one-day course has been held annually in Boston every June since 2009 and was expanded to a two-day format in 2013.

In addition to creating this introductory course, ILM wanted to provide an opportunity for clinicians to focus on physical activity. To meet that need, institute leaders created a two-and one-half day CME course titled Active Doctors, Active Patients: The Science and Experience of Exercise. This course was launched in November 2009 and drew more than 125 participants. It was designed to teach the basic science of exercise and physical activity, provide information about physical activity recommendations, and introduce the principles of health coaching techniques through didactic training. It provided course participants with an opportunity to attend four exercise sessions taught by certified exercise professionals at a local health club. The sessions included aerobic, strength, and flexibility options. The U.S. Surgeon General, Regina Benjamin, MD, MBA, recognized the efforts of the Active Doctors course by presenting the keynote address at the course in 2010. She also led an event titled White Coats, White Sneakers, Walk for a Healthy and Fit Nation on the Boston Common in concert with the Active Doctors course (figure 12.1).

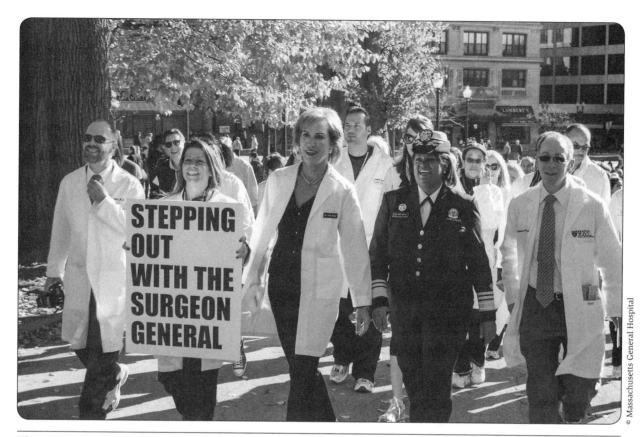

Figure 12.1   Surgeon General Dr. Regina Benjamin leading the White Coats, White Sneakers, Walk for a Fit and Healthy Nation at the 2010 Active Doctors course. She is joined by Drs. Damian Folch, Pamela Peeke, and Edward Phillips, plus more than 100 course attendees.
©MaryKennedy

In response to participant feedback and in recognition of the need to expose the entire health care team (not just physicians) to information about lifestyle medicine, ILM leadership renamed the course Active Lives: Transforming Ourselves and Our Patients. The updated course, in which participants practice the skills of promoting physical activity and prescribing exercise, was introduced in November 2011. The exercise sessions in the revamped course are conducted in an open area next to the conference center rather than within a health club. This change provides an inexpensive and reproducible model for participants to recreate in clinical settings when they return to practice.

Expanding the Foundation

Since the first online course was released in 2005, ILM has developed six additional courses, and several more are in production. To date, more than 6,800 clinicians in more than 115

countries have completed one or more of these courses.

Expansion of the ILM's reach and impact required additional infrastructure to help with research and advocacy for policies to support lifestyle medicine. With limited funding, the ILM has recruited a small army of professionals who volunteer their time and expertise to promote the vision of more healthful behaviors through clinician intervention. A team of researchers also has begun to carve out a specific research agenda for the institute, which will focus on education, and to identify funding opportunities. The goal of the research agenda is to strengthen the institute's education and CME efforts.

Program Evaluation

ILM conducts participant surveys before and after each CME course. The pre-course surveys are sent out approximately one week prior to the course, and the post-course surveys are conducted 90 days after the course ends. These surveys are conducted primarily online. In November 2012, the results of these surveys were published in *Medical Teacher*. The article, "The Impact of Lifestyle Medicine Continuing Education on Provider Knowledge, Attitudes, and Counseling Behaviors," by Dacey and colleagues is summarized here:

> Two hundred participants completed surveys before and 90 days after each CME program. Results indicated that all of the barriers that were targeted during the programs (i.e., lack of knowledge and skills, lack of materials, and perceived poor patient compliance) showed highly significant improvement. Participants also reported significant changes in knowledge, confidence, and counseling behaviors in the areas of exercise and stress management. Some improvements occurred in areas that the CME programs did not target as much, specifically nutrition, smoking, and weight management. The greatest predictor of change was the baseline level of score—those participants who could most benefit from change showed the largest improvements. This work suggests that live CME programs can be effective in educating health care providers about topics within the expanding field of lifestyle medicine.

Further findings not included in the paper reveal the conference was successful in educating participants about physical activity as well as inspiring them to incorporate this knowledge into both their clinical practice and their personal lives. Attendees were asked to rate their current knowledge of exercise and physical activity as well as their confidence in their ability to discuss those subjects with their patients before and after the course. On a scale of 1 to 10 (1 = not knowledgeable; 10 = very knowledgeable), course attendees' knowledge increased from 7.1 precourse to 8.3 at 90 days after the course; their confidence increased from 7.4 to 8.9. Both represent a significant change ($p < .001$). Data suggest that knowledge and confidence translated into practice. The survey found that the percentage of attendees who

prescribed exercise to their patients increased from 41 percent preconference to 63 percent at 90 days after the conference. This represents a significant change ($p = .05$). Surveys following subsequent Active Doctors courses and the Tools for Promoting Healthy Change courses yielded similar results.

Linkage to National Physical Activity Plan

The ILM directly addresses Strategy 5 of the Health Care Sector of the National Physical Activity Plan (NPAP): *Include physical activity education in the training of all health care professionals.* The ILM fulfills this strategy by including physical activity in continuing education programs, using the recommendations from the 2008 Physical Activity Guidelines for Americans. Through the institute's two annual CME courses and the online CME training programs, health care professionals learn why physical activity needs to be an integral part of health care. These programs provide the scientific support for the relationship of physical activity to health and the tools providers need to integrate physical activity measures, prescriptions, and general advice into health care practice.

The ILM has taken this tactic a step further by incorporating physical activity education into the curricula of medical school students and residents in training. For medical students, the ILM started the Lifestyle Medicine Interest Group at HMS in 2009, which HMS formally recognized as an official student group in 2011. The Lifestyle Medicine Interest Group is supported by ILM funds and organized in cooperation with HMS students. In addition, the ILM coordinates a series of lunchtime lifestyle medicine presentations by ILM faculty, staff, and invited guests that is open to all HMS students. This is an initial effort to create a parallel curriculum that focuses on health promotion as ILM works to integrate lifestyle medicine into the formal medical school curriculum. The ILM is working closely with the University of South Carolina School of Medicine at Greenville and ACSM's Exercise Is Medicine campaign to create a national curriculum on physical activity for medical schools.

For residents, the ILM has developed an innovative curriculum in lifestyle medicine for trainees in Yale Medical School's combined Internal Medicine and Preventive Medicine Residency program; the curriculum is based on the lifestyle medicine competencies published in the *Journal of the American Medical Association (JAMA)* in 2010. A Health Resources and Services Administration grant awarded to Yale and the ILM supports this work. Residents participate in all of ILM's online training courses and have the opportunity to attend both of the CME courses. They also have the option to visit Boston for a two-week rotation in lifestyle medicine during their senior year. Finally, speakers give presentations on lifestyle medicine topics, including physical activity, at Yale on an ongoing basis throughout the three-year program.

The residents rotating in Boston gain first-hand experience in physical activity through meeting with an exercise physiologist to assess their personal exercise routine, monitoring their physical activity with an accelerometer, participating in laboratory-based exercise assessments, and providing a final formal presentation that reflects on some aspect of their personal health habits addressed during the rotation.

Evidence Base Used During Program Development

Lifestyle medicine is a relatively new field. Although the competencies necessary to counsel patients on specific health topics (e.g., physical activity, diet) have been described in the literature, only recently have the competencies that address many health topics been brought together using the term *lifestyle medicine*. The first official description of these competencies was published in *JAMA* in a 2010 commentary titled "Physician Competencies for Prescribing Lifestyle Medicine." These competencies were the result of a blue ribbon panel convened in 2009 by the American College of Preventive Medicine, in which members of multiple professional societies—including the American Medical Association, American College of Sports Medicine (ACSM), and American College of Lifestyle Medicine—addressed the knowledge gap that exists for primary care physicians in relation to counseling their patients about lifestyle medicine interventions. Today, the education programs within the ILM address the competencies described in *JAMA*.

The specific physical activity components of the ILM's programs are based on the Physical Activity Guidelines for Americans. The exercise prescription techniques taught by ILM were derived from material created by ACSM over the years. These techniques are detailed in the book *ACSM's Exercise Is Medicine: A Clinician's Guide to Exercise Prescription* (described in the Additional Reading and Resources at the end of this chapter). Dr. Phillips, director of the ILM, is a coauthor of the book, which was published in cooperation with the ILM.

Populations Best Served by the Program

The ILM was created to serve clinicians of all types who have the ability to promote lifestyle medicine interventions with their patients. The institute's education courses were designed originally with the physician in mind; however, clinicians in every area of the health care system have the ability to influence patients' lifestyle habits. As a result, ILM recently made a focused effort to encourage clinicians of all types to attend its courses by expanding the types of continuing education credits offered. Additionally, ILM is working to connect health care providers with exercise professionals to establish a strong referral network. As such, exercise professionals can also benefit from the ILM's programs and from understanding the needs of clinicians.

Lessons Learned

The ILM continues to grow and learn. ILM leaders have learned several lessons that may help other organizations working in related areas.

Work Together

Identify and reach out to people and organizations that are working on similar goals. Although working with other organizations can be time consuming and complex, it can lead to stronger and more enduring results. The most meaningful change will happen when all of the stakeholders are at the same table, working together, and learning how to leverage each other's resources most effectively. For example, in 2011, ILM conducted a survey of sports medicine doctors' attitudes and practices in recommending physical activity and exercise to their patients. This survey resulted from collaboration between ILM, ACSM, and the International Health, Racquet and Sportsclub Association (IHRSA). IHRSA funded the work and ACSM granted ILM access to its member physicians' contact information. The addition of the ACSM contacts expanded the potential number of survey participants and allowed ILM to achieve more robust results. In the end, all three groups benefited from the collaboration. The results of the survey are available at www.instituteoflifestylemedicine.org/file/doc/publications/featured_publications/GlobalSurveySportsMed_FullReport.pdf.

Think Outside the Box

Find ways to move forward despite limited resources. First, cultivate champions. Many people are willing to volunteer time to work toward achieving your goals. Take advantage of these early adopters to help spread the message of your organization. Collect contact information from the people you encounter and build a robust mailing list. ILM collects contact information from all course attendees in order to keep them informed about the institute's work and to encourage them to continue spreading the lifestyle medicine message.

Second, use the media. Public relations is critical and will yield very positive results. Reach out to newspapers, magazines, television, and radio shows that might be interested in learning about and sharing your organization's mission. Apply for local and national awards to highlight the achievements of your organization. Figure 12.2 is an award the ILM applied for, received, and leveraged through media exposure. Even small awards make people take notice of your work. Use the web as much as possible. Create a well-designed website that highlights your organization's mission and provides evidence-based information. Avoid commercial material or links that could cloud your mission or efforts. Create links between your site and related sites to draw in traffic.

Be Patient and Stay Focused

Change is slow, and organizations do not embrace it readily. Although the need for change is urgent, changes may take years to implement and sustain. Be patient and creative in your efforts. If you work within an organization, continually assess new ways in which you can collaborate while staying in sync with their overall mission. If no progress occurs after a sustained effort by two or more organizations, reassess whether the organizations are a good fit for this type of work.

Tips for Working Across Sectors

Working across sectors can be difficult, but it is critical to extending an organization's reach. Reaching across sectors can expand the audience for an organization and its mission. One of the best ways to work with groups in different sectors is to find common ground. Look for ways to attach your organization to an issue that resonates with other groups. For example, when the media reported on the advent of the Medicare Annual Wellness Visits in January 2011, the ILM provided background material for the *Time* magazine article "Wellness: Does Your Doc Know What to Look For?" Dr. Phillips shared his perspective on the Annual Wellness Visits, while also discussing their relationship to lifestyle medicine. It was a win-win and ultimately allowed ILM to get its message to thousands of people who were not familiar with the institute or its mission.

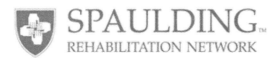

FOR IMMEDIATE RELEASE:
June 11, 2011

CONTACT:
Tim Sullivan, Communications
Spaulding Rehabilitation 1 Network
(617) 573-2918, (617) 573-2909 FAX
tsullivan11@partners.org

Spaulding's Institute of Lifestyle Medicine honored with a President's Council on Fitness, Sports & Nutrition Community Leadership Award

ILM honored for its efforts to encourage health professionals to understand "Exercise is Medicine."

Wellesley, MA—The President's Council on Fitness, Sports & Nutrition (PCFSN) has selected the Institute of Lifestyle Medicine (ILM), based at the Spaulding Rehabilitation Network and Harvard Medical School's Dept. of PM&R, to receive a 2011 PCFSN Community Leadership Award. The award is given annually to a select group of organizations and individuals nationwide who improve the lives of people in their communities by providing or enhancing opportunities to engage in sports, physical activities, fitness or nutrition-related programs.

This year, the PCFSN presented the Community Leadership Award to 33 individuals and 5 organizations across the country for their advocacy in their communities. The ILM was the only award recipient in New England selected.

"We are thrilled to receive the President's Council's recognition of the ILM's accomplishments in promoting healthy lifestyles through clinician intervention," said Eddie Phillips, ILM's Director and Founder.

The PCFSN is a committee of up to 25 volunteer citizens appointed by President Obama to serve in an advisory capacity through the Secretary of Health and Human Services. The PFCSN is comprised of a diverse range of health and fitness advocates such as current and former NFL greats Drew Brees and Tedy Bruschi, NBA stars Chris Paul and Grant Hill and public health experts such as Dr. Risa Lavizzo-Mourey the President and CEO of the Robert Wood Johnson Foundation

"It is our pleasure to present this award to the ILM," says Shellie Pfohl, Executive Director of the President's Council on Fitness, Sports & Nutrition. "Physical activity and good nutrition are important components of living a healthy lifestyle, and we are pleased to recognize organizations such as the Institute

Figure 12.2   Press release for Spaulding's Institute of Lifestyle Medicine. *(continued)*

of Lifestyle Medicine who are committed to making a difference and positively influencing the health of their communities."

A non-profit educational, research and advocacy organization, the ILM is focused on reducing lifestyle-related death and disease through clinician directed interventions with their patients. The PCFSN Community Leadership Award recognizes many of the ILM's innovative methods to assist health professionals expand their knowledge about exercise and nutrition. An example is the "White Coats, White Sneakers" walk, which welcomed US Surgeon General Regina Benjamin and hundreds of health professionals to Boston to advocate prescribing exercise to their patients. Additionally, through Harvard Medical School, the ILM offers a dozen online and live CME courses. These courses, taken by more than 3,000 clinicians in 100 countries, have increased knowledge about exercise and nutrition and engendered positive lifestyle change in healthcare professionals and their patients.

About the Institute of Lifestyle Medicine
We help clinicians get patients healthier. The Institute of Lifestyle Medicine (ILM) was founded in 2007 by Spaulding Rehabilitation Hospital and Harvard Medical School to reduce lifestyle-related death and disease in society through clinician directed interventions with patients. More at www.instituteoflifestylemedicine.org

About the Spaulding Rehabilitation Network

A member of Partners HealthCare, The Spaulding Rehabilitation Network includes Spaulding Rehabilitation Hospital its main campus, a 196-bed facility, located in Boston, as well as Spaulding Rehabilitation Hospital Cape Cod, two long term care facilities Spaulding Hospital Cambridge and Spaulding Hospital North Shore and two skilled nursing facilities, as well as twenty three outpatient sites throughout the Greater Boston area. Spaulding is a teaching hospital of Harvard Medical School as well as the official rehabilitation hospital of the New England Patriots. Spaulding is the only rehabilitation hospital in New England continually ranked since 1995 by *U.S. News and World Report* in its Best Hospitals survey with a #4 ranking in 2010. For more information, please visit www.spauldingrehab.org.

About the President's Council on Fitness, Sports, and Nutrition (PCFSN)
PCFSN promotes healthy lifestyles through fitness, sports and nutrition programs and initiatives that educate, engage and empower all Americans. PCFSN is a committee of volunteer citizens appointed by the President who serve in an advisory capacity through the Secretary of Health and Human Services. For more information about PCFSN, visit www.fitness.gov. For more information about the President's Challenge Physical Activity and Fitness Awards Program or the Presidential Active Lifestyle Award, visit www.presidentschallenge.org.

—End—

Figure 12.2   *(continued)* Press release for Spaulding's Institute of Lifestyle Medicine.

Additional Reading and Resources

ILM website: www.instituteoflifestylemedicine.org

ILM online courses: httwww.harvardlifestylemedicine.org/index.php

Medical Teacher CME article: Dacey, M., F. Arnstein, M.A. Kennedy, J. Wolfe, and E.M. Phillips. 2012. The impact of lifestyle medicine continuing education on provider knowledge, attitudes, and counseling behaviors. *Med Teach.* 35:e1149-56. http://informahealthcare.com/doi/pdf/10.3109/0142159X.2012.733459.

Time magazine article: Russo, F. 2011, January 29. Wellness: Does your doc know what to look for? *TIME.* http:// www.time.com/time/magazine/article/0,9171,2040210,00.html

ACSM's Exercise Is Medicine initiative: http://exerciseismedicine.org/

American College of Preventive Medicine: http://acpm.site-ym.com

JAMA article: Lianov, L., and M. Johnson. 2010. Physician competencies for prescribing lifestyle medicine. *JAMA.* 304(2):202-3.

ACSM's Exercise Is Medicine—A Clinician's Guide to Exercise (Baltimore: Lippincott Williams & Wilkins, 2009). Written by Drs. Steve Jonas and Edward

Phillips (ILM), this book is the essential field guide for health professionals being called upon to promote active lifestyles for their patients and clients and serves as the primary text in support of the ACSM's Exercise Is Medicine program. This book teaches practitioners how to motivate and instruct patients on the importance of exercise and how to design practical exercise programs for patients of all ages and fitness levels, as well as those with special conditions such as pregnancy, obesity, and cancer (http://www.instituteoflifestylemedicine. org/publications/).

CHAPTER 13

Exercise Vital Sign at Kaiser Permanente

Robert Sallis, MD, FAAFP, FACSM
Kaiser Permanente Medical Center

NPAP Tactics and Strategies Used in This Program

Health Care Sector

STRATEGY 1: Make physical activity a "vital sign" that all health care providers assess and discuss with their patients.

The Exercise Vital Sign (EVS) was launched in Kaiser Permanente's Southern California region in October 2009 as a way to make physical activity assessment and exercise prescription a standard of care for all patient visits. Founded in 1945, Kaiser Permanente (KP) is one of the largest health plans in the United States, serving almost 9 million members. KP is a staff model health maintenance organization (HMO) whose members pay a monthly premium and receive all of their health care from KP physicians and staff at KP facilities. Therefore, KP has a tremendous incentive to invest in prevention and keep patients healthy, thereby avoiding the costs associated with caring for more advanced disease. For this reason, helping patients become more active is a key priority in the organization's quest to help them achieve total health.

Program Description

It is customary for patients' vital signs to be measured at almost every visit to a health care provider. Traditional vital signs include blood pressure, pulse, respirations, and temperature. These are most often recorded by a medical assistant or licensed vocational nurse at the beginning of each visit and listed in the patient's chart. The EVS at Kaiser Permanente was designed as a way to assess each patient's physical activity habits at every visit; the EVS provides a numerical value for the amount (in minutes per week) of exercise or physical activity, of moderate or greater intensity, that each patient reports (Sallis 2011).

To accomplish this, patients are asked two questions regarding their typical exercise and physical activity habits, and their responses are recorded in the KP electronic medical record (EMR) (see figure 13.1):

1. On average, how many days each week do you engage in moderate or greater physical activity (like a brisk walk)? Based on the patient's response, the staff member clicks a box that corresponds to the number of days reported, from zero to seven days.

2. On those days, on average, how many minutes do you engage in this physical activity? Again, based on the patient's response, the staff member clicks a box that corresponds to the number of minutes reported (10, 20, 30, 40, 50, 60).

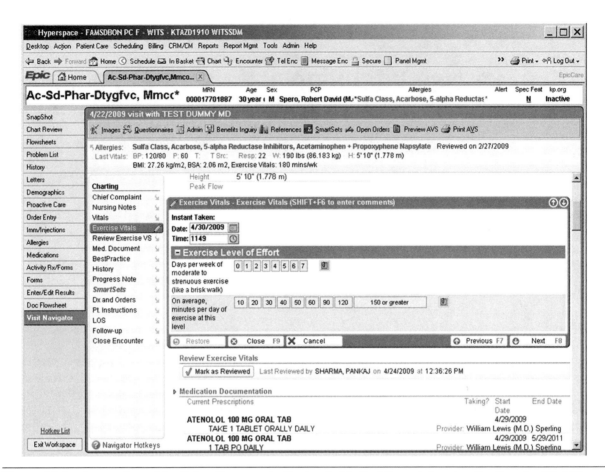

Figure 13.1   Screen shot of the Kaiser Permanente Electronic Medical Record showing the Exercise Vital Sign.
Reprinted, by permission, from Kaiser Permanente.

The computer then multiplies the two responses to calculate the minutes per week of moderate or greater physical activity that the patient has reported that he or she undertakes during a typical week. This number is displayed on the patient's chart in the vital sign header, next to the traditional vital signs (see figure 13.1). The patient's body mass index (BMI) and smoking history also are recorded.

The EVS allows the physician or other health care provider to assess quickly how much physical activity the patient performs. In keeping with the Physical Activity Guidelines for Americans, adult patients who are engaged in less than 150 minutes per week of physical activity and children who are engaged in less than 420 minutes per week are flagged as not meeting optimal levels of physical activity. Most providers will then use this information as a segue into a brief discussion about how physical activity can affect health.

Program Evaluation

After the first year of use, KP conducted a study to evaluate the implementation and validity of the EVS. The study found that 81 percent of adult KP members who had an office visit during the first year of implementation had an EVS recorded on their chart. This was remarkable, given that recording the EVS was not mandatory, and this finding seemed to reflect the acceptance of the EVS among physicians and staff. In reviewing the 1,500,947 adult KP patients who had an EVS recorded between January 1, 2010, and February 28, 2011, the investigators found that 36 percent of these patients were completely inactive (reported no regular exercise or physical activity), 33 percent were insufficiently active (reported 10-149 minutes per week), and 31 percent were meeting public health guidelines (150 or more minutes per week of moderate or greater exercise or physical activity) (Sallis and Coleman 2011).

As in previous studies that used self-reported physical activity, the results varied based on the patient's age, gender, ethnicity, and BMI. Reported physical activity tended to decrease as the age of the patient increased. Men reported doing more physical activity than women, and ethnic minorities reported doing less physical activity than nonminorities, with whites reporting the most, followed by blacks and then Hispanics. Patients with a higher BMI tended to report less physical activity than patients with a lower BMI.

KP compared results from the EVS study with data from the National Health and Nutrition Examination Survey (NHANES) (Tucker et al. 2011), which is generally regarded as one of the best data sets for identifying current trends in the health and nutrition status of Americans, including physical activity status. The NHANES survey reports data on physical activity using both self-report and accelerometry. Typically, the accelerometer reports of physical activity are much lower than the self-reports, reflecting a tendency for respondents to overestimate the amount of physical activity they engage in during a typical week. When compared with the NHANES physical activity measures, the EVS provided a more conservative estimate than the NHANES self-report measure but a higher estimate than the accelerometer report. This suggests that the EVS is, in fact, a valid indicator of patient physical activity levels in this setting. In addition, the NHANES data on physical activity reported similar trends as the KP EVS data, with lower levels of activity reported by older patients, women, ethnic minorities, and patients with higher BMI. The KP results may reflect the willingness of patients to be more truthful about their physical activity habits when being questioned by a medical professional, compared with being questioned by a research surveyor. This offers the potential for the KP EVS to provide information about the relationship between physical activity and health that has not been available previously at the population level.

A survey of physicians and other personnel was conducted two months after the EVS went live at a KP clinic in the Colorado region. This survey revealed that 85 percent of respondents believed that the EVS was easy to use, and 78 percent did not believe that it significantly slowed down their clinic; 67 percent said they were more likely to discuss exercise with their patients since using the EVS, and 65 percent felt more confident about having this discussion with patients. These results indicate that most staff believed the EVS was easy to use and an effective tool to aid in assessing and prescribing exercise to patients.

Although the EVS tool is relatively new, its use has been accepted readily by KP leadership as an effective way to capture information about the exercise and physical activity habits of patients and to bring the topic of physical activity and its importance to health into the exam room. After an initial rollout in the KP Southern California region in October 2009, the KP Northern California region adopted EVS in 2011. Plans are currently in place to roll out the EVS to every KP region.

Linkage to the National Physical Activity Plan

Health care is the largest industry in the United States and currently consumes $2.6 trillion per year, the bulk of which is spent to care for patients who have chronic diseases that are directly related to inactivity (Emanuel 2012). The KP EVS is directly linked to the Heath Care Sector of the National Physical Activity Plan (NPAP), specifically to Strategy 1.

Strategy 1: Make physical activity a "vital sign" that all health care providers assess and discuss with their patients. With the EVS, KP has shown clearly that this strategy can be implemented successfully on a large scale. In developing the EVS, KP followed the NPAP's suggested tactics for this strategy by encouraging KP physicians and staff to assess their patients' physical activity habits and encourage them to make progress toward meeting the Physical Activity Guidelines for Americans. The EVS allows KP providers to accurately identify patients who, by self-report, are not meeting these guidelines. In addition, Kaiser is among the first health care plans to include fields for tracking physical activity in its electronic medical record and has shown that this can be done with minimal disruption to patient flow.

At the same time, KP has encouraged physicians and staff to serve as role models for active lifestyles for their patients. This effort started with the organization's long-running marketing campaign called Thrive. The tag line for this campaign is "At Kaiser Permanente, we want you to live well, be well and thrive." This campaign includes internal and external components and encourages all KP employees to live the brand. In keeping with this message, internal campaigns called Thrive Across America and KP Walk have encouraged staff to join together to become more active and to get out and walk. At the same time, KP Chairman and CEO George Halvorson launched a campaign called Every Body Walk! (see www.everybodywalk.org) in January 2011. This is a nonbranded campaign designed to get Americans walking. Featuring an interactive website as the hub of the campaign, it contains videos and articles designed to inspire and inform patients about how and why they should start walking. The program also includes a helpful Every Body Walk! mobile app that can be downloaded onto smartphones to help people track and personalize their walks (see figure 13.2).

Evidence Base Used During Program Development

The evidence base documenting the health benefits of exercise is incontrovertible. It is clear that a dose-response relationship exists between a patient's activity level and his or her health and longevity (Wen et al. 2011). This relationship exists regardless of the patient's gender, race, or age (*Physical Activity Guidelines for Americans* 2008). There is no disputing the importance of physical activity to health or that it is the single most important lifestyle intervention a person can make to improve his or her health, and clear consensus exists that 150 minutes per week of moderate or greater physical activity (like a brisk walk) is the amount that every adult should strive for (*Physical Activity*

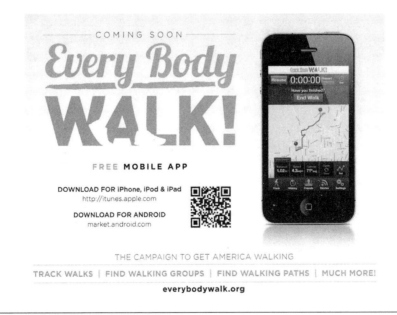

Figure 13.2 The Every Body Walk! mobile app is a useful tool to help patients track and personalize their walking.

Reprinted, by permission, from Kaiser Permanente.

Guidelines for Americans 2008; World Health Organization 2013). For this reason, KP believes that physicians have an obligation to assess the exercise habits of their patients and inform them of the risks of being inactive (Weiler et al. 2012).

The American College of Sports Medicine and American Medical Association have gone so far as to suggest that exercise is similar to a medication that should be prescribed as a first-line therapy for the prevention and treatment of disease (Sallis 2009). In 2007, these organizations launched a campaign called Exercise Is Medicine that calls on all physicians and health care personnel to make exercise assessment and prescription a standard part of the disease prevention and treatment paradigm for all patients (see www.exerciseismedicine.org). The Exercise Is Medicine initiative has developed widespread support among a range of medical organizations around the world, with most calling on their members to assess and prescribe exercise to all their patients. In addition, Healthy People 2020 includes two objectives aimed at increasing the proportion of physician office visits that include counseling or education related to the effects of physical activity on health (Office of Disease Prevention and Health Promotion n.d.).

Unfortunately, the evidence suggesting that health care providers can change the exercise habits of their patients is not as strong. In fact, the U.S. Preventive Services Task Force has said that insufficient evidence exists that physicians prescribing exercise in their practice actually cause a sustained increase in the exercise habits of their patients (Eden et al. 2002). However, this area of research is woefully underfunded, and it is still in its infancy. Similar concerns were expressed almost 50 years ago about the ability of physicians to convince their patients to stop smoking, when the American Medical Association first spoke out about the dangers of smoking. Certainly, as long as physicians resist the call to actively prescribe exercise to patients, it is unlikely that those who are most at risk from inactivity, patients suffering from chronic disease, will ever attempt to change their sedentary ways. For this reason, the KP EVS is a very important step in proving that

physicians can implement exercise assessment and prescription into their routine office visits.

Although progress has been made toward increasing the number of physicians and other health care professionals who recommend exercise or physical activity to their patients, much additional work needs to be done. Data from the National Health Interview Survey in 2000, 2005, and 2010 showed that the percentage of adults receiving advice from their physician or other health care professional to exercise increased by almost 10 percent between 2000 and 2010 (Barnes and Schoenborn 2012). However, only about a third of adults aged 18 and older who had seen a physician or other health professional in the past year had been advised to begin or continue to do exercise or physical activity. Adults who were overweight or who suffered from chronic diseases such as hypertension, cardiovascular disease, cancer, and diabetes were more likely to receive advice on exercise than were adults without these conditions. Kaiser's EVS is an excellent tool that can help increase the percentage of physicians and other health care professionals who counsel their patients on exercise and physical activity.

Populations Best Served by the Program

It is well established that the benefits of exercise apply to everyone, regardless of age, gender, or ethnicity (*Physical Activity Guidelines for Americans* 2008). Further, there is almost no disease or disability that is not improved by regular exercise. In fact, a wide range of established clinical guidelines recommend physical activity promotion as a first-line treatment (Weiler et al. 2012). For conditions as diverse as diabetes, fibromyalgia, and low back pain, regular physical activity is touted as a treatment that generally should be used before prescribing medications. For that reason, KP clinical management recommends that the EVS be used on all populations and by all medical specialties. At KP, the EVS is used in all clinical departments and by every provider who interacts with patients. In keeping with the Physical Activity Guidelines for Americans, children ages 6 to 17 are encouraged to participate in 60 minutes of physical activity daily, and adults age 18 and older are encourage to engage in 150 minutes per week.

Lessons Learned

The first lesson: Ensure that a new program or activity will fit easily into the organization's usual practice. Educate providers and staff about the rationale for the program and how to integrate it into usual practice, and address their questions and concerns. The EVS began as a pilot project in several KP Southern California medical centers in early 2009. The pilot was designed to determine the instrument's ease of use and effect on patient flow. Key concerns were that the EVS might slow down office staff or physicians or that it might not be viewed as valuable information in caring for patients. To ensure that the EVS could be recorded quickly, the two brief questions were selected and more detailed questioning on intensity of exercise was eliminated. Prior to launch of the EVS, the author visited every KP medical center in Southern California to discuss the rationale and importance of assessing and prescribing exercise to patients. This helped set the stage for implementation and was a chance to address physician concerns and encourage physicians and other providers to incorporate exercise prescription into their daily practice.

The second lesson: Test new programs to ensure that they achieve the desired goals, and train providers and staff to implement them properly. Another concern was that responses to the two questions would not accurately reflect patients' true physical activity levels. KP wanted to ensure that physical activity other than traditional exercise, such as vigorous activity or brisk walking done at work or other times in the day, was included in the EVS recorded on each patient's chart. To ensure that these forms of activity were included, KP management held a series of meetings with the department administrators of all KP clinical departments in Southern California to provide training on how to administer and record the EVS properly. The

administrators in turn trained their personnel on how to ask the EVS questions. Educational handouts, videos, and a Wiki page were developed to provide ongoing support and education regarding use of the EVS (see figure 13.3).

The EVS went live in October 2009 for use by every KP provider at every patient visit in Southern California. Since exercise has been proven to be of value to virtually every patient, every clinical department within KP was encouraged to use the EVS, from primary care to specialty care. However, there was no mandate that providers record an EVS as part of their standard routine.

The third lesson: Address push-back and respond to provider and staff concerns about the program. As expected, physicians and clinic staff initially "pushed back" a bit regarding the request to add another task to an already-busy schedule. In today's health care environment, and particularly since the advent of the EMR, there has been a significant increase in the number of issues physicians are asked to discuss with patients at each visit. Although KP physicians acknowledged the importance of exercise to health, they were leery about adding one more item to their already-full plate. Management responded by emphasizing how important exercise is to a patient's health and showing them how to incorporate the EVS information into normal patient flow quickly and easily.

Tips for Working Across Sectors

The EVS is a tool with which health care workers can bring the topic of exercise and physical activity into the examination room for all patients. If the EVS shows that a patient is not meeting guidelines for exercise and physical activity, providers can discuss how the patient can do so. Such a discussion can be made easier and more effective if physicians and other providers are aware of opportunities in their community that are available to increase patients' activity levels. Such opportunities could include park and recreation sites that encourage hiking or other physical activity, community resources such as bike and walking trails, or school-based

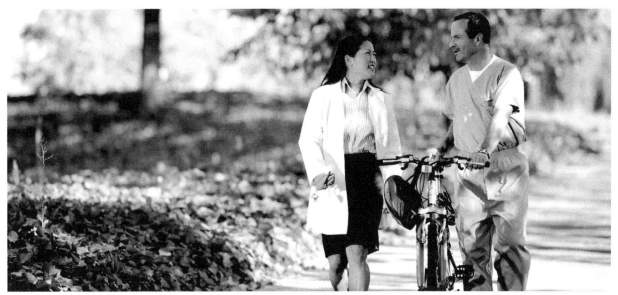

Helping our members understand the importance of exercise

Exercise Is Medicine:
Documenting Exercise Vitals in POE

WHAT IS EXERCISE VITALS?

Exercise Vitals is a KP SCAL initiative to record physical activity as a Vital Sign in our members' care plan. Regular physical activity reduces the risk of many adverse health outcomes. Exercise Vitals sends a clear, consistent message that exercise is an essential part of healthy living.

DOCUMENTING EXERCISE VITALS

Ask two questions:
1. **How many days a week of Moderate to Strenuous exercise?**
2. **On average, how many minutes do you exercise at this level?**

HOW TO ASK PATIENTS ABOUT EXERCISE

1. **What physical activities are you doing now?** Examples are, jogging, running, biking, walking, swimming, dancing, gymnastics, skating, yoga, P.E. class, martial arts, hiking, team sports.
2. **How many days do you spend doing physical activity during a typical week?**

3. **On a typical day, how much time do you spend doing physical activities?**
4. **What counts as exercise?** Moderate physical activity done at work provides the same benefits as moderate recreational exercise. Doing three 10-minute bouts of exercise in a day is the same as doing 30 minutes all at one time.

ACTIVITY LEVELS

Activity	What is it?
Light • not sweating • not breathing hard	Slow walking or dancing, yoga, ping pong, bowling
Moderate • a light sweat • can talk, but can't sing	Dancing, swimming, walking fast, biking, mowing the lawn
Vigorous • sweating • breathing hard • can't talk or sing	Jogging, high-impact aerobic dancing, biking uphill, swimming laps

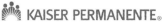 **KAISER PERMANENTE**®

Figure 13.3 Kaiser Permanente handout on documenting the Exercise Vital Sign in adult patients as part of the proactive office encounter.

Reprinted, by permission, from Kaiser Permanente.

programs to help children become more active. For these reasons, it is essential that good communication and idea sharing take place across all of the sectors of the National Physical Activity Plan. Other sectors should develop and publicize resources with an eye toward attracting patients who are most at risk from chronic diseases that are directly attributable to an inactive lifestyle.

Additional Reading and Resources

Learn more about Exercise Is Medicine, the international campaign designed to encourage all health care providers to assess and review every patient's physical activity program at every visit: www.exerciseismedicine.org

Learn more about Every Body Walk!, a national campaign to get Americans walking to achieve better health: www.everybodywalk.org

Learn more about the Kaiser Permanente Thrive campaign, which encourages its members to adopt healthy lifestyles, including regular physical activity, to achieve total health: www.kp.org/thrive

References

Barnes, P.M., and C.A. Schoenborn. 2012. *Trends in Adults Receiving a Recommendation for Exercise or Other Physical Activity From a Physician or Other Health Professional.* NCHS Data Brief, No 86. Hyattsville, MD: National Center for Health Statistics.

Eden, K.B., C.T. Orleans, C.D. Mulrow, et al. 2002. Does counseling by clinicians improve physical activity? A summary of the evidence for the U.S. Preventive Services Task Force. *Ann. Intern. Med.* 137:208-15.

Emanuel, E.J. 2012. Where are the health care cost savings? *JAMA.* 307(1):39-40.

Office of Disease Prevention and Health Promotion. Healthy People 2020 summary of objectives. n.d. www.healthypeople.gov/2020/topicsobjectives2020/pdfs/EducationalPrograms.pdf.

Physical Activity Guidelines for Americans. 2008. Washington, DC: *U.S. Department of Health and Human Services.*

Sallis, R.E. 2011. Developing health care systems to support exercise: Exercise as the fifth vital sign. *Br J Sports Med.* 45:473-4.

Sallis, R.E. 2009. Exercise is medicine and physicians need to prescribe it! *Br. J. Sports Med.* 43:3-4.

Sallis, R.E., and K.J. Coleman. 2011. Self reported exercise in patients using an exercise vital sign. *Med. Sci. Sports Exerc.* 43(5 Suppl):S376.

Tucker, J.M., G.J. Welk, and N.K. Beyler. 2011. Physical activity in US adults: Compliance with physical activity guidelines for Americans. *Am. J. Prev. Med.* 40(4):454-61.

Weiler, R., P. Feldschreiber, and E. Stamatakis. 2012. Medicolegal neglect? The case for physical activity promotion and exercise medicine. *Br. J. Sports Med.* 46:228-32.

Wen, C.P., J.P. Wai, M.K. Tsai, et al. 2011. Minimum amount of physical activity for reduced mortality and extended life expectancy: a prospective cohort study. *Lancet* 378:1244-53.

World Health Organization. Global recommendations on physical activity for health. 2013. www.who.int/dietphysicalactivity/factsheet_recommendations/en/index.html.

CHAPTER 14

Profession MD—Lifestyle Program

Sarah Bilodeau, BSc
Université de Sherbrooke

Marie-France Hivert, MD, MMSc
*Université de Sherbrooke
and Massachusetts General Hospital*

NPAP Tactics and Strategies Used in This Program

Health Care Sector

STRATEGY 5: Include physical activity education in the training of all health care professionals.

The primary preventable causes of death in the world are noncommunicable chronic diseases such as obesity, diabetes, cardiovascular diseases, and cancer. Most of the morbidity and mortality related to those conditions are attributable to lifestyle factors, primarily physical inactivity, poor dietary choices, and tobacco use. Physicians are key health professionals who are highly trusted by the public to provide information about healthy lifestyles and to support patients in modifying their health behaviors. Unfortunately, in most medical doctorate (MD) curricula in North America, very limited education time is devoted to knowledge and skills about physical activity and nutrition counseling. Consequently, physicians feel inadequately prepared to fulfill this role.

In 2008, the Université de Sherbrooke Medical School, in Sherbrooke, Quebec, implemented a new educational program that spans the entire preclinical medical curriculum. This program, known as Profession MD, is divided into several content components, including one that focuses on teaching the benefits of a healthy lifestyle and training future physicians in lifestyle counseling techniques. The principal aims of the Profession MD—Lifestyle program are (1) to raise medical students' awareness about the importance of their own lifestyles and (2) to increase students' knowledge about the benefits of a healthy lifestyle and teach them skills for supporting patients in behavior changes toward a healthier lifestyle.

Early adulthood is a critical period for making personal choices about lifestyle that are likely to last throughout adulthood. It is a favorable time to inform young adults about the benefits of a healthy lifestyle and to demonstrate how daily choices can affect their personal health significantly in the short term (e.g., physical activity for stress management and improved concentration for studying) and long term (e.g., physical activity for maintenance of a healthy weight and prevention of cardiovascular diseases). As part of the academic program, students monitor their own lifestyle in order to learn that aspects of their lifestyle might need to be improved and that behaviors such as dietary intake and physical activity levels are not easy to measure. Students choose one lifestyle habit they would like to improve or one behavior they would like to modify. By doing so, students learn that changing is not easy, which should help them approach with empathy their patients who are struggling to change behaviors. Physicians serve as role models for their patients, and physicians who practice healthier lifestyles are more credible and inspiring for their patients (Hash et al. 2003). In addition, studies have shown that physicians with healthier personal habits are more likely to discuss related preventive behaviors with their patients (Frank et al. 2004; Frank et al. 2010).

Despite the fact that most physicians and patients believe in the importance of a healthier lifestyle, the frequency of lifestyle counseling by physicians remains low; physician self-reported rates of lifestyle counseling are approximately 34 percent (Lobelo et al. 2009). A much smaller percentage of patients, 20.5 percent, report that they have been counseled about physical activity by their physician (Bleich et al. 2011). Barriers that may explain the low levels of physician counseling include physicians' lack of knowledge about physical activity, nutrition, and other lifestyle habits and lack of confidence

in their counseling skills. Prior to 2008, the MD curriculum at Université de Sherbrooke included almost no information or training about physical activity, nutrition, and behavior modification, and the situation is similar at most other medical schools.

This chapter presents the content and format of the Profession MD—Lifestyle program, the lessons learned through the process of implementation, and preliminary results of a formal program evaluation.

Program Description

Figure 14.1 shows the current MD curriculum at the Université de Sherbrooke Medical School. The Profession MD—Lifestyle curriculum, which received an award from the Minister of Education of Quebec for its innovative approach and the quality of the academic material, is

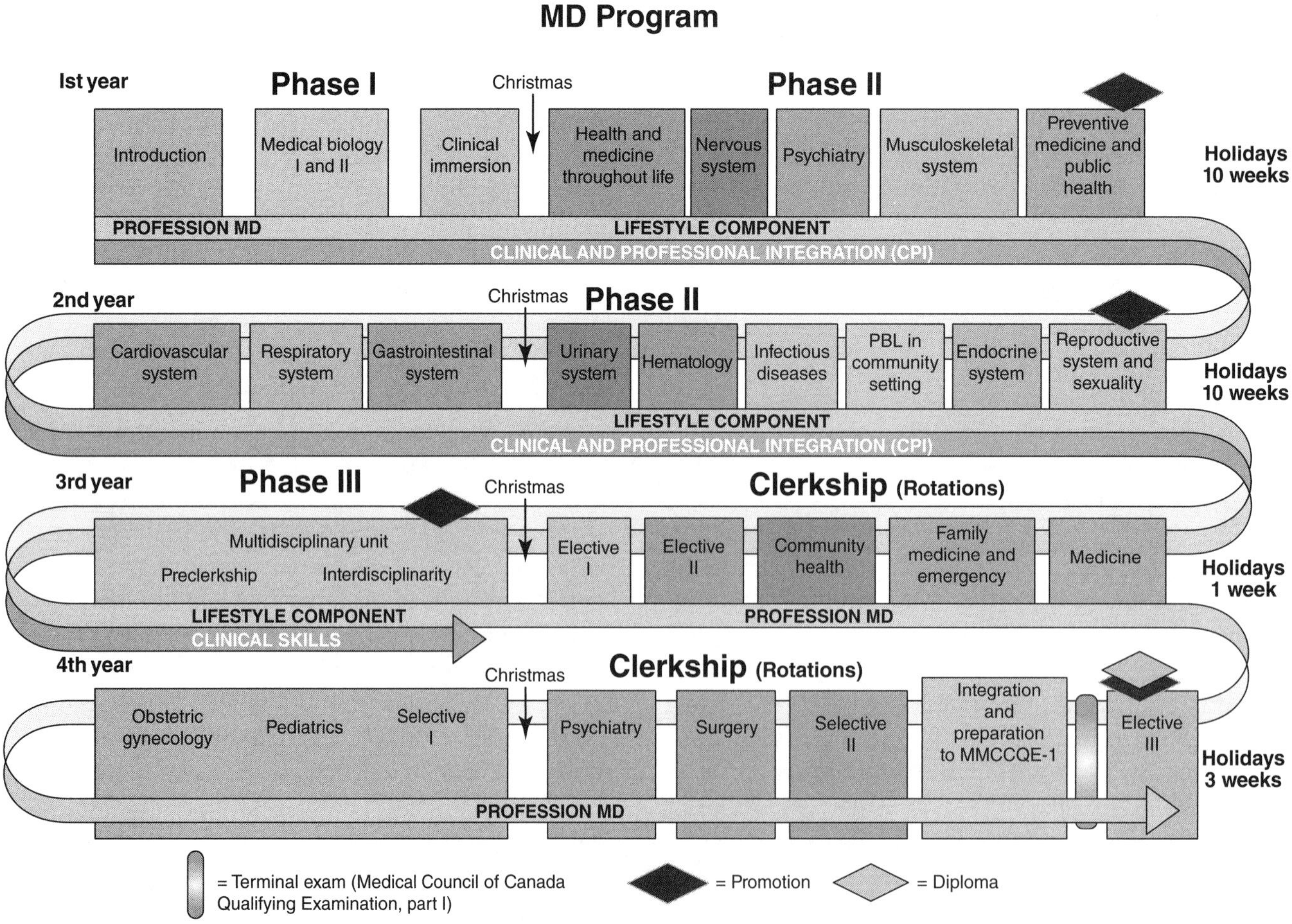

MD Program

Figure 14.1 Profession MD—Lifestyle throughout the preclinical medical curriculum.

Reprinted, by permission, from Université de Sherbrooke MD Program.

represented by the red ribbon. Components of the curriculum are described next.

Self-Monitoring Exercises

First-year students complete several self-monitoring exercises, including keeping a three-day food diary and a three-day physical activity diary and wearing a pedometer. Students are not evaluated on their results but are informed that the self-monitoring is required and that they will use some of their data in future educational exercises. Students repeat the self-monitoring exercises in the fall of the second year in order to assess the evolution of their health habits over time.

Students also learn to conduct anthropometric measurements, including waist circumference. The goal of training future physicians in these skills is that it will lead to higher frequency of measuring weight and waist circumference in the future, something that is often overlooked in clinical practice.

Introductory Lecture

In December of the first year, students attend a three-hour introductory class. The topics covered in this class include epidemiology of lifestyle and its consequences on the health of the population and the health care system, basic physiologic concepts related to nutrition and physical activity, and public health recommendations (from Health Canada) regarding physical activity and nutrition. This introductory lecture is provided in a large-group setting (the entire first-year class), but the format is structured so that students actively participating in many of the educational activities during the class.

Small-Group Seminars

Beginning in January of the first year and continuing through the end of second year, the program is built on small-group seminars, aligned with preclinical modules (see figure 14.1). The seminars last for 60 minutes and take place about once a month, with five seminars in the first year and eight in the second year. The small groups are composed of 12 students and one professor to optimize interaction. Seminar themes include benefits of physical activity, concepts of nutrition for clinical practice, tools to help with smoking cessation, psychological aspects of behavior modification, and basic concepts of motivational interviewing. The complete list of seminar topics is shown in table 14.1.

The seminars are led by professors from the medical school faculty who have received specific training (for standardization of educational

Table 14.1 Brief Description of Profession MD—Lifestyle Program

First year: Auto-monitoring Introductory session (large group, three hours)	Second year: Auto-monitoring	Third year: Auto-monitoring
Interactive sessions (small group, 45 minutes) Lifestyle and society Basics of healthy eating Psychological aspects of lifestyle change Physical activity (part I) Nutraceuticals and functional foods	Interactive sessions (small group, 45 minutes) Smoking cessation Motivational interviewing Environmental influences on nutrition Food labeling Physical activity (part II) Demystifying diets Sleep: management and repercussions on health Impact of family on lifestyle	Clinical integrations session on lifestyle counseling (simulated patients, two hours)

content). Didactic documents were developed for professors and students to facilitate comprehension and to standardize key messages taught to students. The student workbook contains references and reflection exercises as well as space to take notes on the educational activities during the seminars. The professors' guide includes the same items presented in the student workbook as well as key messages from selected references (often complementary to mandatory readings). Professors receive a detailed animation guide for the educational activities so that they can easily lead the seminars.

Students are required to complete educational activities in preparation for the seminars, which usually include reading one or more scientific articles related to the main theme and completing a related activity. The seminars often begin with a discussion based on the readings or activities. Educational content is presented through short case studies, quizzes, or other forms of interactive activities. Students often work in smaller groups and then share what they have learned with the larger group. To conclude the seminar, the professor and students discuss the relevance of the seminar topic to clinical practice.

Physical Activity Seminars

Several of the seminars are devoted to topics related to physical activity. The first seminar addresses the impact of sedentary time on health and introduces the concept of nonexercise activity thermogenesis (NEAT). The importance of NEAT in the total energy expenditure calculation and as a key component of energy balance is presented, as is its potential impact on the population trend in obesity. During the seminar, students learn ways to increase NEAT in daily living, for their personal application and for future counseling. Students also learn about the importance of physical activity for promoting concentration and optimizing learning.

Two seminars cover specific benefits of physical activity in prevention, treatment, and management of medical conditions. Assessment tools are presented, and basic recommendations regarding physical activity planning and goal setting are reviewed. In the first year, students learn about the benefits of physical activity for

obesity, stroke, and musculoskeletal problems (in line with the modules in the MD curriculum). In the second year, they learn about physical activity as it relates to myocardial infarction, chronic pulmonary obstructive disorders, peripheral vascular disorders (claudication), and cancer. Students learn about the American College of Sports Medicine's statements related to various diseases, and they study relevant readings. They examine case studies of patients with these medical conditions and identify the specific benefits of physical activity for each case. In addition, students learn to take into account special considerations related to each condition (such as potential limitations and common medications).

Physical activity content is also covered in other seminars, including those that focus on stages of change, motivational interviewing, sleep, and pregnancy.

Counseling Skills and Practical Integration Session

During the fall of the third year (before students begin clinical rotations), the Profession MD—Lifestyle program includes a session that integrates knowledge and skills about lifestyle counseling into clinical practice. This educational activity uses simulated patients who are trained to role-play a case, receive lifestyle counseling, and then give personalized feedback about their perceptions while receiving the counseling. This type of activity requires integration of knowledge, skills, and attitudes (including interview techniques). By practicing lifestyle counseling on simulated patients, students experience how to use counseling tools and learn to understand the patient's point of view. This activity is a very good preparation for the objective structured clinical examination (OSCE), an evaluation of clinical skills.

Academic Evaluation

Academic evaluation is based on professor evaluation, written exams, and performance at the OSCE. Professors give an assessment of each student based on level of preparation (including completion of the self-monitoring exercises) and participation during the seminars. Written exams at the end of each of the two first years cover the content of the introductory class and seminars. The third-year OSCE already included one case that involved counseling skills; it was modified to incorporate content that Profession MD—Lifestyle brought to the overall curriculum.

Program Evaluation

In addition to collecting feedback from students and professors, the medical school is conducting a research project to evaluate the curriculum. The study compares the students receiving the new program (intervention cohort, 2008-2012) to a group of volunteers recruited from the preceding academic year who did not receive the program (control cohort, 2007-2011). The goal of the study is to evaluate the impact of the program on students' knowledge and counseling skills. Data were collected longitudinally every year in the two groups, including results of the written and oral (OSCE) exams (see table 14.2). In brief, the students in the 2008 cohort had higher knowledge concerning lifestyle on the written exams and better specific skills for behavior counseling during the OSCE. The study also collected data about dietary habits, physical activity levels, and anthropometric measures in participating students. A modified version of the Canadian Community Health Survey, which assesses food habits, leisure physical activity, study time, sedentary activities, sleep, and transportation, was completed every year (Statistique Canada 2002). Complete analysis of data from the two cohorts is underway.

Linkage to the National Physical Activity Plan

The Profession MD—Lifestyle curriculum addresses Strategy 5 of the Health Care Sector of the National Physical Activity Plan: *Include physical activity education in the training of all health care professionals.* The program trains all medical students to incorporate education

Table 14.2 Students Results of Written Exam 1 and 2, OSCE Exam

Evaluation	Intervention cohort (*N* = 200)*	Control cohort (*N* = 31)*	*p*
Written exam year 1 (median for grade over 100 points)	86.4 (81.5-90.1)	58.6 (53.1-68.6)	<.0001**
Written exam year 2 (median for grade over 100 points)	87.7 (87.7-91.1)	51.6 (43.9-57.0)	<.0001**
OSCE exam year 2			
Global note (mean [SD] for grade over 100 points)	57.3 ± 14.5	52.8 ±12.3	.22***
Assessment of physical activity level Proportion (%) of students with grade A	24.2	12.9	.70****
Use of motivational interviewing skills Proportion (%) of students with grade A	32.0	12.9	.0005****
Follow-up and monitoring Proportion (%) of students with grade A	80.8	0.0	<.0001****

*Values are percentages. **Mann-Whitney. ***Independent *t* test. ****Fisher exact test.

and counseling about physical activity into their medical practices and to adopt physical activity habits that allow them to model positive health behaviors. A shorter, adapted version of the program is also included in the nurse practitioner training program at the Université de Sherbrooke.

Evidence Base Used During Program Development

The Profession MD—Lifestyle program was based on a pilot study conducted by Marie-France Hivert from 2002 until 2005. This randomized controlled study, which used small-group interactive seminars on healthy lifestyles, demonstrated prevention of weight gain over the first two years of university in 115 volunteer medical students (Hivert et al. 2007). The intervention successfully prevented weight gain in normal-weight medical students and provided some of the rationale that convinced the medical school administration to include a lifestyle component in the new Profession MD curriculum in 2008.

Other publications also provided evidence demonstrating the importance of increasing education about lifestyle and counseling in the medical curriculum. Numerous studies show that the percentage of patients receiving counseling about nutrition and physical activity is low (Bleich et al. 2011). Clear evidence also exists to show that health professionals' own lifestyles influence their counseling practice. Attending a medical school that promotes healthy personal practices and following these practices significantly predict whether physicians will counsel patients about preventive medicine (Frank et al. 2008). Furthermore, physicians' personal health behaviors appear to affect patients' attitudes and motivation to make lifestyle changes (Frank 2004).

Because the fields of physical activity and nutrition change rapidly, the content of the program is based on the latest guidelines and input from experts in each field. For example, one of the seminars focuses on functional foods, defined as a food given an additional function (often one related to health promo-

tion or disease prevention) by adding new ingredients or more of existing ingredients. For example, "vitamin-enriched" products are functional foods. (Agriculture and Agri-food Canada , 2012). The seminar material includes tables with the level of scientific evidence and recommended intakes for vitamin D, omega-3, and dietary fiber in diverse conditions, so that professors can refer to the latest scientific data when students have further questions.

Lessons Learned

Using the formal feedback collected from both students and professors, the faculty revised some of the seminars, adding or deleting references, refining some of the themes, and modifying some of the activities. Overall, both students and professors reported that the material was very complete and highly pertinent and that they enjoyed the sessions.

One of the seminars that is still a challenge is the one that covers motivational interviewing (MI). MI is not an easy concept to teach; few of the professors learned about this approach as part of their clinical training. For second-year students, it is hard to grasp the importance of this kind of approach, as they have had very limited clinical exposure. The program coordinator simplified the educational activities included in the MI seminar but kept MI as one of the main themes. The aim of the seminar is not to have students master the MI approach but rather to introduce the basic concepts that support it. Given experience with the curriculum to date, the program coordinator advises adding another MI session later in the curriculum, possibly at the end of the clinical rotations (fourth year) or during residency (especially for primary care specialties).

Scheduling Issues

Initially, the curriculum developers allocated only 45 minutes per seminar, and both students and professors believed that it was too little time. Consequently, beginning in 2011, they allocated 60 minutes for each seminar. The seminars are scheduled during lunchtime on the same days that the students have to be on campus for the clinical and professional integration sessions; this arrangement was chosen to minimize students' travel time. This schedule received mixed reviews from professors and students, and the medical school administration is considering other possible schedules.

Feedback From Professors

Professors who choose to teach the Profession MD—Lifestyle component come from very diverse specialties (anesthesiology, orthopedics, cardiology, endocrinology, nephrology, family medicine) and some are non-MD health professionals (dietitian, social worker). Because most of the professors had little knowledge about the actual content of the program, the curriculum developers had to ensure that the didactic material was very clear and complete. The feedback from the professors has confirmed that the intensive effort that was devoted to developing the didactic material was necessary and appreciated. The professors' guide highlights all key messages and summarizes the main references to ensure that all professors communicate the same take-home messages. Moreover, professors reported that they learned a lot and could apply the knowledge to both their own lives and their clinical practices.

Populations Best Served by the Program

The program is designed for medical students, and a shorter version is provided to nurse practitioner students. The program could be adapted for other health professional training programs. This type of program is needed in other medical schools in Canada and the United States and will become increasingly important as the prevalence of chronic diseases increases.

Tips for Working Across Sectors

Many health professionals, including kinesiologists, dieticians, behavioral scientists, and physicians, provided input into the development of the curriculum. In addition, experts in medical education and pedagogy reviewed the format of some of the educational activities and offered recommendations.

Summary

Profession MD—Lifestyle program has added great value to the MD curriculum at the Université de Sherbrooke. Both students and professors believe that the material is very pertinent and of high quality. The faculty see the difference in the approach that the medical students take with patients in the current clinical rotations compared with previous cohorts of medical students. Faculty are confident that the curriculum will lead clinicians to become more aware of and more likely to address prevention in their practices, which in turn will lead to adoption of healthier behavior in the population and, it is hoped, to a reduction in chronic diseases over the long term.

References

Agriculture and Agri-food Canada, What are functional foods and neutraceutics?, 2012 www.agr.gc.ca/eng/industry-markets-and-trade/statistics-and-market-information/by-product-sector/functional-foods-and-natural-health-products/functional-foods-and-nutraceuticals-canadian-industry/what-are-functional-foods-and-nutraceuticals-/?id=1171305207040, Consulted 2013-07-25.

Bleich, S.N., O. Pickett-Blakely, and L.A. Cooper. 2011. Physician practice patterns of obesity diagnosis and weight-related counseling. *Patient Educ. Couns.* 82(1):123-9.

Frank, E. et al., 2010. Predictors of Canadian physicians' prevention counseling practices. *Can. J. Public Health* 101(5):390-5.

Frank, E. 2004. Physician health and patient care. *JAMA.* 291(5):637.

Frank, E., E. Tong, F. Lobelo, J. Carrera, and J. Duperly. 2008. Physical activity levels and counseling practices of U.S. medical students. *Med. Sci. Sports Exerc.* 40(3):413-21.

Hash, R.B. et al., 2003. Does physician weight affect perception of health advice? *Prev. Med.* 36(1):41-4.

Hivert, M.F., et al. 2007. Prevention of weight gain in young adults through a seminar-based intervention program. *Int. J. Obes.* 31:1262.

Lobelo F., et al. 2009. Physical activity habits of doctors and medical students influence their counseling practices. *Br. J. Sports Med.* 43(2):89.

Statistique Canada. (2002). Enquête sur la santé dans les collectivités canadiennes: Premier coup d'oeil. www.statcan.gc.ca/daily-quotidien/020508/dq020508a-fra.htm.

CHAPTER 15

Development and Implementation of the Physical Activity Vital Sign (PAVS)

Elizabeth A. Joy, MD, MPH, FACSM
Intermountain Healthcare

Janet M. Shaw, PhD, FACSM
University of Utah College of Health

Trever Ball, MS
University of Utah College of Health

NPAP Tactics and Strategies Used in This Program

Health Care Sector

STRATEGY 1: Make physical activity a patient "vital" sign that all health care providers assess and discuss with their patients.

Brief physical activity (PA) counseling during every routine medical visit has the potential to increase physical activity among a large segment of the American population. To implement this type of counseling, health care providers need a simple tool that can be administered at every visit, similar to assessment of vital signs. To provide physicians and other providers with such a tool, primary care physicians and public health faculty at the University of Utah created a measure called the Physical Activity Vital Sign (PAVS), designed specifically for use in primary care settings. The PAVS tool helps providers assess physical activity levels in their adult patients. It consists of two questions that a nurse or medical assistant asks each patient (adults and older adolescents) at the beginning of every office visit:

1. How many days during the past week have you performed physical activity during which your heart beats faster and you breathe harder than normal for 30 minutes or more? (in three 10-minute bouts, or one 30-minute bout)

2. How many days in a typical week do you perform a similar activity?

Answers to these two questions generate a PAVS score ranging from a minimum of 0/0 to a maximum of 7/7. The answers provided by patients and reviewed by physicians begin the process of patient education with respect to PA. The PAVS is designed to provide reliable information about PA within the constraints of a busy office practice.

Program Description

Intervention trials that have evaluated the effects of PA counseling have found a direct relationship between the frequency of counseling and patient PA levels (Calfas et al. 1996). Implementing such counseling, however, is difficult without a system for assessing current physical activity levels. The PAVS is designed for use in busy primary care practices. It builds on assessments that are already familiar to providers and patients, such as checking weight and blood pressure at every office visit. The developers of the PAVS intend for it to become as accepted as other measurements of vital signs during office or clinic visits.

Despite the mounting evidence supporting office-based PA counseling by physicians, an inadequate number of physicians regularly assess and counsel their patients about PA (Anis et al. 2004). To increase this number, medical practices need to adopt a systematic approach to help physicians acquire information about their patients' PA levels. This approach should include participation of other members of the health care team in data collection. Technological advances, such as devoted data fields in electronic health records, can ensure that staff and providers collect and record PA data for every patient.

The PAVS is designed to be administered and recorded by a nurse or medical assistant before the physician enters the examination room. Taking only 30 seconds to complete, the PAVS does not consume a significant amount of time in the outpatient encounter. The score is interpreted by the physician and discussed with the patient during that visit. For patients who need additional help to become physically active, future visits can be scheduled for counseling and development of an exercise prescription that meets the patients' needs.

Program Evaluation

The PAVS has been evaluated against constructs related to PA, such as obesity determined by body mass index (BMI) (Greenwood et al. 2010), and against PA measured objectively by accelerometry (Ball 2011; Ball et al. 2012). Greenwood and colleagues (2010) found in a sample of 261 primary care patients that BMI was 0.91 units lower for each day in a typical week during which a patient engaged in 30 minutes of activity, as reported on the PAVS. BMI was 2.90 units lower in patients who reported five or more days of physical

activity in a typical week. In the same sample, the odds of obesity were significantly lower for each day that included PA, as reported on the PAVS (Greenwood et al. 2010).

One study assessed the criterion validity of the PAVS in a small sample (N = 45) of predominantly female, primary care clinic staff. Ball and colleagues (2011) gathered participants' responses to the PAVS and compared these with the same participants' results from seven days of objectively measured PA by accelerometry. This homogenous sample was chosen primarily to familiarize clinic staff with the PAVS and facilitate implementation of PAVS into regular clinical use.

In this sample of clinic staff, the PAVS correctly identified 92% of the respondents who were not sufficiently active. This suggests a strong ability for the PAVS to identify people most in need of counseling for PA. The PAVS responses were significantly correlated with number of days measured by accelerometry with 30 minutes or more of moderate to vigorous PA performed in cumulative bouts of 10 minutes or more (r = .52, p < .001). The PAVS was 91% accurate overall in assessing whether respondents did or did not meet current PA recommendations (kappa = .46, p < .001).

The PAVS has demonstrated preliminary evidence of effectiveness in identifying insufficiently active patients who would most benefit from PA counseling. The ability of the PAVS to accurately assess changes in PA behavior over time, or its repeatability, is still unknown.

Linkage to National Physical Activity Plan

The PAVS addresses the first strategy of the Health Care Sector of the National Physical Activity Plan.

Strategy 1: Make physical activity a patient "vital" sign that all health care providers assess and discuss with their patients. The process of developing and implementing the PAVS links directly to this strategy. When the PAVS is integrated into patient care visits, it provides a patient's health care provider with valuable information. Assessing PA during office or clinic visits brings PA into the discussion between patient and physician and allows the physician to more completely address chronic disease risk. Under the premise that "you manage what you measure," physicians and patients both benefit from a systematic approach to PA assessment. In addition, documenting patient physical activity levels in the medical record contributes to clinical epidemiology concerning the relationship between PA and health outcomes. Finally, the PAVS is a tool that can improve the quality of health care delivery.

Evidence Base Used in Program Development

The more often a physician discusses the importance of PA with a patient, the greater the likelihood the patient will change his or her behavior (Lewis et al. 1991; Manson et al. 2004). A survey of 1,818 U.S. adults found that the frequency of exercise advice increased with the number of physician visits over the course of a year: 24.5% for zero or one visit per year versus 40.9% for four or more visits per year (Glasgow et al. 2001). This finding raises important issues that can be addressed by implementing the PAVS in a medical practice. Individuals who visit a physician frequently are more likely to have chronic conditions that require regular monitoring, compared with those who see a physician zero or one time per year (Van Den Bussche et al. 2011). The former are also more likely to need assistance with developing a regular PA program.

Populations Best Served by Program

The Physical Activity Vital Sign is designed for use with older adolescents and adults. Written at the eighth-grade reading level, the PAVS can be understood by the majority of patients for whom it is intended. A medical assistant or nurse administers the PAVS before the patient is seen by a physician. The PAVS is recorded in the medical record along with other vital signs such as weight and blood pressure.

The PAVS aligns with recommendations that adults should achieve 30 minutes of moderate to vigorous intensity physical activity on at least 5 days of the week, en route to a minimum of 150 minutes per week (U.S. Department of Health and Human Services 2012).

The PAVS was designed with busy primary care clinicians in mind. Taking only seconds to administer, it fits into clinic workflow without disruption. The scale of 0/0 to 7/7 resembles a blood pressure recording, taking advantage of pattern recognition by physicians. Pattern recognition is a cornerstone of clinical practice, often guiding further diagnostic testing and therapeutic decision making. A physician's approach to medical care is often predicated on his or her ability to rapidly assess patterns in a patient's clinical presentation. In the primary care setting, where face-to-face time with the patient is limited, both standardization of care and well-designed workflows are key factors in the delivery of comprehensive and cost-effective care.

Implementation of the PAVS also helps health care systems meet established quality improvement metrics. The National Committee on Quality Assurance maintains the Healthcare Effectiveness Data Information Set (HEDIS), which includes measures that are used to determine the quality of health care provided. Two HEDIS measures are designed to assess how well health care systems assess physical activity assessment and counseling in older adults ($\geq$65 years old) and children and adolescents (2-17 years old) (Agency for Healthcare Research and Quality 2012; National Committee for Quality Assurance 2010). Although not designed for use in children, the PAVS has been used in older adults and adolescents.

Lessons Learned

The PAVS has been used for more than six years in both academic and community-based primary care clinics. Anecdotal reports from providers indicate mixed support for regularly assessing patient PA. However, assessing and counseling for physical activity require more than a discrete field in an electronic medical record. This process requires a cultural shift among clinic providers and staff, which generally requires the presence of an enthusiastic leader who strongly supports this shift in practice. Further, providers cannot be the only source of information for patients concerning the importance of physical activity for health. The shift in practice must occur in all aspects of the clinic.

In recent clinic-based research that used accelerometry to examine the criterion validity of PAVS, very few clinic staff (primarily medical assistants) achieved 150 minutes per week of moderate to vigorous physical activity, as recommended by the Physical Activity Guidelines for Americans (Ball et al. 2011). In the study, participants who were trying to lose weight had similar PA levels (approximately 17 accumulated daily minutes of moderate PA) as those who were not trying to lose weight (Goh et al. 2012). Therefore, the majority of the clinic staff in the sample were not engaging in ideal PA behaviors for health or for weight loss. Interestingly, some participants in the study were medical assistants who were familiar with and had administered the PAVS. Clearly, having knowledge of PA guidelines and working in a medical setting, even one that addresses PA with patients, are not always sufficient to help a person change his or her PA behavior.

Although the literature shows that a physician's personal PA level is a predictor of his or her PA counseling behaviors (Lobelo et al. 2009), much less is known about the role of clinic staff in promoting PA behavior though modeling. Preliminary data suggest that much more research on clinic culture and patient PA is needed.

Tips for Working Across Sectors

Implementation of PAVS links with the strategies and tactics developed by other sectors of the National Physical Activity Plan (NPAP). One of the main advantages of the PAVS is that it highlights the importance of physical activity as a significant component of health. Likewise, it links to the overarching strategies of the NPAP: raising awareness about the health benefits of regular PA, providing an opportunity for physicians to educate patients about these benefits, and promoting development of a best-practice approach to office-based PA promotion as providers learn what works and doesn't work in real-world environments (National Physical Activity Plan 2012).

Implementation of the PAVS has been dependent on the assistance and support of the other NPAP sectors. In turn, a physical activity vital sign also supports the efforts of other sectors.

• Public Health: Dissemination of the PAVS into various health care settings (e.g., academic health care clinics, community health centers) has occurred with the support of public health professionals and funding.

• Education: The Education Sector encourages postsecondary institutions to incorporate population-focused PA promotion in relevant disciplines such as nursing, medicine, and physical therapy. The integration of the PAVS into clinical care has led to efforts to educate health care professionals about the importance of PA on health, ways to assess PA, and methods for counseling patients and families about PA.

• Transportation, Land Use, and Community Design, and Parks, Recreation, Fitness, and Sports: PAVS prompts health care providers to discuss with their patients environmental strategies to promote increased physical activity, linking to strategies in the Transportation, Land Use, and Community Design Sector and the Parks, Recreation, Fitness, and Sports Sector. For example, a PA assessment prompt like the PAVS may lead providers to discuss with patients both their activity preferences and local resources provided by parks and fitness facilities.

• Business and Industry: Discussion of PA during clinical visits can prompt discussions between physicians and patients about strategies to improve PA levels in the workplace, such as taking the stairs, using standing or walking desks, and participating in active transportation to work.

Summary

Given the shift in public health recommendations for PA in adults, which have changed from 30 minutes of moderate physical activity on most days of the week to 150 minutes per week of at least moderate intensity activity, the PAVS has been reworded to be consistent with this change. Now three questions long, the PAVS asks,

1. On average, how many days a week do you perform physical activity or exercise?

2. On average, how many total minutes of physical activity or exercise do you perform on those days?

   Days per Week × Minutes per Day
   = Total Minutes per Week.

3. Describe the intensity of your physical activity or exercise:

   light = casual walk

   moderate = brisk walk

   vigorous = jogging

In a recent pilot project within a primary care clinic in Salt Lake City, researchers reviewed medical records from nearly 600 clinic visits. Physical activity assessment and counseling increased from a mean of 44% (range, 22%-69%) of visits at baseline to a mean of 78% (range, 57%-93%) of visits in just four weeks. At six months, 79% of all visits included PA assessment (Joy and Briesacher 2012).

Integrating the PAVS into clinical workflow is essential to making the information available in a way that allows providers to act on it. Likewise, providers and office staff need both knowledge and skills to use the PAVS to counsel patients regarding the benefits of PA in promoting health and preventing disease.

References

Agency for Healthcare Research and Quality. Physical activity in older adults: percentage of Medicare members 65 years of age and older who had a doctor's visit in the past 12 months and who received advice to start, increase or maintain their level of exercise or physical activity. http://qualitymeasures.ahrq.gov/content.aspx?id = 32405.

Anis, N.A., R.E. Lee, E.F. Ellerbeck, N. Nazir, K.A. Greiner, and J.S. Ahluwalia. 2004. Direct observation of physician counseling on dietary habits and exercise: Patient, physician, and office correlates. *Prev. Med.* 38(2):198-202.

Ball, T., E.A. Joy, T.L. Goh, J.M. Shaw, and J.C. Hannon. 2011. Validity of two brief physical activity self-report assessments used in primary care. Presented at the 2011 Annual American College of Sports Medicine Conference, Denver, CO.

Ball, T., E.A. Joy, J. Greenwood, and J.M. Shaw. 2012. Agreement of a repeated primary care physical activity measure with accelerometry. Presented at 2012 Annual American College of Sports Medicine Conference, San Francisco, CA.

Calfas, K.J., B.J. Long, J.F. Sallis, W.J. Wooten, M. Pratt, and K. Patrick. 1996. A controlled trial of physician counseling to promote the adoption of physical activity. *Prev. Med.* 25:225-33.

Glasgow, R.E., E.G. Eakin, E.B. Fisher, S.J. Bacak, and R.C. Brownson. 2001. Physician advice and support for physical activity: Results from a national survey. *Am. J. Prev. Med.* 21:189-96.

Goh, T.L., T. Ball, J.M. Shaw, and J.C. Hannon. 2012. Physical activity and dietary behaviors of health clinic workers trying to lose weight. *Health.*

Greenwood, J.L., E.A. Joy, and J.B. Stanford. 2010. The Physical Activity Vital Sign: A primary care tool to guide counseling for obesity. *J. Phys. Act. Health* 7(5):571-6.

Joy, E.A., and M. Briesacher. 2012. Implementation of the physical activity vital sign (PAVS). Presented at the FIMS Annual Meeting, Rome, Italy, September 28, 2012.

Lewis, C.E., C. Clancy, B. Leake, and J.S. Schwartz. 1991. The counseling practices of internists. *Ann. Intern. Med.* 114:54-8.

Lobelo, F., J. Duperly, and E. Frank. 2009. Physical activity habits of doctors and medical students influence their counseling practices. *Br. J. Sports Med.* 43(2):89-92.

Manson, J.E., P.J. Skerrett, P. Greenland, and T.B. VanItalie. 2004. The escalating pandemics of obesity and sedentary lifestyle. *Arch. Intern. Med.* 164:249-58.

National Physical Activity Plan: Overarching Strategies. 2012. www.physicalactivityplan.org/theplan_overarching.php.

U.S. Department of Health and Human Services. 2012. Physical Activity Guidelines for Americans. www.health.gov/paguidelines/guidelines/summary.aspx.

Van Den Bussche, H., G. Schön, T. Kolonko, H. Hansen, K. Wegscheider, G. Glaeske, and D. Koller. 2011. Patterns of ambulatory medical care utilization in elderly patients with special reference to chronic diseases and multimorbidity—Results from a claims data based observational study in Germany. *BMC Geriatr.* 13;11:54.

Weight Assessment and Counseling for Nutrition and Physical Activity for Children/Adolescents. 2010. National Committee for Quality Assurance (NCQA). www.ncqa.org/portals/0/Weight%20Assessment%20and%20Counseling.pdf

CHAPTER 16

Strides to Strength Exercise Program for Cancer Survivors

Tara Ballard, CET, MES

Novant Health: Presbyterian Medical Center Cancer Care

NPAP Tactics and Strategies Used in This Program

Health Care Sector

STRATEGY 1: Make physical activity a patient "vital sign" that all health care providers assess and discuss with their patients.

STRATEGY 3: Use a health care systems approach to promote physical activity and to prevent and treat physical inactivity.

STRATEGY 4: Reduce disparities in access to physical services in health care.

STRATEGY 5: Include physical activity education in the training of all health care professionals.

STRATEGY 6: Advocate at the local, state, and institutional level for policies and programs that promote physical activity.

The purpose of the Strides to Strength program is to maintain or improve the quality of life of cancer survivors through a medically supervised exercise program.

Program Description

Nearly 12 million cancer survivors are living in the United States, and this number increases each year (Hewitt et al. 2006; Horner et al. 2006.). The term *cancer survivor,* as defined by the National Coalition for Cancer Survivorship, includes people from the time of diagnosis until the end of life. The American Cancer Society recommends exercise for cancer prevention, for symptom management, and to increase quality of life. Research also suggests that exercise may decrease the chance of recurrence up to 50 percent. However, little research has examined approaches to implementing exercise rehabilitation in cancer survivors (Mina et al. 2012). In

2000, in response to the clear evidence demonstrating the positive impact of exercise on cancer survivors, Novant Health: Presbyterian Medical Center Cancer Care began investigating the structure, staffing, and other resources that would be required to provide a medically supervised exercise program to its survivors.

Strides to Strength is a personalized exercise therapy, fatigue management, nutritional counseling, education, and support program for cancer survivors. Novant Health: Presbyterian Medical Center Cancer Care began the program by adding one class to the hospital's cardiac rehabilitation program. The program then increased to four classes a week, offered on a private floor in the community's YMCA. It now includes 14 one-hour classes per week, offered by the hospital's cancer rehabilitation department (which also includes services such as yoga, massage, nutrition, physical therapy, and lymphedema therapy). The hospital began developing the program by creating an advisory board, with clinical direction from physicians (surgical oncologist, medical oncologist, radiation oncologist) and staff. It then created a mission and vision, setting guidelines on staffing requirements and training and establishing short- and long-term goals. All participants are assessed before and upon completion of the program by an oncology registered nurse, clinical exercise physiologist (certified cancer exercise trainer), oncology social worker, and oncology nutrition specialist. Assessments include fitness, quality of life, function, fatigue, pain, distress, nutrition, and goals.

Exercise

Strides to Strength is tailored to benefit all cancer survivors, from nonexercisers to athletes, through a medically driven, personalized exercise program. Data on program participants show that supervised exercise not only improves strength, endurance, and flexibility but also reduces cancer-related fatigue and improves quality of life. Activities include a variety of cardiovascular exercises, strength training, and flexibility exercises. Classes are limited to 10 survivors and include warm-up, individual exercise prescription (e.g., treadmill, arm ergometer, recumbent bike), group functional strength training, relaxation, and monitoring of heart rate, rate of perceived exertion, oxygen saturation, and blood pressure.

Nutrition

Strides to Strength survivors learn about the latest trends in cancer nutrition. Each survivor receives individual consultation, a personalized nutritional plan, periodic monitoring with feedback, and formal nutrition classes. Classes include topics such as nutrition during cancer treatment, herbs and nutritional supplements, and interactive cooking classes. Each survivor completes a three-day food diary and MedGem analysis (a simple breathing test that measures oxygen consumption and calculates resting metabolic rate [the number of calories burned at rest]), allowing the oncology nutrition specialist to create a nutrition plan that meets the survivor's and the physician's goals.

Education

Strides to Strength offers classes that present state-of-the-art information on stress management, lymphedema, nutrition, osteoporosis, exercise and medication, home exercise programs, genetic counseling, and fear of recurrence. The program focuses on the research that links exercise and nutrition with lowered risk factors for cancer, obesity, stroke, heart disease, and many more health conditions. Strides to Strength staff members believe strongly in providing participants with the knowledge, tools, and skills they need to manage their recovery and health.

Support

Strides to Strength offers regular contact and monitoring by a licensed oncology social worker through weekly support groups and individual counseling. Survivors are empowered by learning to understand and manage emotions commonly experienced by cancer survivors. Through education and discussion, participants learn to take an active role in their emotional, psychological, and spiritual health, creating a feeling of safety, support, and peace of mind. This service also allows for direct referrals for the survivor, caregiver, and other family members to additional services offered through the hospital's cancer psychosocial department, the Buddy Kemp Cancer Support Center.

Program Team

Cancer survivors typically have one or more other health issues or chronic diseases prior to diagnosis, and these must be addressed along with cancer treatment side effects. To help survivors address these issues, the Strides to Strength team includes a wide range of highly qualified and trained oncology staff:

- Oncology registered nurses
- Exercise physiologists, certified cancer exercise trainers
- Registered dieticians, certified in oncology nutrition
- Licensed clinical social workers, certified in oncology

Program Evaluation

Strides to Strength collects program and clinical outcomes data both subjectively and objectively. Over the years the program diagnosis mix has included more breast cancer survivors, averaging 62 percent, followed by people with urologic diagnoses at 16 percent and a mix of other diagnoses. The diagnosis percentages for program participation reflect the hospital's patient population (figure 16.1).

Participants include the full range of treatment statuses, including pre- and postsurgery, current chemotherapy, post chemotherapy, current radiation therapy, and post radiation therapy. These numbers show that all types of survivors have a desire to feel better and improve their quality of life. These same outcomes support the need for staffing qualified and trained professionals (figures 16.2 and 16.3).

Eighteen percent of program graduates achieve the exercise guideline of 150 minutes a week, months after completing the program,

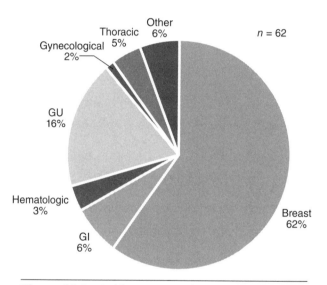

Figure 16.1 Strides to Strength cancer diagnosis 2011-2012.

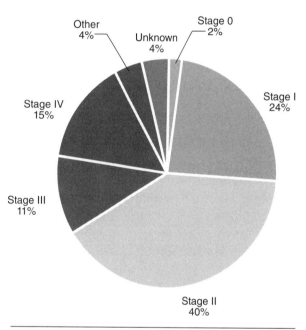

Figure 16.2 Staging for cancer survivors, 2010-2011.

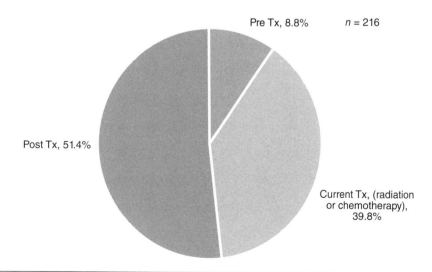

Figure 16.3 Treatment status during Strides to Strength.

similar to the 19 percent of the U.S. adult population who meet the goal (CDC National Center for Health Statistics 2013). The most impressive assessments are the clinical outcomes, which surprise both the survivors and their physicians. Results vary, but improvements are consistently observed in all areas measured. In a group of participants who completed all 24 exercise sessions and a postprogram evaluation ($N = 56$), the quality-of-life measurement, FACT-G, improved from 81 to 86.7 (average improvement, 5.7; "important difference" noted, 3-7). FACIT-Fatigue improved from 36.6 to 41.4 (average improvement, 4.8; important difference, 3-4). Fitness (as assessed with a six-minute walk) improved from 1,761 to 1,903 feet (average improvement, 142 feet; figure 16.4) (Ballard et al. 2010).

Linkage to National Physical Activity Plan

Strides to Strength supports six of the Health Care Sector strategies of the National Physical Activity Plan (NPAP).

Strategy 1: Make physical activity a patient "vital sign" that all health care providers assess and discuss with their patients. Strides to Strength encourages physician partners and staff to assess and discuss with all survivors the benefits of physical activity, both during and after treatment. The cancer center's navigators and the second opinion clinic give educational material to survivors and initiate referrals upon diagnosis. Many physicians have established

criteria (based on diagnosis, treatment status, and other factors) to generate an automatic referral to Strides to Strength. Strides to Strength also is listed on the Comprehensive Oncology Referral form that is used by all staff and MDs for referrals to services within the cancer center.

Strategy 3: Use a health care systems approach to promote physical activity and to prevent and treat physical inactivity. Novant Health Presbyterian Medical Center, the health care system, and its physicians support and promote physical activity for cancer survivors through the Strides to Strength program. This health care system promotes the program because of the value it brings to the survivors, the hospital downstream revenue, and cost savings for the hospital and survivors resulting from decreased hospital admissions and emergency room visits attributable to healthier patients. The Strides to Strength program is based on the successful cardiac and pulmonary rehabilitation models that have come to be standard programs within hospitals. Although hospital systems rely on insurance to cover services, this health care system sees the current and future benefits for survivors, hospitals, and community.

Strategy 4: Reduce disparities in access to physical services in health care. The program provides scholarships for survivors who have financial barriers to participation, to ensure that people at high risk for chronic disease and side effects related to their cancer diagnosis have equal or better access to services.

Strategy 5: Include physical activity education in the training of all health care professionals. New employees at the cancer center tour the Strides to Strength program to learn about the benefits of physical activity for survivors. All cancer center nursing employees take an educational course that addresses the importance of cancer rehabilitation services, including physical activity, for symptom management. American College of Sports Medicine (ACSM) cancer exercise guidelines and updates are given to the physicians on an annual basis during tumor board conferences.

Strategy 6: Advocate at the local, state, and institutional level for policies and programs that promote physical activity. At the institutional level, the program complies with the Commission on Cancer and the Association of Com-

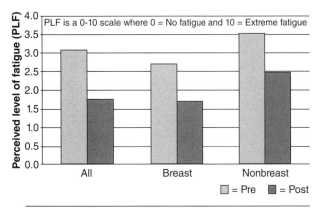

Figure 16.4 Perceived level of fatigue (PLF) comparison: patients with versus without breast cancer.

munity Cancer Centers standards and program guidelines. Strides to Strength staff advocate for cancer and physical activity programs at the state and national level. Such promotions have included presentation at the North Carolina Cancer Control Plan's Navigators annual conferences and state survivorship summits. Staff members also have presented both posters and colloquiums on the survivors' outcomes at national conferences, such as ACSM. The author advocates for physical activity programs for cancer survivors at the state level by sitting on the Survivorship Subcommittee and at the national level as chair of the Cancer Exercise Interest Group with ACSM.

Evidence Base Used During Program Development

During the development of the Strides to Strength program, very few similar programs existed nationally, little research was available, and cancer exercise guidelines had not been developed. The information and programs that did exist focused on breast cancer and fatigue (NCCN Guidelines 2012.). The evidence base used to develop Strides to Strength came from the model of cardiac rehabilitation, with input from oncology nursing, reviews of the literature, physician direction, and research on the benefits of exercise as it relates to symptoms (nausea, osteoporosis, heart health, balance). Research on the benefits of exercise for cancer survivors undergirded the program. These benefits include the following (Schmitz et al. 2010):

- Improved physical function and physical fitness
- Improved aerobic fitness
- Increased muscular strength
- Improved flexibility
- Improved or maintained ideal body size (weight, body mass index, muscle mass, and body composition)
- Increased bone health
- Help with lymphedema-related outcomes (Schmitz et al. 2009)
- Improved physiological outcomes (e.g., hemoglobin, blood lipids, IGF pathway hormones, oxidative stress, inflammation, immune parameters)
- Improved sleep patterns
- Decreased depression
- Decreased anxiety
- Decreased symptoms and adverse effects (including pain)
- Improved quality of life
- Increased adherence and compliance to treatment
- Decreased chance of recurrence

The ACSM released the 2010 guidelines for exercise and cancer (http://journals.lww.com/acsm-msse/Fulltext/2010/07000/American_College_of_Sports_Medicine_Roundtable_on.23.aspx#) after a number of experts in cancer and exercise science reviewed the current status of safety and efficacy of exercise training during and after adjuvant cancer therapy and research on physical activity and cancer survivorship. The general guidelines for cancer survivors were to avoid inactivity (some activity is better than none) and be as physically active as possible, considering abilities and conditions. Recommendations were made for weekly amounts of activity for cancer survivors:

- Aerobic: 150 minutes of moderate-intensity or 75 minutes of vigorous-intensity exercise
- Strength training: two or three sessions that involve the major muscle groups
- Flexibility: stretching of major muscle groups on days that other exercises are performed (Schmitz et al. 2010)

Lessons Learned

Strides to Strength staff recommend the following:

- Create a strong foundation and infrastructure to gain the confidence of the hospital administration, referring physicians, and survivors. Key components include hiring highly trained professionals, modeling the program after successful programs, complying with hospital policies and standards, and communicating and working closely with clinical care teams.

- Track program and clinical outcomes. Examples of data that should be collected include age, diagnosis, stage, treatment status, baseline physical assessments (six-minute walk, body mass index, balance, weight), subjective assessment tools, satisfaction with program, adherence, income, compliance to exercise, completion of program, and barriers.
- Cancer survivors want and need this type of program. If it is available, they will come.

Populations Best Served by the Program

Research has shown that exercise for cancer survivors is safe and beneficial (Schmitz et al. 2010). For that reason, Strides to Strength is available to any cancer survivor over the age of 18. Survivors may participate with any diagnosis, at any stage, at any phase of treatment or recovery. The program truly best serves all cancer survivors.

Tips for Working Across Sectors

The Strides to Strength program is open and receptive to working across sectors and building relationships. As a department within the nonprofit health care sector, the marketing and community relations department works with the media to inform and educate the public about the program. It also collaborates with educational institutions, working with local universities to provide internship opportunities within the program.

Exploring collaboration with other sectors of the National Physical Activity Plan would enhance opportunities for cancer survivors to be more active. Examples could include working with the Transportation, Land Use, and Community Design Sector to facilitate access to and safety within environments that promote walking and cycling or with the Parks, Recreation, Fitness, and Sports Sector to provide access to additional physical activity opportunities.

Additional Readings and Resources

Doyle, C., L. Kushi, T. Byers, et al. 2006. Nutrition and physical activity during and after cancer treatment: An American Cancer Society guide for informed choices. *CA Cancer J. Clin.* 56:323-53.

Holmes, M., W. Chen, D. Feskanich, et al. 2005. Physical activity and survival after breast cancer diagnosis. *JAMA.* 293:2479-86.

Ligibel, J., W. Demark-Wahnfried, P. Goodwin, et al. 2009. Diet, exercise, and supplements: Guidelines for cancer survivors. *Am. Soc. Clin. Oncol.* Educational Book. Alexandria, VA: ASCO, 2009, pp.541-547.

Meyerhardt, J., E. Giovannucci, M. Holmes, et al. 2006. Physical activity and survival after colorectal cancer diagnosis. *J. Clin. Oncol.* 24:3527-34.

References

Ballard, T., P. Downey, P. Nebus, et al. 2010. Rehabilitation: Group exercise is beneficial for improving quality of life, reducing fatigue and increasing fitness. Poster abstract presented at ACSM. American College of Sports Medicine, 57th Annual Meeting & 1st World Congress on Exercise is Medicine June 1-5, 2010, Baltimore, Maryland.

CDC National Center for Health Statistics. 2013. Summary health statistics for U.S. adults: National Health Interview Survey. www.cdc.gov/nchs/fastats/exercise.htm.

Hewitt, M., S. Greenfield, E. Stovall, Eds. 2006. *From Cancer Patients to Cancer Survivor: Lost in Transition.* Washington, DC: National Academies Press.

Horner, M.J., L.A. Ries, M. Krapcho, et al. 2006. SEER cancer statistics review, 1975-2006. Bethesda, MD: National Cancer Institute. www.seer.cancer.gov/csr/1975_2006/.

Mina, D., S. Alibhai, A. Matthew, et al. 2012. Exercise in clinical cancer care: A call to action and program development description. *Curr Oncol.* 19(3):e136-144.

NCCN Guidelines. 2012. Cancer-related fatigue. NCCN Version 1. Schmitz, K.H., R.L. Ahmed, A. Troxel, et al. 2009. Weight lifting in women with breast cancer-related lymphedema. *N. Engl. J. Med.* 361:664-73.

Schmitz, K., K. Courneya, C. Matthew, et al. 2010. American College of Sports Medicine roundtable on exercise guidelines for cancer survivors. *Med. Sci. Sports Exerc.* 2010; 42 (7):1409-1426.

Parks, Recreation, Fitness, and Sports

Andrew Mowen, PhD

Pennsylvania State University

The Parks, Recreation, Fitness, and Sports (PRFS) Sector is a critical partner in efforts to address the physical inactivity crisis in the United States. This sector is represented by a wide range of public, nonprofit, and corporate organizations whose mission is to provide healthy recreational opportunities to their constituents. PRFS services exist in practically every American community and often are available at low or no cost to participants. Although these services have been available for more than a century, the increasingly sedentary lifestyles of most Americans are compelling PRFS providers to increase the physical activity impact of those services, particularly for those at greatest risk for inactivity and its associated health consequences (e.g., low-income families). This sector is quickly recognizing the need to partner with other sectors (e.g., education, health care, business and industry) and is actively engaged in initiatives to combat physical inactivity. This sector also recognizes that no single approach is likely to be as effective as multiple strategies working in unison. Indeed, model programs that have achieved success typically involve a combination of efforts, including policy changes, environmental changes, programming, and promotional strategies.

Model programs selected for this section include a cross section of approaches, illustrate the potential of emerging strategies, and reinforce the notion that solving America's inactivity crisis requires collaborative and adaptive efforts to make both short-term and long-term gains in increasing physical activity. These programs were selected based on their ability to reach broad segments of the population, use of diverse strategies, and availability of effectiveness data. For example, chapters focus on program interventions in after-school

(chapter 18, Hanson and Rea) and summer day camp programs (chapter 19, Baker and McGregor) and in a professional sports setting (chapter 22, Yancey et al.). Other chapters focus on environmental (chapter 20, Shores) and policy approaches (chapter 17, Harnik and Mowen) that improve access to physically active spaces. Finally, chapter 21 (by Vinluan) provides an overview of the YMCA of the USA's campaign to engage in community-wide collaboration through multiple active living strategies. Each chapter provides an overview of core approaches used and acknowledges the challenges faced in implementation.

Collectively, these programs illustrate the importance and potential of the Parks, Recreation, Fitness, and Sports Sector to other sectors in their quest to increase active living in the United States. Despite the early promise and success illustrated by these and other model programs, challenges and concerns lie ahead. For example, there remains a need to document the effectiveness of interventions in terms of their long-term physical activity effects. Today's PRFS organizations also must move beyond their sector "silos" to identify, pool, and leverage resources with organizations in other sectors. Indeed, the current budgetary situation has forced many in the sector to ally with non-traditional partners (e.g., insurance companies, businesses) that can provide complementary skills and assets, alliances that not only ensure the continuation of existing initiatives but also provide expanded reach to a greater cross section of the nation. Despite these challenges, readers are encouraged to consider and adopt the approaches discussed in this section for their own initiatives. The future health and vitality of the next generation are at stake.

CHAPTER 17

ParK–12 and Beyond

Converting Schoolyards Into Community Play Space in Crowded Cities

Peter Harnik
*Center for City Park Excellence,
The Trust for Public Land*

Andrew Mowen, PhD
Pennsylvania State University

NPAP Tactics and Strategies Used in This Program

Parks, Recreation, Fitness, and Sports Sector

STRATEGY 1: Promote programs and facilities where people work, learn, live, play, and worship (i.e., workplace, public, private, and non-profit recreational sites) to provide easy access to safe and affordable physical activity opportunities.

Parks provide many opportunities for Americans to lead active, healthy lives. In fact, a number of studies have found a positive connection between people's access to parks and their physical activity levels (Kaczynski and Henderson 2007). Communities that provide residents with easy access to parks, recreation, sport, and fitness facilities also have more active and healthier residents. However, many communities lack convenient access to these types of environments. For example, a study of California youth found that one in four reported having no access to a safe park in his or her neighborhood (Babey et al. 2008). The problem is particularly severe in crowded, built-up urban areas where lack of open land makes it difficult and expensive to develop new park, recreation, sport, and fitness facilities.

One way to increase park capacity and accessibility is to make better use of existing open space through policy changes—for example, increasing the utility and benefits of existing schoolyards. In many urban communities, schoolyards are fenced, and they are locked when school is not in session. Converting these K-12 school spaces into public parks that community members can access during nonschool hours is a promising approach that can lead to higher physical activity levels for the whole community.

Commonly referred to as *schoolyard parks*, these facilities represent a cooperative venture between a board of education and a parks and recreation department. The movement to create schoolyard parks has undergone precipitous growth in recent years, as New York, Denver, Boston, Chicago, and Houston have made schoolyard conversions a central strategy in their efforts to increase recreational space capacity.

Linkage to the National Physical Activity Plan

Converting schoolyards to public parks during nonschool hours supports Strategy 1 of the Parks, Recreation, Fitness, and Sports Sector of the National Physical Activity Plan: *Promote programs and facilities where people work, learn, live, play, and worship (i.e., workplace, public, private, and non-profit recreational sites) to provide easy access to safe and affordable physical activity opportunities.* These conversions represent the kind of joint use agreements to increase operating hours that are specifically recommended by the national plan. In addition, schoolyard parks meet one of the evidence-based recommendations of the Guide to Community Preventive Services' Systematic Review for Promoting Physical Activity (CDC 2001).

Not surprisingly, creating a schoolyard park is not a simple task. However, a significant number of cities have taken on the challenge, and more are following suit. What follows is an overview of the substantial progress made in New York City and a discussion of common barriers and tips for overcoming them.

Program Description

Converting schoolyards into community playgrounds is not an entirely new concept. The first such transformation occurred in 1938 at Fort Hamilton High School in New York City (and the agreement is still in effect today). However, within the past decade, as cities have been driven by the increasing demand for athletic fields and playgrounds in heavily populated urban areas, the number of schoolyard parks has mushroomed. New York City has taken the concept the furthest. Working with the Trust for Public Land (TPL), a U.S. national nonprofit with a mission of parks for people, the New York Board of Education piloted joint-use agreements that leveraged private sector funding for high school sport fields (Dolesh 2009). The success of this pilot program led TPL to begin a schoolyard-to-playground initiative in 25 of the city's most underserved neighborhoods.

After his election in 2001, Mayor Michael Bloomberg announced PlaNYC, the massive process of adopting a new comprehensive plan for the city. A review of park capacity data revealed that New York lagged behind other cities, with only 4.6 acres of parkland per 1,000 residents (below the median of 6.8 acres per 1,000 for 13 densely populated cities). To address this deficiency, PlaNYC set a goal of providing a public park or playground within a 10-minute walk of every New Yorker. Planners quickly calculated that schoolyard parks could provide about 1,170 acres of additional recreation space and that they would be an essential component of reaching this goal (Brewer 2006).

The Schoolyards to Playgrounds initiative, a partnership between the city's Department of Education, Department of Parks and Recreation, and the TPL (as well as private funders MetLife, Credit Suisse, Deutsche Bank, and the Michael and Susan Dell Foundation) was formally announced in July 2007. The goal was to spend $110 million to transform 290 decrepit and uninviting schoolyards into showcase parks by 2010 (Harnik 2010). Not all the conversions involved the Department of Parks and Recreation, but all involved TPL and the Department of Education.

Despite having a strong mayoral system of government, New York does not have a political culture in which top-down decrees are sent from headquarters. Rather, the decision-making process is a bottom-up approach and, in the case of schoolyard parks, includes the voices of school principals, parent-teacher associations, and community stakeholders. Indeed, schoolyard park proposals can be derailed by teachers who don't want to lose parking spaces, by custodians who don't want to handle park maintenance, or by communities that don't want kids out late playing basketball. Moreover, although New York school recreation grounds are owned by the Department of Education, the schoolyard conversions have been overseen by TPL and the Department of Parks and Recreation.

"This program is community-run," says Mary Alice Lee, director of TPL's New York City Playground Program (as cited by Dolesh 2009). Although all properties are fenced and have locks, in some places the school custodial staff have the only key, whereas in others the key is held by the neighborhood sponsoring organization or a block association. A few of the parks are permanently unlocked. Each community sets its own hours, with a typical schedule of 8 a.m. to dusk seven days a week except when school is in session. In some neighborhoods,

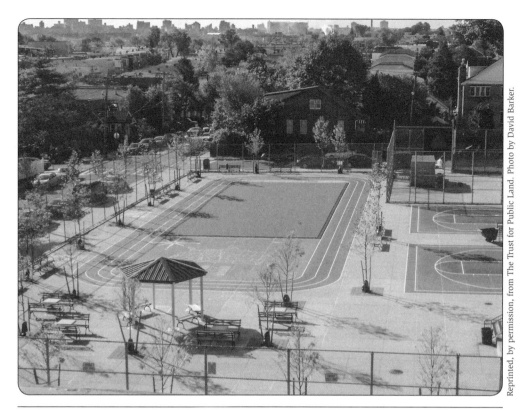

Reprinted, by permission, from The Trust for Public Land. Photo by David Barker.

P.S. 129Q's schoolyard in Queens, after it opened to the public in fall 2009. The New York Schoolyards to Playgrounds program has added more than 100 acres of open space since its launch in 2007

the community wants the park closed earlier; the most restrictive schedule is 3 p.m. to 6 p.m. weekdays, 10 a.m. to 2 p.m. Saturdays, and closed on Sundays. Maintenance is the responsibility of the school custodial staff, so it is important that they are involved in all design decisions from the beginning. Often they turn down a particular piece of equipment; in some cases they have nixed the playground entirely. As for natural grass, it has proven impossible to maintain under intense use, and TPL now uses only artificial turf for the playgrounds' ballfields (Harnik 2010).

Designing a schoolyard park can take up to three months. Children are the lead designers, responding to a set of questions and opportunities posed by TPL. Certain realities, however, including liability, equipment breakability, horticultural survivability, cost, and lessons from previous schoolyard park conversions, affect decision making (Harnik 2010). The children work hard, learning how to innovate, compromise, and reach a consensus when their initial ideas turn out to be too expensive or require too much space. "Because of the kids," says Lee, "we've created murals and mosaics, a hair-braiding area, a jump-rope zone, planting gardens, performance stages, outdoor classrooms, rain gardens, and bowling lanes—as well as the usual soccer fields, running tracks, basketball and tennis courts, and play equipment" (Harnik 2010, p. 114).

Populations Best Served by the Program

Unlike schoolyards, schoolyard parks serve a wide range of ages and have the potential to provide significant physical activity benefits to the whole community. In addition to school-age children, teenagers and adults of all ages can enjoy recreation activities within these spaces. However, communities can limit who can be served (and when). Many communities are opposed to nighttime use because of noise and possible questionable activities. In some cases, the community may decide to limit recreation options (such as mandating basketball courts with one hoop rather than two) in order to discourage overuse. In some instances, schoolyard park conversions take away parking opportunities from school staff and neighbors. At one Boston site, a conflict broke out when parents proposed converting a school parking lot into a soccer field; ultimately, the parents raised enough money in private funds to complete the conversion (Harnik 2010).

Program Evaluation

Although schoolyard park conversions are an increasing phenomenon, and several evaluations have looked at the condition of play and support features as well as the presence of on-site supervision, few systematic evaluations have examined their impact on visitation and activity. One evaluation, by the Office of the New York City Public Advocate, found that 16 (23 percent) of the first 69 converted schoolyards continued to be locked or inaccessible to the public on weekdays and 28 (40 percent) were inaccessible on weekends (Gotbaum 2008). Of those that were accessible, 94 percent did not have a Department of Education staff member present during nonschool operating hours, and few schoolyard parks had adequate activity and support features such as playground climbing features, swings, shade provision, and benches, even though most were judged to be in good overall condition (Gotbaum 2008). The review concluded that schoolyards without play features and support amenities were unlikely to provide an environment conducive to youth physical activity, and it recommended that sites without such amenities be slated for capital improvements.

As additional schoolyard parks are created, a more systematic evaluation of use and physical activity will be needed. A simple starting point is to determine the percentage of schools in each jurisdiction that allow the general public to use school facilities during nonschool hours (Keener, et al. 2009). Proven methods and measurements exist for assessing park features and conditions as well as on-site levels of physical activity within these converted spaces. Many of these monitoring tools (and instructions for using them) are available from Active Living Research at www.activelivingresearch.org/resourcesearch/toolsandmeasures.

Lessons Learned

Since there are a large number of real and perceived barriers to opening school facilities to the general public, success in schoolyard conversions requires a strong commitment from elected officials and unit administrators. Ideally, both the school system and the park system are under the direction of the mayor; without this kind of singular authority, one partner can simply withdraw from the key shared agreements when obstacles arise (Harnik 2010). The success rate increases when the community is warmly invited to participate and engage in the process. Residents and schoolyard users (particularly the affected children) should have a direct role in design and policy development—they are, after all, the primary users and beneficiaries.

Naturally, initial capital costs can be significant in cases where the old schoolyard had little or no parklike infrastructure, such as benches, backstops, play equipment, or grass. In New York, playground parks routinely cost $1 million or more each, including the cost of artificial turf.

Maintenance costs and responsibility are other major challenges. Many school administrators are reluctant to invest school funds in upkeep when those funds are needed for core educational programs. At the same time, school officials may be reluctant to hand off maintenance to the parks department, fearing a loss of control. There is also the question of who should be responsible for locking and unlocking these schoolyards and monitoring their use. This is a particular problem if no custodian or attendant works on the premises during nonschool hours.

Concerns over user liability can derail joint-use schoolyard agreements. In a U.S. nation-wide survey of school principals in low-income and minority communities, although 69 percent of respondents reported that their school recreational facilities were already open to the public after hours, the primary barriers to additional openings included issues of liability, safety, and insurance (table 17.1).

In several cities, including Houston, this concern has been addressed in part through state indemnity clauses that protect schools and cities from certain incidents that occur on public grounds (aside from incidents related to inadequate maintenance). Moreover, joint use policies that allow schools to maintain site operational control and guarantee the ability to convert the space back to school use entirely may promote buy-in from school administrators.

Tips for Working Across Sectors

Although the challenges associated with converting schoolyards to public use are significant, key tips and strategies may enhance the success of these joint use endeavors.

Table 17.1   Perceived Barriers to Opening School Facilities

	Perceived barriers	% Extremely important barrier
Liability and security	Liability	61
	Insurance	61
	Safety	58
	Vandalism	46
	Burglary and theft	41
	Graffiti	37
Resources	Cost of running activities and programs	60
	Staffing for security	56
	Cost of maintenance	56
	Staffing for maintenance	54
	Scope of maintenance responsibilities	54
	Staffing for activities and programs	53
	Limited space and facilities (availability)	49
	Hours of operation	36
Social support	Priority of use	36
	Opens facilities to controversial groups	33
	Lack of school support	28
	Lack of community support	28

Reprinted, by permission, from J.O. Spengler, J.Y. Ko, and D. Connaughton, 2011, "An analysis of perceived barriers to after hours use of schools in under-resourced communities." *Eighth Active Living Research Annual Conference* (San Diego, CA).

- Ensure that the highest levels of local government support this type of facility sharing. (If the mayor controls both the school system and the park system, so much the better.)
- Ensure that the planning and design of specific schoolyards are delegated at the local level and use participatory decision making. The process should include teachers, students, parents, maintenance staff, and local residents.
- Establish clear schedules for community use and school use, and ensure that these schedules match the staffing and security resources available.
- Consider working with local businesses and private foundations to raise funds and engage community members.
- Develop a clear plan for who will be responsible for long-term maintenance.
- Consider using nonprofit "friends groups," both school-by-school and citywide, to advocate for schoolyard conversions and keep school and park officials focused on the project.
- Avoid a one-size-fits-all approach to school conversions. Locking policies, hours of operation, and maintenance responsibility will vary from site to site.
- Focus on developing schoolyard parks in areas where real deficiencies in park access and opportunity exist, particularly for children's after-school play.

Additional Reading and Resources

The National Policy & Legal Analysis Network to Prevent Childhood Obesity (NPLAN) has developed resources and a toolkit to assist cities through model joint-use policies; these resources are available at www.changelabsolutions.org/childhood-obesity/joint-use. More information on New York's School-yards to Playgrounds initiative, including progress reports, is available at www.nycgovparks.org/sub_about/planyc/playgrounds.html.

References

Babey, S., T. Hastert, H. Yu, et al. 2008. Physical activity among adolescents: When do parks matter? *Am. J. Prev. Med.* 34(4):345-8.

Brewer, G.A. 2006. Accessible schoolyards: A report by the Office of Council Member Gale A. Brewer on the public accessibility of New York City schoolyards. Council of the City of New York. www.publicadvocategotbaum.com/policy/documents/sy2pgreportfinal.pdf.

Centers for Disease Control and Prevention. 2001. Increasing physical activity: A report on recommendations of the Task Force on Community Preventive Services. *MMWR Morbid. Mortal. Wkly. Rep.* 50(RR-18):1-16.

Dolesh, R. 2009. School of thought: Schoolyards as playgrounds is not a radical concept. Putting it into practice, however, takes cooperation. *Parks and Recreation* 44(8): 14-18.

Gotbaum, B. 2008. Space to play, room for improvement: An evaluation of the schoolyards to playgrounds program. Public Advocate for the City of New York. http://publicadvocategotbaum.com/policy/documents/sy2pgreportfinal.pdf.

Harnik, P. 2010. *Urban Green: Innovative Parks for Resurgent Cities.* Washington, DC: Island Press.

Kaczynski, A.T., & K.A. Henderson. 2007. Environmental correlates of physical activity: A review of evidence about parks and recreation. *Leisure Sciences* 29(4):315-54.

Keener, D., K. Goodman, A. Lowry, S. Zaro, & L. Kettel Khan. (2009). Recommended community strategies and measurements to prevent obesity in the United States: Implementation and measurement guide. Atlanta, GA: U.S. Department of Health and Human Services, Centers for Disease Control and Prevention.

Spengler, J.O., J.Y. Ko, and D. Connaughton. 2011. An analysis of perceived barriers to after hours use of schools in under-resourced communities. Eighth Active Living Research Annual Conference, San Diego, CA, February 2011.

CHAPTER 18

Learning to be Healthy and Active in After-School Time

The Säjai Foundation's Wise Kids Program

Melissa Hanson, BS, MBA
Säjai Foundation

Amy Rea, BA
Säjai Foundation

NPAP Tactics and Strategies Used in This Program

Parks, Recreation, Fitness, and Sports Sector

STRATEGY 1: Promote programs and facilities where people work, learn, live, play and worship (i.e., workplace, public, private, and non-profit recreational sites) to provide easy access to safe and affordable physical activity opportunities.

STRATEGY 5: Improve physical activity monitoring and surveillance capacity to gauge program effectiveness in parks, recreation, fitness, and sports settings based on geographic population representation and physical activity levels, not merely numbers served.

Childhood obesity is a national crisis in the United States. In more than 30 states, the percentage of overweight and obese children is 30 percent or higher. One in three children born after the year 2000 is projected to develop diabetes, physicians prescribe cholesterol medications for children as young as 8 years, and more than 23 percent of children ages 9 to 13 get no physical activity. Long-term risks for these children include type 2 diabetes, cancer, and heart disease, leading to predictions that this generation will be the first in two centuries to have a shorter life span than its parents. A poll by the Nature Conservancy found that only about 10 percent of children spend time outdoors every day. More than ever, today's children need to make smart nutrition and activity decisions and spend more time outdoors, improving their health and developing a greater appreciation for the world around them.

Research suggests that purposeful after-school programming promotes success in three important areas that combat obesity and health problems: healthy eating, physical activity, and connection to the natural world. Interventions that increase time spent in outdoor physical activity and promote healthy eating boost emotional skills, improve children's social skills, and increase their ability to focus in the classroom. First Lady Michelle Obama's Let's Move campaign calls for community partnerships to effectively curb childhood obesity trends. The Säjai Foundation and its Wise Kids program have taken a big step forward in helping youth-serving agencies and their community partners do just that.

Program Description

The Säjai Foundation, a nonprofit organization that focuses on providing preventive education that promotes healthy living (nutrition, physical activity, and outdoors), developed the Wise Kids program to provide youth leaders and caregivers with easy-to-use tools for teaching children about wellness. The Wise Kids program is designed to be fun, experiential, and educational while promoting nutritional awareness and increasing physical activity and outdoor involvement in youth ages 6 to 11. By using after-school hours to weave in preventive messages and provide opportunities to be physically active, both indoors and outdoors, organizations that work with children can help them develop positive attitudes and healthy habits.

Wise Kids is a nine-lesson preventive wellness program that teaches children ages 6 to 11 about healthy living. The Wise Kids program follows a learn–do–play format to introduce children to the concept of energy balance (calories in = calories out), provide them with hands-on opportunities to apply the concepts, and help them increase physical activity. Children spend 15 minutes learning about the energy balance concept through workbooks and discussion. They then transition into learning activities to help them understand the concept in a hands-on way. Finally, participants spend 30 minutes in physical activities designed to get them moving. Activities encourage everyone to participate, not just those who are athletically inclined. Because the program uses games and techniques that make physical activity less skill-based, more children feel comfortable participating, thereby increasing time spent being active. Some of the key topics covered include energy balance, food labels, the heart, and activity.

The Säjai Foundation initially worked with beta sites to implement and test the program in multiple settings across the United States. The foundation assessed process implementation and impact of the Wise Kids program at four recreation centers in St. Paul, Minnesota. A total of 96 youth ages 7 to 12, from diverse socioeconomic and cultural backgrounds, participated in the program. Program implementation spanned 8 weeks, with the formal testing spanning a 10-week period in winter-spring 2007. Park and recreation locations in the cities of Minneapolis, Minnesota, Tampa, Florida, and East Hartford, Connecticut, also implemented the program and provided weekly feedback to help refine it for broader use. A total of 394 children in these communities participated before the program was rolled out on a national level.

The Theory of Planned Behavior (TPB) was applied to the evaluation of the program. TPB is based on the concept that individuals are

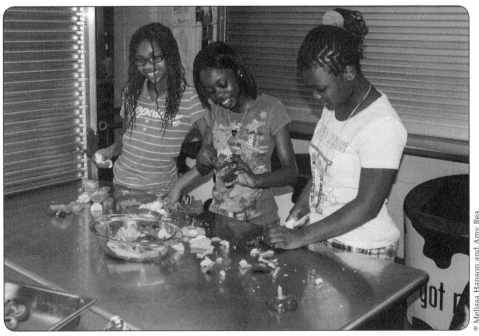

© Melissa Hanson and Amy Rea.

more likely to *intend* to participate in physical activity and adopt healthy eating habits if they are positively disposed toward those behaviors, if they perceive social pressure to do so, and if they believe they will be successful. Because intention plays such a critical role in understanding behavior in the TPB model, it serves as a mediator between attitudes, values, norms, and perceived behavioral control.

Having formal and informal testing locations enabled the Säjai Foundation to receive input from diverse communities and program formats. Program leaders in all locations provided input to help build a program that is easy to lead and easy to replicate. Qualitative feedback was used to modify workbook activities and leader training materials and to provide enhancements to some of the physical activities. For example, some activities were simplified to ensure that more activity was involved, and the program developers added messages to leaders, encouraging them to customize and localize the program to meet the needs of their children and location.

Program Evaluation

An initial evaluation conducted by Recreation, Parks, and Leisure Studies and the School of Kinesiology faculty at the University of Minnesota in St. Paul demonstrated that Wise Kids had positive and significant impacts on attitudes and behaviors that influence healthy eating and physical activity behaviors in youth. In addition, the results suggested that Wise Kids positively affected children's trends in body mass index (BMI) and has the potential to stem increases in BMI (figure 18.2). Finally, the evaluation highlighted that it is feasible to implement this type of program in after-school environments that serve youth, such as recreation centers, and that such programs welcome structured and purposeful programs that focus on physical activity and nutrition.

Since the formal studies were conducted, Wise Kids has been used in agencies in 40 states to reach nearly 15,000 children. The Säjai Foundation is conducting ongoing research

into the effectiveness of the program. Pre-to-post testing in key areas used during the initial study helped to create the Wise Kids Evaluation tool, which is an integral part of each program kit. Communities are encouraged to conduct pre- and postprogram testing with participating children. To date, 48 of the 130 participating agencies have conducted such tests. The testing results continue to indicate positive changes in children's attitudes and behaviors, including physical activity (see figures 18.3 and 18.4).

Linkage to the National Physical Activity Plan

The Wise Kids program aligns with the National Physical Activity Plan under two primary strategy areas of the Parks, Recreation, Fitness, and Sports Sector:

Strategy 1: Promote programs and facilities where people work, learn, live, play and worship (i.e., workplace, public, private, and non-profit recreational sites) to provide easy access to safe and affordable physical activity opportunities. Wise Kids is designed for after-school and summer camp programs. Because it was developed to be easy to lead, youth leaders of all abilities and experience levels, from novice teenagers to experienced adults, have success-

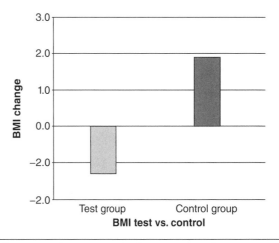

Figure 18.2 Wise Kids shows potential to positively affect participants' BMI.

© The Säjai Foundation.

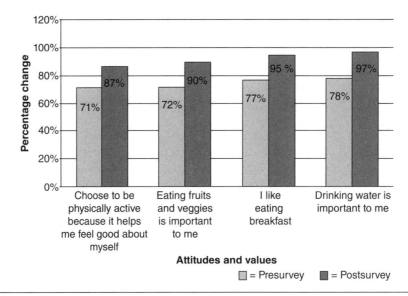

Figure 18.3   Change in attitudes and values from pre- to postprogram testing.
© The Säjai Foundation.

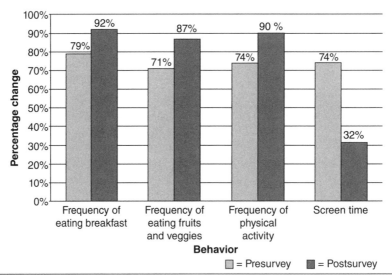

Figure 18.4   Change in behavior from pre- to postprogram testing.
© The Säjai Foundation.

fully implemented the program. More than 8.4 million children participate in after-school programs, providing an excellent opportunity to teach them about the value of physical activity. After-school care encompasses a large portion of a child's day, so programs that enable them to learn about activity and be physically active meet the intent of Strategy 1.

Strategy 5: Improve physical activity monitoring and surveillance capacity to gauge program *effectiveness in parks, recreation, fitness, and sports settings based on geographic population representation and physical activity levels, not merely numbers served.* Wise Kids addresses Strategy 5 by offering agencies a way to ensure consistency in program delivery and to measure changes in values, beliefs, and behaviors regarding physical activity and healthy living. Ensuring that evaluation is part of the program helps agencies to track program effects over

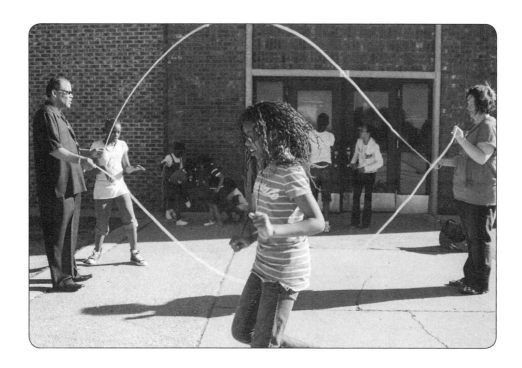

time and quantify efforts to increase physical activity. Pre-to-post testing is also a great way to determine how children feel about being physically active and to determine how their behaviors are changing. Wise Kids encourages collaborative efforts between the Säjai Foundation, youth-serving agencies, and third parties, such as grant makers, volunteer groups, and local businesses, that agree to participate in functions related to the program (e.g., grocery stores that provide food for Wise Kids family nights).

Parent evaluations show that wellness learning goes home. Sixty-four percent of parents in one community noted that their children brought information on Wise Kids home on a weekly basis. As one parent noted, "Wise Kids

has had a profound impact on how my son views food as well as exercise. He now actively makes healthier choices on his own. . . . It has provided a mindset about food and exercise that he will carry with him throughout his life. . . . The key was teaching him at a young age." Creating changes in the home can help improve both the child's and the family's physical activity levels.

Populations Best Served by the Program

Wise Kids has been implemented and evaluated in numerous environments, including after-school programs, parks and recreation settings, YMCA camps, school programs, and faith and community-based programs. Children ages 6 to 11 respond best to the program; the materials and activities are designed for their interests and developmental stage. Childhood obesity affects children in all demographic groups, and the program can be successful in both urban and suburban settings and a variety of economic conditions. Research on Wise Kids indicates that the earlier the program reaches children, the greater their interest in learning more (figure 18.6).

Table 18.1   Wise Kids Results Attitudes, Norms, and Behaviors Test vs. Control

	% Change
Attitudes	5.5
Norms	2.6
Behaviors	4.1

© The Säjai Foundation.

Table 18.2   Highlights from Pre-to-Post Testing in Milwaukee

Participating children—Milwaukee Public Schools	Pre	Post	% Change
Healthy eating (true or very true for me)			
Choose foods that are good for me	55.9%	69.4%	24.2%
Healthy snacking (almost every day or every day)			
Last week's behavior: choosing healthy snacks	68.6%	73.9%	7.7%
Physical activity (almost every day or every day)			
Last week's behavior: physical activeness	70.2%	84.7%	20.7%
Knowledge of 5 health concepts			
Junk foods	47.6%	74.5%	56.5%
Nutritious foods	43.5%	70.7%	62.5%
Food labels	38.2%	69.4%	81.7%
Physical activity	31.9%	66.2%	107.5%
Energy balance	21.5%	62.4%	190.2%

Highlights from Milwaukee Public Schools/Milwaukee Recreation Services—Wise Kids 2009.
© The Säjai Foundation.

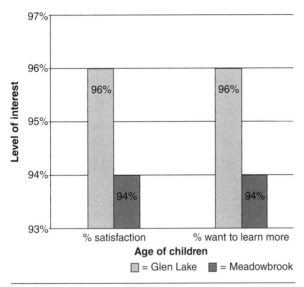

Figure 18.6 Kids in Hopkins, Minnesota, completed the Wise Kids program and wanted to learn more.
Wise Kids Evaluation tool © Melissa Hanson and Amy Rea.

Lessons Learned

The program developers and participating agencies learned a number of lessons while creating and implementing Wise Kids:

- A high level of support within the implementing organization increases the effectiveness of Wise Kids with children and the broader community. For example, if the organization has a strategic plan that calls for increased levels of physical activity for the children it serves, directors or supervisors are likely to push for incorporating these elements into the after-school or summer camp hours and to support staff in doing so in order to meet the overarching plan.

- The level of youth leader engagement directly affects overall success with participating children. For example, if the leader participates in games and activities along with the children or openly shares his or her success with and enjoyment of physical activity, the children are more likely to participate and feel comfortable talking about their experiences.

- Agencies can engage community partners to support efforts. For instance, one agency working with the Wise Kids program invited a local university dance team to

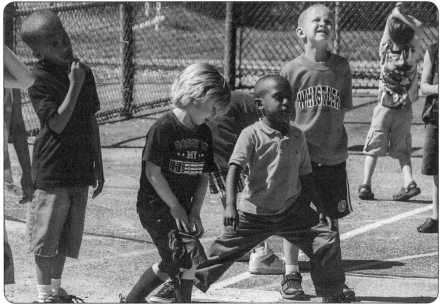

© Melissa Hanson and Amy Rea.

demonstrate and teach children some easy dance moves. Another invited a local grocer to bring in healthy foods for the kids to try. To increase effectiveness, agencies should invite dance and karate studios, health clubs, fishing groups, gardening clubs, health organizations, and similar organizations to send representatives to add additional education and interest to the program.

- Tracking mechanisms can help motivate children to become involved and to continue the program. For example, pedometers provide children with an easy-to-understand way of measuring their activity levels. Likewise, posters or charts that track things like steps taken or minutes running can be a fun way to motivate children.

Tips for Working Across Sectors

Park, recreation, fitness, and sports agencies and programs play a central role in promoting physical activity, especially with children. Often, these organizations rely on funding and support from multiple sectors (business, nonprofit, health care, and schools) in order to provide quality programs. The Säjai Foundation has helped connect financial resources with deserving after-school agencies, creating successful partnerships involving all of these sectors to bring the Wise Kids program to agencies across the country. To be successful in securing funding, agencies should seek out organizations that have a vested interest in healthy living or overall community health. As the community becomes involved in Wise Kids and similar programs, efforts to help children be active will become easier to sustain. Beyond financial resources, other sectors can bring their expertise or services to an after-school agency and the children it serves to demonstrate physical activity opportunities. This help can be as simple as inviting local businesses to demonstrate wellness-related concepts, such as providing opportunities for children to try new activities (yoga, karate, lacrosse, tennis, hiking, running), or it can be as complex as asking a business to provide adult volunteers who serve as physical activity role models. Finally, agencies should collaborate with other sectors in developing programs that combine physical activity with information about health and wellness. For example, an introductory running program combined with learning about physical activity and health is more likely to promote long-term change than is either activity in isolation. A YMCA might want to incorporate a nutrition or physical activity component into an outdoor camp but may need expertise from another organization or a business to develop that component. Among the barriers to these kinds of partnerships are lack of full commitment by one partner, divergent goals of the participating organizations, funding difficulties, and changing values. Frequent, clear communication can help overcome some of these barriers. All sectors should find ways to collaborate in encouraging children and families to become active and should saturate the community with positive health messages. No single physical activity program or venue provides a magic solution. Rather, agencies, organizations, and businesses should look for ways to promote learning and create physical activity opportunities across sectors.

Additional Reading and Resources

Physical Activity for Everyone: The CDC Guidelines: www.cdc.gov/physicalactivity/everyone/guidelines/children.html

Physical Activity and Children (from the American Heart Association): www.heart.org/HEARTORG/GettingHealthy/Physical-Activity-and-Children_UCM_304053_Article.jsp

Moving and Learning: www.movingandlearning.com

Physical Activity Guidelines for Children: www.pbrc.edu/pdf/PNS-physicalactivity.pdf

Children and Physical Activity (PBS Teachers): www.pbs.org/teachers/earlychildhood/articles/physical.html

Indoor Physical Activity Ideas for Kids: www.foodlinkny.org/pdfs/Physical_Activity_Ideas_for_Kids.pdf

Physical Activity (American Academy of Pediatrics): www.healthychildren.org/english/healthy-living/fitness/Pages/default.aspx

CHAPTER 19

Moovin' and Groovin' in the Bayou
Summer Camps Increase Youth Physical Activity Through Intentional Design

Birgitta L. Baker, PhD
Louisiana State University at Baton Rouge

Andrew McGregor, MS
Louisiana State University at Baton Rouge

NPAP Tactics and Strategies Used in This Program

Parks, Recreation, Fitness, and Sports Sector

STRATEGY 1: Promote programs and facilities where people work, learn, live, play and worship (i.e., workplace, public, private, and non-profit recreational sites) to provide easy access to safe and affordable physical activity opportunities.

STRATEGY 2: Enhance the existing parks, recreation, fitness, and sports infrastructure to build capacity to disseminate policy and environmental interventions that promote physical activity.

STRATEGY 6: Increase social marketing efforts to maximize use of recreation programs and facilities and promote co-benefits with environmental and other related approaches.

Less than 49 percent of boys and 35 percent of girls ages 6 to 11 in the United States meet the guidelines that recommend 60 minutes of physical activity on all or most days of the week (Troiano et al. 2008). Evidence also suggests that children's patterns of change in body mass index are less healthy during the summer than during the school year (Downey and Boughton 2007). Summer camp settings may provide an opportunity for children to attain recommended levels of physical activity and promote healthy growth patterns. One such program, Moovin' and Groovin', integrates physical activity into summer camp programs through intentional design. The goal of Moovin' and Groovin' is to increase physical activity levels of children participating in a summer day camp. The design, implementation, and evaluation of this program involve a partnership between a municipal park and recreation agency (the Recreation and Park Commission for the Parish of East Baton Rouge; BREC) and a university kinesiology department (Louisiana State University Department of Kinesiology; LSU). The pilot test of the program, described in this chapter, involved three camps that implemented Moovin' and Groovin' and three comparison camps. Since the pilot test, many of the other summer camps run by BREC have implemented the program. The program design incorporates several strategies and tactics from the U.S. National Physical Activity Plan.

Program Description

The Moovin' and Groovin' program is a component of BREC's initiative to address low activity levels in children and is part of a wider partnership between BREC and the LSU Department of Kinesiology. The partnership also includes Family Fitness Fun Days and an after-school program. In initiating the Moovin' and Groovin' program, summer camp organizers asked faculty and students from LSU to partner with them to design, implement, and evaluate the program. The program included four key strategies: (1) add additional designated physical activity times to the schedule of an existing program, (2) train staff and build excitement about the program, (3) provide staff with a variety of activity options, and (4) evaluate the program. The first three strategies are described next. The fourth strategy, program evaluation, is described in a later section.

Add Additional Designated Physical Activity Times to the Schedule of an Existing Program

The BREC summer camps run for eight weeks, and participants ages 6 to 12 years can attend all or part of the eight weeks. The camps are located at BREC park facilities throughout the parish. Each of the six facilities that took part in the pilot project have a recreation center, most of which include an indoor gym. Camp activities include outdoor and indoor games, arts and crafts, and field trips. Field trips occur one or two times per week and include trips to the zoo, swimming pools, "exergaming" facilities, and museums. Camp prices range from $12.50 to $73 per week depending on the camp location and the participant's family income. Camps run from 8 a.m. to 5 p.m., and pre- and postcamp activities are offered from 7 to 8 a.m. and from 5 to 6 p.m. for an additional fee of $12 per week. All of the camps offer some opportunities for physical activity. Moovin' and Groovin' was designed to supplement the existing summer camp program by incorporating an additional 30-minute activity break on non–field trip days. An LSU student hired by BREC was responsible for coordinating the Moovin' and Groovin' pilot program and providing support for the camp staff.

Train Staff and Build Excitement About the Program

Moovin' and Groovin' training occurs during precamp staff training attended by all of BREC's summer camp staff. The Moovin' and Groovin' training includes information about the program goals, activities, and evaluation. To build excitement and buy-in among program staff, training includes discussions of the potential benefits of the program for the children and a description of the program design, which was intended to minimize additional work for the staff. The majority of the camp staff in the pilot project were K-12 teachers or college students, and many of them had previous experience facilitating children's physical activity.

Provide Staff With a Variety of Activity Options

Staff receive a list of activities with descriptions and instructions. They are instructed to implement a variety of activities in their camps during the designated Moovin' and Groovin' time slots. Some of the activities are suitable for specific age groups and some are suitable for the full group. This allows camp staff to tailor the program to times when all the campers are together and times when they are divided into age groups.

Activities are designed to enhance a range of physical fitness outcomes, including cardiovascular fitness, muscular strength and endurance, and flexibility. The aerobic and muscular fitness activities are games designed to maximize participation and enjoyment. Activities also are designed to be easy to set up and explain. This minimizes transition time and maximizes time spent engaged in the activity. Examples of activities included small side soccer (three to five players per team with cones used as goals), obstacle courses (set up either in the gym or outside using the playground equipment), jump rope, and push-up tag (similar to freeze tag but instead of standing still while waiting to be "unfrozen" after being tagged, the player does push-ups until touched by someone other than "it").

During the pilot project, program staff encouraged camp staff members to select activities they believed their campers would enjoy, to adapt the activities to the needs and abilities of their campers, and to incorporate alternative activities in consultation with the program coordinator. Staff who were physical education teachers during the school year were particularly effective in identifying alternative activities and in structuring activity sessions to provide quick, active transitions.

Program Evaluation

Evaluation of the pilot program focused on accelerometer-measured moderate to vigorous physical activity (MVPA). Data were collected by faculty and students from LSU. Six camps were grouped into pairs based on location and participant demographics. One camp in each pair was then randomly assigned to the Moovin' and Groovin' group and the other camp served as a control. Participants at each camp wore accelerometers for four days during the eight-week program. Accelerometer data between the hours of 8 a.m. and 4 p.m. were used in the analyses. This eliminated variability resulting when campers arrived late or left early. As a result, some campers, particularly those who participated in the extended pre- and postcamp activities, would have accumulated additional physical activity that was not included in the evaluation results.

The campers at the Moovin' and Groovin camps participated in an average of 64 minutes of MVPA per day, whereas those in the regular camps participated in about 54 minutes per day. These results were statistically significant and indicate that (1) summer day camp programming can create an environment in which children can accumulate the recommended 60 minutes of MVPA per day and (2) physical activity levels can be increased in camp settings through structured activity time.

Process evaluation indicated that most camp staff found the program easy to implement and that staff believed that the children enjoyed and benefitted from the activities. Challenges included identifying activities that all campers, regardless of age and ability, could enjoy and ensuring that campers did not overheat in the Louisiana summer weather. Physical activity times were alternated with lower activity times, children had unrestricted access to water, and, on very hot and humid days, activities took

place indoors rather than outdoors to ensure the safety of the participants.

Reports from the campers support the staff perceptions. Campers reported that the activities were fun and that they wanted to do more. A few of the younger campers indicated that when activities were not structured, they were excluded by the older campers. This appeared to be particularly relevant when informal basketball games occurred during free-play time.

Linkage to National Physical Activity Plan

Moovin' and Groovin' addresses several strategies of the Parks, Recreation, Fitness, and Sports Sector of the National Physical Activity Plan:

Strategy 1: Promote programs and facilities where people work, learn, live, play and worship (i.e., workplace, public, private, and non-profit recreational sites) to provide easy access to safe and affordable physical activity opportunities. Programs in summer day camps address a key tactic of this strategy—provide programs in parks, recreation, fitness, and sports that have demonstrated positive physical activity outcomes that are appropriate for children of both genders, those from diverse cultures, and those with different abilities, developmental stages, and needs. The Moovin' and Groovin' program serves children ages 6 to 12 years. The program design allows staff to adapt the program to a range of ages and ability levels. It includes games and activities appropriate for only the younger age group (ages 6-9), only the older age group (ages 10-12), or all ages, allowing camp staff to select developmentally appropriate options. The day camp setting allows the program to reach racially and socioeconomically diverse groups of participants. Summer camps are located throughout the parish (county), allowing children to attend camps close to their homes or where their parents work. The program evaluation provided evidence that program participants obtained at least 60 minutes of physical activity on more than half the days.

Strategy 2: Enhance the existing parks, recreation, fitness, and sports infrastructure to build capacity to disseminate policy and environmental interventions that promote physical activity. Moovin' and Groovin' addresses one of the tactics recommended as part of this strategy—use volunteers and education entities to increase the sector's ability to execute the National Physical Activity Plan. The partnership between BREC and LSU's Department of Kinesiology allowed program development and evaluation at minimal cost, enabling BREC to direct program funds toward providing camp experiences. The partnership also provided LSU undergraduate and graduate students with valuable hands-on experiences in program design and evaluation.

Strategy 6: Increase social marketing efforts to maximize use of recreation programs and facilities and promote co-benefits with environmental and other related approaches. The program increased physical activity opportunities for less active groups (e.g., girls, children with mental or physical disabilities, and low-income youth) through increased programming, social marketing, and transportation assistance. Two of the three parks in which Moovin' and Groovin' was piloted were reduced-fee camps located in low-income areas. These camps served high proportions of campers from low socioeconomic backgrounds who were at increased risk for low levels of physical activity. The expansion of the program following the successful pilot project also reaches camps in low income areas.

Evidence Base Used During Program Development

A 2004 Institute of Medicine report, Preventing Childhood Obesity: Health in the Balance, highlighted the importance of community-based programs (including programs that provide physical activity opportunities) that target groups at higher risk for obesity. The Moovin' and Groovin' program targets children from low income families through community-based programming in the neighborhoods in which they live.

The 2008 Physical Activity Guidelines for Americans recommend that individuals ages 6 to 17 accumulate 60 minutes of physical activity, primarily aerobic, on all or most days of the week, and that at least three days include muscle-strengthening activities. The Moovin' and Groovin' program incorporates three 30-minute activity sessions into the daily camp schedule to ensure that participants have sufficient opportunities to accumulate 60 minutes of activity while allowing for activity transitions and down time.

Research indicates that enjoyment (Vierling et al. 2007; Wilson and Rodgers 2004) and a sense of competence (Sollerhed et al. 2008; Trost et al. 1997; Welk and Schaben 2004) are important factors in maintaining physical activity behaviors. The Moovin' and Groovin' program was designed to be fun, with a focus on games rather than on exercise. The program includes a variety of activities for all ages to help participants develop feelings of competence.

Populations Best Served by Program

Moovin' and Groovin' is designed for and implemented with children ages 6 to 12 years. The basic components of Moovin' and Groovin'—incorporating additional physical activity opportunities into existing programs, training staff, and providing staff with a variety of activity options—could be applied to a range of additional age groups, with the time and activities appropriately modified. This program is effective in reaching children from groups at risk for low levels of physical activity. Existing camps and after-school programs could incorporate similar strategies to increase physical activity levels among their participants.

Lessons Learned

Partnerships between parks and recreation agencies and local higher education providers can benefit both parties. In the case of Moovin' and Groovin', the parks and recreation agency benefits from physical activity programming and evaluation expertise provided by the university, whereas faculty and students from the university gain opportunities to apply concepts in real-world settings and to hone their practical skills.

Quality programs require quality staff. Providing camp staff with autonomy to choose activities worked well during the pilot project. Staff reported that they appreciated the option to select activities that matched the skill and ability level of their campers. As camp staff implemented the program, they identified activities that were suitable for younger campers, older campers, or all campers and tailored activity choices to the makeup of the group. Variability in the specific physical activities chosen by the camps was evident from observations and from camp schedules. Different camps favored different activities, and staff selected different activities in the same camp setting when they were programming activity time with younger versus older participants. In addition, staff who worked at the camps during the summer and as physical education teachers during the school year were very effective. Actively recruiting local physical education teachers provided BREC with a source of highly skilled day camp staff who were seeking summer-only rather than year-round employment.

Tips for
Working Across Sectors

Identify the benefits for each partner in advance of program design and implementation. In the implementation of the pilot program, benefits to BREC included the expertise of LSU students and faculty, particularly in the areas of designing evidence-based programs and measuring physical activity and physical fitness. The LSU students benefitted from the practical experience. The opportunity to apply concepts from their course work to a setting in which things did not run as smoothly as they do in theory was invaluable. While designing and implementing the program, LSU students learned that it can be challenging to ensure that a program is carried out consistently across sites and that quality staff are crucial to the success of a program. Students involved in program evaluation learned that fitness testing is more challenging when you are testing 6- to 12-year-olds than when you are testing your college classmates and that the logistics of measuring physical activity in the field are complicated.

Allow extra lead time to negotiate challenges. Policies and procedures of both the university and the parks and recreation agency often extended planning and approval time beyond what would have been required by either entity working alone. University requirements included institutional review board approval for collecting data and the constraints of semester schedules. BREC requirements included approval processes for programming and advertising and timing of parent meetings and staff training. Negotiating these challenges required intensive communication, anticipation of potential sticking points, and a willingness of both partners to adjust to the timelines and requirements of the other.

Summary

The success of the Moovin' and Groovin' program was facilitated by the partnership between BREC and LSU and by enhancement of an existing program rather than creation of a new program. For agencies looking to implement similar programs, partnering with a local college or university can provide access to expertise and person power to enhance programming, particularly through service-learning partnerships. Increasing physical activity opportunities in an existing program allowed Moovin' and Groovin' to increase physical activity without the challenges of staffing, marketing, and development that would have been required to start a new program. Relatively short activity breaks could be integrated into a variety of existing programs, including summer camps, after-school programs, and cultural education programs. The summer camps that implemented Moovin' and Groovin' already provided opportunities for physical activity, and the program increased the physical activity levels compared to the existing format.

Additional Reading and Resources

More information on the Moovin' and Groovin' program can be obtained by contacting the Recreation and Park Commission for the Parish of East Baton Rouge.

References

Downey, D.B., and H.R. Boughton. 2007. Childhood body mass index gain during the summer versus during the school year. *New Dir. Youth Dev.* 114:33-43.

Sollerhed, A.C., E. Apitzsch, L. Rastam, and G. Ejlertsson. 2008. Factors associated with young children's self-perceived physical competence and self-reported physical activity. *Health Educ. Res.* 23:125-36.

Troiano, R.P., D. Berrigan, K.W. Dodd, L.C. Masse, T. Tilert, and M. McDowell. 2008. Physical activity in the United States measured by accelerometer. *Med. Sci. Sports Exerc.* 40(1):181-8.

Trost, S., R. Pate, R. Saunders, D.S. Ward, M. Dowda, and G. Felton. 1997. A prospective study of the determinants of physical activity in rural fifth-grade children. *Prev. Med.* 26:257-63.

Vierling, K.K., M. Standage, and D.C. Treasure. 2007. Predicting attitudes and physical activity in an "at-risk" minority youth sample: A test of self-determination theory. *Psychol. Sport Exerc.* 8:795-817.

Welk, G.J., and J.A. Schaben. 2004. Psychosocial correlates of physical activity in children: A study of relationships when children have similar opportunities to be active. *Meas. Phys. Educ. Exerc. Sci.* 8(2):63-81.

Wilson, P.M., and W.M. Rodgers. 2004. The relationship between perceived autonomy support, exercise regulations and behavioral intentions in women. *Psychol. Sport Exerc.* 5(3):229-42.

CHAPTER 20

Finding Common Ground
Play Space Modifications Can Increase Physical Activity for All Children

Kindal A. Shores, PhD
East Carolina University

NPAP Tactics and Strategies Used in This Program

Parks, Recreation, Fitness, and Sports Sector

STRATEGY 2: Enhance the existing parks, recreation, fitness, and sports infrastructure to build capacity to disseminate policy and environmental interventions that promote physical activity.

STRATEGY 5: Improve physical activity monitoring and surveillance capacity to gauge program effectiveness in parks, recreation, fitness, and sports settings based on geographic population representation and physical activity levels, not merely numbers served.

Play is essential to development, because it contributes to the cognitive, physical, social, and emotional well-being of children and youth (Burdette and Whitaker 2005). Play promotes healthy development and reduces childhood obesity (Brown and Vaughn 2009; Sothern 2007). The American Academy of Pediatrics, Centers for Disease Control and Prevention, and American Public Health Association have all linked a lack of gross motor playtime to the current childhood obesity epidemic (Centers for Disease Control and Prevention 2009). Indeed, play is so essential that the United Nations Convention on the Rights of the Child states that the right to play is a fundamental human right that must be guaranteed for all children.

Children's play can occur in many places. Local parks and school playgrounds are prime locations for play. However, the vast majority of playgrounds in the United States and around the world are geared to the needs of children without disabilities. According to national surveillance data from 2005, approximately 19 percent of children ages 5 to 17 have some type of disability (Brault 2008), including social, emotional, and cognitive developmental delays, as well as physical disabilities. Although no clearinghouse of U.S. playgrounds exists, it is clear that far fewer than 19 percent of playgrounds meet the needs of children with disabilities. A national registry that tracks accessible play spaces in the United States has identified 403 accessible park playgrounds in the 50 states (not including the more than 100 inclusive playgrounds in New York City) (www.accessibleplayground. net). This discrepancy is problematic. Children with disabilities tend to have higher body mass indices and lower levels of physical activity than their peers who are developing typically (Hardy et al. 2004). Formative research also suggests that children with disabilities can make greater developmental gains when playing outdoors or at playgrounds, compared with their typically developing peers (Hobbs et al. 2011).

To address concerns about the lack of play spaces for children with disabilities and to provide universally accessible play spaces, communities are now working to build or alter the physical play environment to accommodate all children through play opportunities. These inclusive playgrounds are designed to help children with and without disabilities interact informally and play together. This provides social benefits for both groups. Further, inclusive playgrounds often are a favorite among all children because these spaces provide more diverse play activities than do typical modular playgrounds. A typical playground will focus almost exclusively on physical challenges (climbing, sliding), whereas inclusive playgrounds provide new physical challenges (hand trikes, sand backhoe manipulation) as well as sensory challenges (multiple textures, use of water and sounds) and intellectual challenges (riddles, word games).

The community of Greenville, North Carolina, hosts an inclusive playground. Greenville is a community of approximately 72,000 residents (2010 Census) that wanted to improve the quantity and quality of play opportunities for youth. In 2008, the Greenville Recreation and Parks Department removed a traditional toddler park and installed an inclusive playground, designed for children with and without disabilities to play actively and cooperatively. At the same time, the city converted a grass softball field to a fully accessible baseball field. These initiatives are in line with the National Physical Activity Plan (NPAP)'s, Recreation, Fitness, and Sports Sector, Strategies 2 and 5. Strategy 2 seeks to *Enhance the existing parks, recreation, fitness, and sports infrastructure to build capacity to disseminate policy and environmental interventions that promote physical activity.* By removing the existing toddler playground for children without disabilities and installing an accessible playground, the community gained infrastructure that allowed more children to engage in active play. Since the city elected to evaluate this renovation, using observations of youth activity, it demonstrated the ability of existing surveillance tools to monitor the effectiveness of this environmental change. The playground renovation also serves as an example of small-scale actions that contribute to Strategy 5: *Improve physical activity monitoring and surveillance capacity to gauge program effectiveness in parks, recreation, fitness, and sports settings based on geographic population representation and physical activity levels, not merely numbers served.* Specifically, this is an example of one of the tactics of Strategy 5 that calls for assessing physical activity levels associated with use of these facilities and services and evaluating cases of major improvement.

Program Description

In 2007, Elm Street Park was a well-loved and busy city park. The 12-acre green space housed one large parking lot, a lighted youth baseball field, grass softball field, two playgrounds (one for children 2-5 years of age, the other for children 6 years and older), six lighted tennis courts, community center, gymnasium, open space, and picnic shelters with grills. Much of Elm Street Park remains the same today. However, the city made two substantial changes to enhance youth play and physical activity. First, it converted the grassy softball diamond to an accessible baseball and softball diamond. Second, it removed the playground for children ages 2 to 5 and replaced it with a new playground structure designed for all children ages 2 to 12.

The softball field is named in honor of Sarah Vaughn. Sarah is a young woman with mobility impairments who, together with her family, catalyzed the community into action. In 2008, the Sarah Vaughn Field of Dreams, a fully accessible baseball field, was built at the Elm Street Park (figure 20.1). The accessible ball field features a flat cushioned synthetic turf, embedded bases, spacious field-level dugouts, and an audiovisual score sign. This field is used for unplanned play, family events, and game days as well as for spring, summer, and fall baseball leagues for children and adults with disabilities.

Upon installation of the Vaughn field, the city started a Challenger baseball league for children ages 5 to 18 (see figure 20.2). More than 50 youth participated in the Challenger league in its inaugural year, and 80 participated in 2009. In 2010, the Exceptional Community Baseball League (ECBL) was formed with the cooperation of the Greenville Recreations and Parks

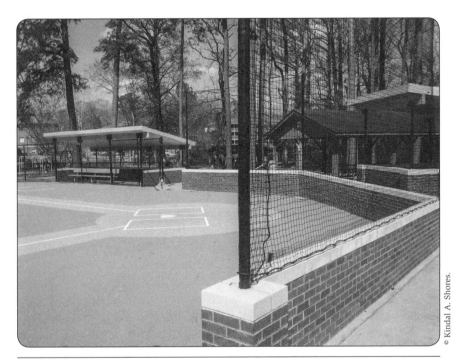

Figure 20.1 Sarah Vaughn Field of Dreams.

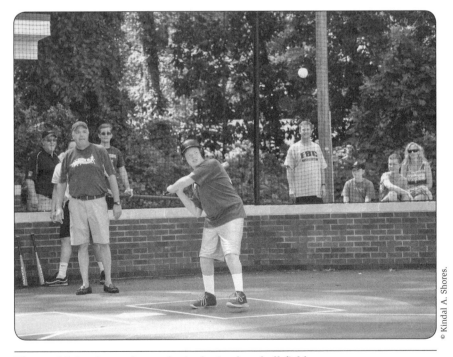

Figure 20.2 Game day at the inclusive baseball field.

Department and a grant from the Cal Ripken Sr. Foundation. The ECBL formed three divisions: youth (ages 5-14), senior youth (ages 15-24), and adult (ages 25 and up). In the first spring season in 2010, the ECBL increased from 80 youth players to more than 150 participants of all ages.

The same community group that advocated for the inclusive baseball field also championed an inclusive playground. The group's momentum and success in fund-raising allowed the ball field and the inclusive playground, the Common Ground Playground for All, to open in the same year. The inclusive playground consists of approximately 2,500 square feet (762 square meters) of play space (see figure 20.3). The fenced space is anchored on each end by a set of four swings and is divided roughly in half by an entrance arch and ramp. One half features an approximately 1,100-square-foot (102-square-meter) play structure that includes three types of slides, three climbers, one step entrance that is in compliance with the Americans with Disabilities Act (ADA), two separate ramp entry and exits, and four play panels in the structure. An open area on the other side of the play space offers additional play panels, spring riders, a large raised sandbox, hand trikes, and an in-ground sandbox with an ADA-compliant backhoe.

The evolution of the Vaughn Field of Dreams and the Common Ground Playground for All in Greenville resulted from a grassroots initiative that local officials and corporate partners embraced. A conversation between Sarah Vaughn's parents and other parents of children with disabilities sparked a movement to benefit the more than 6,500 residents of Greenville who have disabilities. A working group for inclusive recreation was established in Greenville in early 2006, and the group coordinated its efforts with the Greenville Recreation and Parks Department. Local contractors, private donors, a county priority fund, and a grant from the North Carolina Parks and Recreation Trust Fund provided funding. Ongoing programs and services at these facilities are sponsored primarily by local businesses, regional sport teams, and individual gifts. No single source contributed more than $100,000 toward the

more than $300,000 in total renovations. The accessible field and play space were both open by summer 2008.

Populations Best Served by the Program

Communities of almost every size can install accessible playgrounds. Costs of these facilities (surfacing, fencing, equipment) vary widely but begin at around $15,000 for a small installed play set. Extensive structures with towers and custom components can cost upward of $100,000. Individual play components such as toddler bouncers or a raised, wheelchair-accessible sand and water table can be purchased at prices beginning at $500 per component. Ideally, rural communities and cities with limited formal resources for children with disabilities will benefit the most. Data from Greenville, however, suggest that children with and without disabilities stand to benefit from this environmental change.

Communities must determine the philosophy that will guide development of their playground before they can design an appropriate facility. This chapter uses the term *accessible playground*, which is a global term that encompasses several types of playgrounds. *Accessibility* is a general term that refers to the degree to which a service or environment can be used (accessed) by as many people as possible. In the context of an accessible playground, the play space should allow any child to play without barriers. The words *accessible, inclusive, universal, boundless*, and *ADA compliant* are often used interchangeably in conversation; however, each term refers to a specific type of playground and reflects the targeted population and goals for that space. For example, accessible playgrounds can be designed for children with disabilities, for interactive play between children with and without disabilities, for simultaneous but separate play, and, at a minimum, to allow children with disabilities physical access to a space. In contrast, an ADA-compliant playground must meet minimal federal guidelines related to access and mobility within a space but is not specifically designed to meet the needs of people with emotional and social disabilities. Universal playgrounds, in contrast, are playgrounds that have been designed using the seven design principals of Universal Design for Learning. In these spaces, the playground is not designed for children with disabilities but is designed so that all of the equipment works for people with and without disabilities. An inclusive playground takes the design one step further and encourages children of multiple abilities to play *together*—not just in close proximity to each other.

It may be helpful for communities to identify a target population for the play space. Playground equipment manufacturers are now creating highly specialized play components that encourage play for children with limited upper-body mobility, challenge children to problem solve, or engage children with autism spectrum disorders in sensory play. For example, the Common Ground Playground at Elm Street Park incorporates a hand trike for upper-body exercises for children with upper-body mobility and inclusive swing seats that provide stability for children with limited upper-body control or strength (figure 20.4). With regard to problem-solving challenges, a play panel asks children a riddle and then provides the answer in braille. However, the braille station to "decode" the answer requires the child to run or push up a ramp to match the braille letters with alphabetical letters. Finally, a play panel with texture is incorporated into the play structure. These sensory experiences are fun for all children but critical for the development of children with autism spectrum disorders. Each play panel provides space for the child to roll up and place his or her legs under the station. This allows for play by children without disabilities and by children who use a wheelchair. However, if park space is limited, a community may place a premium on the needs of one group of special needs in the design plan.

Program Evaluation

To gauge the impact of the environmental changes, it is important to collect empirical data. For three consecutive summer seasons (2007, 2008, 2009), the city evaluated park visitation outcomes at Greenville's Elm Street Park. To document use and physical activity at the playground site before and after renovation, the city adopted the protocol outlined in the System for Observing Play and Recreation in Communities (SOPARC). Developed and tested by McKenzie, Cohen, Sehgal, and colleagues (2006), SOPARC relies on momentary time sampling techniques in which trained researchers undertake systematic and periodic scans of park environments. The evaluation focused on the playground and the softball field.

Data were collected during June and July each year using systematic scans of target areas at four time intervals throughout the day (7:30-8:30 a.m., 12-1 p.m., 3:30-4:30 p.m., and 6:30-7:30 p.m.). During each scan, the number of participants and their observable personal characteristics and physical activity intensity were recorded. Two observations were taken for each time point, at each target area, on each of the seven days of the week. Thus, a total of 56 scans of the two target areas were obtained each year.

Prior to renovation, when Elm Street Park still had an enclosed toddler playground and a grass field with a softball backstop, the evaluation found that 206 people visited these two areas over seven summer days (table 20.1). The playground had 96 visits, most of which included moderate or vigorous physical activity. The open field had 110 visitors; only 16 of these visits were vigorous physical activity. In late spring 2008, the playground and new ballfield opened to the public. During summer 2008, 290 visits were observed at these sites. Total visits increased and physical activity at the ball field increased modestly. Three-quarters of playground visitors were physically active before the renovation; 78 percent were active after the renovation. Prior to the renovation, 53 percent of visits to the softball field were active; 72 percent were active immediately following the renovation. More than one year after the renovations were completed, use had risen again. In 2009, the evaluation recorded 215 visits at the playground and 148 visits at the ball field. Although the percentage of active users in 2009 was similar to that in 2008, the overall increase in visitation resulted in significantly more people engaged in physical activity after the accessibility renovations. Prior to the renovations, 129 visitors were engaged in moderate and vigorous physical activity in this part of the park. One year after the renovations, 281 visitors were engaged in physical activity in these park spaces. This represents a considerable percent increase in physical activity.

Tips for Working Across Sectors

The first challenge to overcome in developing an accessible play space is the need to recruit a passionate and dedicated group of residents to advocate for resources. Success stories from around the United States have a common theme: local champions. Of the documented accessible playgrounds in the United States, one in five is named for a child or family who inspired and advocated for the play space. Many play areas have been successful in achieving funding when a local child or family can provide a human face to raise the consciousness of donors, granting agencies, and local government officials.

Once a team of dedicated residents is assembled, the most common challenges to creating an accessible playground are typically site selection and funding. Accessible playgrounds tend to include larger physical components than

some traditional playground structures and require adequate space to access and maneuver around each element. Ideally, the play space should provide access to nature or natural elements, since many children with sensory processing disorders are comforted by green and natural elements. Best practices in inclusive playgrounds also call for quiet spaces within the more chaotic play area. For all visitors, shade is an important consideration, and the site must be well graded and level. Wide ramps that integrate and match the entire play structure should be provided for children to access the play area, and a child should be able to enter and exit the playground using more than one approach. In other words, the structure should draw the child into and through the play area by engaging him or her physically and mentally. Finally, sites must be large enough to allow for the addition of accessible parking for convenient park use.

Site selection and playground design are, of course, influenced by financial considerations as well. As described previously, a range of options exists for accessible playgrounds, from simply ADA-compliant to interactive, inclusive play spaces. For the most successful play areas, the more inclusive components should be selected. However, this decision has to be ratified consistently by those championing the effort at each point in the design process. One of the first decisions that must be made is the surface for the playground. According to ADA legislation,

Table 20.1   Physical Activity Levels at Elm Street Park Before and After Renovation

	2007: BEFORE RENOVATION (N = 216)		2008: NEWLY RENOVATED (N = 290)		2009: 1 YEAR AFTER RENOVATION (N = 363)	
	Playground	Field	Playground	Field	Playground	Field
Sedentary visits	24 (25%)	52 (47%)	36 (12%)	34 (28%)	42 (20%)	40 (27%)
Moderate/walking visits	31 (32%)	42 (38%)	55 (33%)	74 (60%)	72 (33%)	80 (54%)
Vigorous visits	41 (43%)	16 (15%)	76 (45%)	15 (12%)	101 (47%)	28 (19%)
Totals	96	110	167	123	215	148

loose fill (engineered wood, shredded rubber), pea gravel, and sand are appropriate options for surfacing the play area. "Pour in place" recycled rubber and polymer surfacing, rubber mats or tiles, and artificial grass with rubber underneath are more durable, are easier to maintain, and provide a more functional surface for a greater number of park visitors; however, these surfaces are more expensive. Maintaining a consistent design philosophy in the face of budget challenges is difficult.

Changing existing playground spaces or creating new ones can be an expensive proposition. In most communities in the United States, public playgrounds are built and maintained by a local parks and recreation department. As leaders of a city or county entity, parks and recreation administrators must make the case for the health, environmental, and social value of parks and playgrounds in order to receive a portion of the city's general fund, pass a bond resolution, or receive grants and donations toward the environmental change. To advocate effectively for the value of parks to communities, local officials have partnered with researchers to collect monitoring and change data on the outcomes that park spaces may achieve. The observation and documentation of visitors to Elm Street Park before and after renovations is an example of this process. Objective scientific data are a valuable tool that can be used to make the case for government funding for an inclusive playground.

Unfortunately, this type of monitoring data cannot be achieved until funds have been committed to a site. To achieve an initial investment for playgrounds, park and recreation professionals typically rely on a piecemeal approach. This was the case for the renovations at Elm Street Park. David Vaughn, the father of Sarah Vaughn, initiated the redevelopment process for the inclusive baseball field as a grassroots movement. An avid baseball fan and Little League coach to Sarah's brothers, David Vaughn thought that his daughter and other children deserved a place to play. He established a working group of recreation, business, and political leaders who acquired significant donations of in-kind materials and labor. The city council matched the donations. The Vaughn family story has been echoed across the United States in the development of almost every inclusive facility. Although difficult to finance, a renovated play area for children with and without disabilities is a relatively small investment on the scale of community spending. For this reason, grassroots advocacy and an individual champion can make a considerable impact on a city or county government's decision to fund this type of project. If local funding is not achieved or remains inadequate, the business sector can be approached: Most major playground manufacturing companies offer competitive grants for inclusive playgrounds. Without exception, matching funds and sweat equity are required of the awarded grantees.

Finally, a less common but equally important psychological barrier exists to building an inclusive playground or ball field. Residents (often parents) who have never seen or used an accessible playground are sometimes hesitant to support these efforts. Residents worry that extensive community resources will be spent on inclusive playgrounds that will serve only a few select children. Despite assurances that inclusive playgrounds are for everyone, a field trip, active video, and images of other successful sites are often required so that parents can see that the play space is available and attractive to children with and without special needs. Evaluation data that track use can also help make the case that inclusive play spaces can increase the use of a park area by children with and without disabilities.

Additional Reading and Resources

If you are interested in working toward an accessible play space in your community, the following resources, organizations, and websites serve as valuable starting points:

Boundless Playgrounds is a nonprofit organization that works with communities to develop playgrounds accessible by all children, with or without disabilities: www.boundlessplaygrounds.org

KaBOOM! is a nonprofit agency that seeks to provide a play space within walking distance of every child in America: www.kaboom.org

National Institute for Play is a nonprofit agency that promotes play to improve human health, imagination, and intellect: http://nifplay.org

National Program for Playground Safety is a clearinghouse of information on safety regulations and recommendations for outdoor playgrounds in the United States.

National Recreation and Park Association is the leading advocacy and professional organization dedicated to the advancement of public park and recreation opportunities: www.nrpa.org

References

Brault, M. 2008. Americans with disabilities: 2005. Current populations reports. U.S Bureau of the Census. www.census.gov/prod/2008pubs/p70-117.pdf.

Brown, S., and C. Vaughan. 2009. *Play: How It Shapes the Brain, Opens the Imagination, and Invigorates the Soul.* New York: Penguin Books.

Burdette, H.L., and R.C. Whitaker. 2005. Resurrecting free play in young children: Looking beyond fitness and fatness to attention, affiliation, and affect. *Arch. Pediatr. Adolesc. Med.* 159:46-50.

Centers for Disease Control and Prevention. 2009. Prevalence of no leisure-time physical activity--35 States and the District of Columbia, 1988-2008. *Morbidity and Mortality Weekly Report*, 53(4), 82-86.

Hardy, K.R., J.S. Harrell, and L.A. Bell. 2004. Overweight in children: Definitions, measurements, confounding factors, and health consequences. *J. Pediatr. Nurs.* 19(6):376-84.

Hobbs, T., L. Bruch, J. Sanko, and C. Astolfi. 2001. Friendship on the inclusive playground. *Teaching Exceptional Children* 33(6):46-51.

McKenzie, T.L., D.A. Cohen, A. Sehgal, S. Williamson, and D. Golinelli. 2006. System for Observing Play and Recreation in Communities (SOPARC): Reliability and Feasibility Measures. *Journal of Physical Activity and Health* 3(S1), S208-S222.

Sothern, M.S. 2007. Obesity prevention in children: physical activity and nutrition. *Pediatrics* 119(1):182-91.

CHAPTER 21

Pioneering Physically Active Communities
YMCA of the USA's Healthier Communities Initiatives

Monica Hobbs Vinluan, JD
YMCA of the USA

NPAP Tactics and Strategies Used in This Program

Public Health

STRATEGY 3: Engage in advocacy and policy development to elevate the priority of physical activity in public health practice, policy, and research.

STRATEGY 5: Expand monitoring of policy and environmental determinants of physical activity and the levels of physical activity in communities (surveillance), and monitor the implementation of public health approaches to promoting active lifestyles (evaluation).

Education

STRATEGY 1: Provide access to and opportunities for high-quality, comprehensive physical activity programs, anchored by physical education, in pre-kindergarten through grade 12 educational settings. Ensure that the programs are physically active, inclusive, safe, and developmentally and culturally appropriate.

STRATEGY 5: Provide access to and opportunities for physical activity before and after school.

Health Care

STRATEGY 1: Make physical activity a patient "vital sign" that all health care providers assess and discuss with their patients.

STRATEGY 3: Use a health care systems approach to promote physical activity and to prevent and treat physical inactivity.

STRATEGY 4: Reduce disparities in access to physical activity services in health care.

STRATEGY 5: Include physical activity education in the training of all health care professionals.

Business and Industry

STRATEGY 1: Identify, summarize, and disseminate best practices, models, and evidence-based physical activity interventions in the workplace.

STRATEGY 2: Encourage business and industry to interact with all other sectors to identify opportunities to promote physical activity within the workplace and throughout society.

Parks, Recreation, Fitness, and Sports

STRATEGY 1: Promote programs and facilities where people work, learn, live, play and worship (i.e., workplace, public, private, and non-profit recreational sites) to provide easy access to safe and affordable physical activity opportunities.

Mass Media

STRATEGY 3: Develop consistent mass communication messages that promote physical activity, have a clear and standardized "brand," and are consistent with the most current *Physical Activity Guidelines for Americans.*

STRATEGY 5: Sequence, plan, and provide campaign activities in a prospective, coordinated manner. Support and link campaign messages to community-level programs, policies, and environmental supports.

Transportation, Land Use, and Community Design

STRATEGY 3: Integrate land-use, transportation, community design and economic development planning with public health planning to increase active transportation and other physical activity.

STRATEGY 4: Increase connectivity and accessibility to essential community destinations to increase active transportation and other physical activity.

Volunteer and Nonprofit Sector

STRATEGY 1: Advocate to local, state and national decision makers for policies and system changes identified in the National Physical Activity Plan that promote physical activity.

STRATEGY 2: Convene multi-sector stakeholders at local, state, and national levels in strategic collaborations to advance the goals of the National Physical Activity Plan.

* * *

Community-based organizations play a crucial role in providing opportunities for individuals to engage in physical activity. Thousands of organizations provide not only venues for physical activity but also programs that support physical activity. The YMCA is one of these organizations; it is the largest nonprofit provider of youth sports and after-school activities in the United States.

The Y is helping to improve the nation's health and well-being through efforts to promote community-based healthy living and prevent chronic disease. The Y is influencing and motivating positive lifestyle behavior changes among children, adults, and families who need ongoing support to make healthy living a reality in their lives. Local YMCAs accomplish this by creating opportunities for individuals, families, and communities nationwide to make and sustain healthier choices.

The Y is strengthening communities through youth development, healthy living, and social responsibility. For nearly 160 years, YMCAs have helped improve physical, social, emotional, and spiritual health and well-being for millions of people in diverse communities across the United States. Today, YMCAs continue to promote healthy living by providing people with the support they need to take control of their health. YMCAs not only are changing the way they work inside their facilities to influence and motivate individuals and families to make positive changes but also are working in their communities to support approaches that help people overcome barriers to healthier living.

Program Description

In nearly 200 communities across the United States, Ys are collaborating with other community organizations to ensure that healthy living is within reach of the people who live in those communities. Ys that are engaged in Y-USA's Healthier Communities Initiatives (Pioneering Healthier Communities; statewide Pioneering Healthier Communities; and ACHIEVE) are creating active communities by using Complete Streets initiatives to make streets safer for all users; developing safe routes to schools to give parents peace of mind when their kids walk to school; working with schools to increase physical education and physical activity during the school day; and conducting many related activities.

Y-USA's Healthier Communities Initiatives (HCIs) engage community leaders, convened by local YMCAs, in policy, systems, and environmental change efforts that support and promote healthy lifestyles. These initiatives empower local communities by providing them with proven strategies and models to create and sustain positive, lasting change for healthy living.

The chief strategic objectives of these initiatives include the following:

- Communicating the importance of a healthy lifestyle
- Building relationships within communities by focusing on the leading health issues facing the United States
- Strengthening the capacity for coalition building in communities
- Attracting a new set of volunteers to the effort to build a healthy community
- Increasing the community's ability to promote policy and environmental changes that encourage and support healthy living

Y-USA's Healthier Communities Initiatives include three distinct initiatives: Pioneering

Healthier Communities, Statewide Pioneering Healthier Communities, and ACHIEVE.

Pioneering Healthier Communities

Pioneering Healthier Communities (PHC, launched in 2004) focuses on local YMCAs' engagement with community leaders, working together to create an environment that promotes health and developing policies that promote and sustain healthy changes. With support from the Centers for Disease Control and Prevention (CDC) and corporate and foundation donors, more than 100 communities are participating in PHC.

Statewide Pioneering Healthier Communities

Y-USA received funding from the Robert Wood Johnson Foundation (RWJF) to launch a statewide PHC policy change initiative at the local and state levels in six states and 32 communities over five years, starting in 2009. This initiative addresses the childhood obesity epidemic through policy and environmental changes that will have implications for communities, states, and the nation. The work is taking place in Connecticut, Illinois, Kentucky, Michigan, Ohio, and Tennessee.

Action Communities for Health, Innovation, and Environmental Change

The Action Communities for Health, Innovation, and Environmental Change (ACHIEVE) initiative was launched in 2008 to support local health departments and YMCAs in advancing community leadership in the nation's efforts to prevent chronic diseases. ACHIEVE was inspired, in part, by YMCA of the USA's PHC initiative. The goals of ACHIEVE are to build on the success of PHC and to formalize the relationship between YMCAs, local and state health departments, parks and recreation departments, and other community-based organizations. ACHIEVE is supported by the CDC and is a partnership between the National Association of Chronic Disease Directors, the National Association of County and City Health Officials,

the National Recreation and Park Association, and Y-USA.

Several key efforts undergird all three initiatives:

- High-level community leaders are involved at every step, using their positions, influence, and ability to make changes within their organization and the greater community.

- Multiple sectors and diverse organizations are involved to maximize experience, assets, resources, and skills.

- Participating organizations work to influence policy and environmental changes to improve community environments.

- Local initiatives are organically grown, with strategies specific to the needs of each community.

- YMCA serves as convener in the community and co-leads the initiative with partner organizations.

By September 2011, 190 YMCAs and their communities were participating in these initiatives. Participating communities include a variety of sizes (urban, suburban, rural), hard-to-reach populations (low-income, underserved, and racial and ethnic minority populations), and geographic areas.

HCI sites are selected through a competitive application process. Preference is given to communities with demonstrated capacity to engage in policy change work and a proven history of collaboration with multiple sectors of their community. For example, applicants that have engaged in policy change work in one school and now want to address policy change with the entire school district would be considered competitive applicants. Communities that are selected to participate in an HCI initiative are supported by Y-USA through a variety of learning experiences. The leadership team of each community receives technical assistance to learn about innovative strategies to influence policy, systems, and environmental (PSE) changes. Each community team learns how to engage community members, develop a shared vision, and design and implement a community action plan.

The HCI model consists of the following key actions by a Y and a partner coach:

- Build a multisectoral community leadership team.
- Understand the importance of a policy approach to community change.
- Conduct a community assessment to understand community needs.
- Develop a community action plan to create policy and environmental changes that promote a healthier community.
- Implement the community action plan.
- Evaluate progress and update plans based on results.
- Sustain the collaboration within the community to generate more PSE changes.

Y-USA provides funding and technical assistance to each community leadership team to ensure that the community accomplishes its goals. YMCAs participating in HCI initiatives receive funding for planning, traveling to meetings, and implementing the activities identified in their community action plans.

The exact makeup of each community leadership team is different from community to community. Typically, members of the leadership team come from schools, after-school programs, public agencies, and private industry. Community leadership teams are very deliberate in considering who is included on the team.

An essential component of the technical assistance that Y-USA provides to local community teams is the Community Healthy Living Index. This tool was developed to measure opportunities for physical activity and healthy eating for an entire community, including after-school child care sites, early childhood programs, neighborhoods, schools, work sites, and the community at large. Communities that use this index indicate that it helps them focus their efforts, strengthen or create partnerships, build consensus, and gain early wins. In addition to the Community Healthy Living Index, many other data collection processes are available to help communities in their assessment activities. Typically, these include city or county health department data as well as GIS (Geographic Information Systems) and U.S. census data. By gathering and analyzing these data, Ys and their partner agencies can prioritize the needs of the community, inform the decision-making process, and build awareness of opportunities within the community.

A community action plan is designed to help capture the strategic directions for a leadership team and provide a way for coaches to track and monitor progress in the team's PSE efforts. The community action plan is designed to be a living document and is meant to reflect shifting priorities for the team and capture shifts in implementation timelines.

Each community team creates a community action plan that establishes the vision and mission of the team, identifies specific efforts to increase opportunities for physical activity, lays out action plans for accomplishing these objectives, and identifies strategies for measuring the objectives. Community action plans focus on a variety of sectors and a number of policy interventions, equally divided between physical activity and healthy eating focus areas.

Program Evaluation

HCI communities and states move through five steps that improve health outcomes.

- Step 1: HCI communities and states build their capacity to effect change by building a high-functioning and multisectoral leadership team.
- Step 2: Each team creates and implements a plan and makes PSE changes that promote healthy eating and active living.
- Step 3: PSE changes lead to environmental improvements that support healthy eating and physical activity.
- Step 4: Individuals increase healthy eating and active living behaviors.
- Step 5: Individuals attain improved health.

Through Healthier Communities Initiatives, community leaders from public health, government, education, business, and philanthropy can work together to plan and implement policies that support healthy living, such as these:

- Increasing access to and use of attractive and safe locations for physical activity

- Developing supportive environments to complement and support individual and family efforts to make healthy decisions

- Providing all students with adequate opportunities for physical activity before, during, and after school through recess, intramural activities, and other offerings

- Influencing work site policies and implementing work site wellness programs

- Influencing policies such as requiring sidewalks and countdown cross signals in neighborhoods and ensuring that school food contracts include more fruits and vegetables and whole grain foods

- Reducing the disparities in health and access to opportunities for physical activity and healthy eating in low-income communities

In a recent survey of 91 of Y-USA's HCI sites, local leaders reported that they influenced 14,459 changes to support healthy living within their communities, affecting 34.3 million lives.

Following are some of the highlights related to physical activity interventions from this survey:

Leaders advanced 318 strategies and encouraged changes in the physical environments of their neighborhoods to provide greater access to physical activity, including creating the following:

- 112 sidewalks designed or improved to increase physical activity options

- 71 traffic safety improvements or enhancements to increase physical activity options

- 52 "complete streets" that are open and accessible to all users, including bicyclists, pedestrians, and people with disabilities

In schools and after-school programs, HCI communities advanced 3,223 changes designed to promote physical activity before, during, and after the school day:

- 1,261 after-school sites added physical activity or increased the amount of physical activity they provide.

- 172 schools added or enhanced a Safe Routes to School program.

- 618 schools added or improved physical education criteria.

- 594 schools instituted classroom physical activity breaks during the day.

- 242 schools added or expanded recess during the day.

- 336 sports-related programs were added to the after-school setting.

In commercial work sites, HCI communities advanced 2,091 changes that helped employers incorporate healthier food and beverage options or expand opportunities for physical activity into their work sites:

- 386 work sites improved vending options.

- 368 work sites improved food choices available in meetings.

- 866 work sites incentivized their employees to engage in physical activity or nutrition education.

- 211 work sites promoted commuting options that include physical activity.

- 260 work sites promoted physical activity breaks during the workday.

In community-based organizations and public agencies, HCI communities advanced 1,277 changes that helped incorporate healthier food and beverage options or expanded opportunities for physical activity into their settings:

- 218 organizations and agencies improved vending options in their work sites.

- 343 organizations and agencies improved food choices available in meetings.

- 239 organizations and agencies incentivized their employees to engage in physical activity or nutrition education.
- 238 organizations and agencies promoted commuting options that include physical activity.
- 239 organizations and agencies promoted physical activity breaks during the workday.

The goal of the Healthier Communities Initiatives is to create long-term cultural shifts that promote health. Although it is too early to evaluate changes in health status, community leaders should look for signs that HCI teams are on course. Signs of early-stage success include these:

- New policies, systems, and environmental changes: These types of changes are being put into place across virtually all HCIs. Many of these changes have a strong research basis to suggest that they will produce lasting behavioral changes that lead to health improvements.
- Behavioral change and health outcomes: A large number of HCI teams are measuring and observing behavior changes in favor of healthy living. To support behavior changes, HCI sites are working to make the healthy choice the easy choice.
- Growth of collaborative culture: Although this is difficult to measure, signs indicate that a truly collaborative culture is starting to form across the traditional community sectors that typically focus only on their own agendas. Evidence includes heightened community engagement, increased cooperation among partners, and renewed interest by involved organizations to strengthen community.

Linkage to National Physical Activity Plan

HCI communities are engaging in hundreds of policy interventions, many of which align with the National Physical Activity Plan.

Specifically, sites are engaging in policy, systems, and environmental changes in each of the National Physical Activity Plan sectors. Following are examples of some of the strategies that HCI sites are pursuing:

Public Health

- *Strategy 3: Engage in advocacy and policy development to elevate the priority of physical activity in public health practice, policy, and research.*
- *Strategy 5: Expand monitoring of policy and environmental determinants of physical activity and the levels of physical activity in communities (surveillance), and monitor the implementation of public health approaches to promoting active lifestyles (evaluation).*

Education

- *Strategy 1: Provide access to and opportunities for high-quality, comprehensive physical activity programs, anchored by physical education, in pre-kindergarten through grade 12 educational settings. Ensure that the programs are physically active, inclusive, safe, and developmentally and culturally appropriate.*
- *Strategy 5: Provide access to and opportunities for physical activity before and after school.*

Health Care

- *Strategy 1: Make physical activity a patient "vital sign" that all health care providers assess and discuss with their patients.*
- *Strategy 3: Use a health care systems approach to promote physical activity and to prevent and treat physical inactivity.*
- *Strategy 4: Reduce disparities in access to physical activity services in health care.*
- *Strategy 5: Include physical activity education in the training of all health care professionals.*

Business and Industry

- *Strategy 1: Identify, summarize, and disseminate best practices, models, and evidence-based physical activity interventions in the workplace.*

- *Strategy 2: Encourage business and industry to interact with all other sectors to identify opportunities to promote physical activity within the workplace and throughout society.*

Parks, Recreation, Fitness, and Sports

- *Strategy 1: Promote programs and facilities where people work, learn, live, play and worship (i.e., workplace, public, private, and non-profit recreational sites) to provide easy access to safe and affordable physical activity opportunities.*

Mass Media

- *Strategy 3: Develop consistent mass communication messages that promote physical activity, have a clear and standardized "brand," and are consistent with the most current Physical Activity Guidelines for Americans.*

- *Strategy 5: Sequence, plan, and provide campaign activities in a prospective, coordinated manner. Support and link campaign messages to community-level programs, policies, and environmental supports.*

Transportation, Land Use, and Community Design

- *Strategy 3: Integrate land-use, transportation, community design and economic development planning with public health planning to increase active transportation and other physical activity.*

- *Strategy 4: Increase connectivity and accessibility to essential community destinations to increase active transportation and other physical activity.*

Volunteer and Nonprofit

- *Strategy 1: Advocate to local, state and national decision makers for policies and system changes identified in the National Physical Activity Plan that promote physical activity.*

- *Strategy 2: Convene multi-sector stakeholders at local, state, and national levels in*

strategic collaborations to advance the goals of the National Physical Activity Plan.

Tips for Working Across Sectors

During eight years of working to engage communities in the Healthier Communities Initiatives, Y-USA leaders have identified practices that are the key to implementing this model successfully:

1. Start with a shared, compelling vision and spirit of inquiry: Like others involved in collaborative efforts, HCI teams have found that identifying shared values and creating a compelling vision provide a strong foundation upon which they can address subsequent opportunities and challenges. By developing an end goal that is bigger than the goal any organization or group can achieve on its own, HCI teams open a door to new, often unexpected, opportunities for learning and collaboration.

2. Adapt to emerging opportunities: Given the speed at which the world changes around us, most detailed plans won't remain relevant for very long. By developing a shared vision and an opportunistic mind-set, HCI leaders are better able to adapt their efforts to emerging opportunities, while still staying on track.

3. Borrow from others and build your own: Believability is a big part of change. When people believe that the desired change is possible, they are more likely to help create the change in their own communities. Many HCI participants are inspired to move into action because they see what members of another community have done and the results they have achieved.

4. Engage cross-boundary leaders who care: A key to the success of HCI teams has been their ability to build cross-sectoral teams of action-oriented community decision makers for whom community well-being is a core motivation. HCI teams typically include leadership from Ys, schools and academic institutions, government agencies and elected officials, hospitals, health insurance companies, public health

organizations, businesses, community- and health-focused foundations, faith-based groups, media, and other community sectors.

5. Serve in multiple roles: HCI leadership teams have discovered that the role the community needs them to play varies over time, depending on the needs of a particular action area. At different times, HCI teams may find themselves serving as conveners, promoters, policy advocates, educators, or implementers. Most have found this role versatility to be essential, and they have found it important to be clear about these roles with partners.

6. Use data to guide, not drive, the effort: HCI sites use various types of data throughout their process. However, they also recognize that HCI is about creating change, not collecting data. Having limited time and resources means that data collection and analysis need to be focused primarily on identifying, understanding, and acting on strategic opportunities. Perhaps less important is a traditional comprehensive needs assessment at the beginning of the process. How the data are collected and used depends on the availability of the data, current understanding of issues among stakeholders, and the scope of the initiative.

7. Develop leadership structures that distribute ownership and action: Leading an initiative with ambitious aims, limited staffing, and busy volunteers requires a well-designed structure and effective processes. The structure and processes have a great influence on how team members use their talents and time and whether they stay engaged. In some cases, HCI teams are designed to complement the structure of existing initiatives, and in other cases they work more independently.

Although there is no single model for organizing an effective HCI structure, these seven common elements characterize the most effective ones.

Summary

Across America, innovative collaborations, such as Y-USA's Healthier Communities Initiatives, are adapting to the changing needs of their members and communities. Through changes in programming, staffing, and the physical environment, Ys are seeking to foster and support sustained relationships with individuals and families who want to experience greater total health and well-being. As a result, members are becoming more engaged and are having better success reaching their goals.

No single organization can effectively solve the chronic disease crisis in the United States; YMCAs are leading a national movement to mobilize communities to respond to this public health crisis. Collectively, all sectors of our communities and nation must come together to advance a common strategy to remove the barriers and increase the opportunities for physical activity for all.

Community organizations and local agencies can connect with their local Ys to find out whether they are engaged in Healthier Communities Initiatives. If they are already involved, organization leaders can ask to be included on the leadership team to complement its efforts to make policy changes to create a healthier community. In communities that are not yet participating in HCI, community organizations can encourage their local Ys to get involved.

CHAPTER 22

Professional Sport Venues as Opportunities for Physical Activity Breaks
The San Diego Padres' FriarFit Instant Recess

Antronette (Toni) K. Yancey, MD, MPH
UCLA School of Public Health

Portia Jackson, DrPH, MPH
UCLA School of Public Health

David Winfield, BA
San Diego Padres

Sally Lawrence Bullock, MPH
*University of North Carolina
Gillings School of Global Public Health*

Mariah Lafleur, MPH
*The Sarah Samuels Center
for Public Health Research & Evaluation*

Sarah Samuels, DrPH
*The Sarah Samuels Center
for Public Health Research & Evaluation*

Andrew Mowen, PhD
Pennsylvania State University

NPAP Tactics and Strategies Used in This Program

Parks, Recreation, Fitness, and Sports Sector

STRATEGY 1: Promote programs and facilities where people work, learn, live, play and worship (i.e., workplace, public, private, and nonprofit recreational sites) to provide easy access to safe and affordable physical activity opportunities.

STRATEGY 3: Use existing professional, amateur (Amateur Athletics Union, Olympics), and college (National Collegiate Athletics Association) athletics and sports infrastructures and programs to enhance physical activity opportunities in communities.

Few Americans participate in physical activity at recommended levels, and most Americans do not enjoy the many benefits of a physically active lifestyle. Children are not exempt from this trend, and many experts believe that societal norms must shift if we are to arrest the epidemic of childhood obesity (Institute of Medicine 2004, 2006, 2009). New and innovative ways to reengineer physical activity back into daily life will be needed to shift the American paradigm from primarily sedentary to significantly active. Changes in policies and practices within a broad range of institutions and organizations may help to expand opportunities for physical activity (Mittelmark 1999).

Regular and sustained participation in physical activity may be enhanced by making physical activity the default option, or path of least resistance, requiring people to consciously avoid physical activity, or "opt out." Integrating short activity bouts into organizational routine is such an "active by default" policy, one that incorporates experiential learning and facilitates fitness conditioning in an organization's normal routines and practices. This type of policy has been implemented across a number of settings, including work sites, schools, and religious institutions. The activity bouts (typically 10 minutes or less) have taken the form of brief aerobic routines held during meetings or events or at certain times during the day, walking meetings, and restrictions on nearby parking and elevator use. Engaging captive audiences (i.e., those convened for other purposes) in structured group physical activity provides built-in social support and activates peer (social conformity) pressure, a strategy that relies less on individual initiative and motivation than do traditional "pull" strategies (e.g., gym membership subsidies, exercise classes, on-site fitness and shower facilities).

One example of an intervention that focuses on short bouts of physical activity is Instant Recess (IR), an evidence-based, technology-driven approach designed to integrate enjoyable 10-minute group physical activity breaks into the routine daily conduct of business. Instant Recess aims to create a fitness-promoting cultural and social norm change and render prolonged sitting as socially unacceptable as drinking and driving or smoking (Yancey 2009; Yancey et al. 2009). Instant Recess break movements are simple and low impact, usually choreographed from sports or ethnic dance traditions and performed to music, and are captured on CDs and DVDs that can be used in a variety of settings. The breaks are scientifically designed to maximize energy expenditure while minimizing injury risk and perceived exertion, permitting individuals of differing levels of fitness and agility to participate together (Yancey et al. 2004, 2006; Yancey 2010).

One of the more innovative applications of IR has been its use in sports arenas as pregame, time-out, and half-time entertainment. Professional sports organizations are natural allies in the quest to increase physical activity, and sports arenas are natural settings for short-duration physical activity breaks for several reasons: (1) athletes serve as high-profile models for fitness, (2) communities identify with teams, (3) teams and arenas provide opportunities to share

media messages that promote physical activity, (4) spectator physical activity experiences drive attendance and fosters experiential learning, and (5) teams can continue their tradition of youth-targeted philanthropic involvement by promoting physical activity for young fans.

Program Description

The FriarVision Fitness Fanatics Initiative (FriarFit) is a multiyear healthy food and physical activity initiative developed by the San Diego Padres and the California Endowment, in partnership with the San Diego Childhood Obesity Initiative, UCLA, and SportService (Petco Park concessionaire) (The Sarah Samuels Center for Public Research & Evaluation 2009). In response to the alarming increase in childhood obesity, FriarFit's long-term goal is to improve the health of all San Diegans through collaborative community efforts to improve physical activity and healthy eating in schools and by providing appealing opportunities for physical activity and healthier food and beverage options at the ballpark. Working with schools and the community, FriarFit aims to create momentum for widespread changes in sociocultural norms, policies, and practices that will contain and ultimately reverse the obesity epidemic for all San Diego residents.

In collaboration with public health expert Dr. Toni Yancey and the Professional Athletes Council, the Padres adopted IR as the primary physical activity component of FriarFit. The team developed an IR break that was choreographed and set to original music (commissioned by an outside artist), with nine baseball moves representing each of the nine innings in a baseball game (or nine players on the field). The break is implemented during the pregame show at family-focused Sunday games and other youth events, for example, as a warm-up or cool-down during baseball clinics (Yancey et al. 2009). The featured moves include these:

1. Batter on Deck (warm-up)
2. Batter Up
3. Fast Ball
4. The Wave
5. Foul Ball

6. Celebration

7. Seventh Inning Stretch

8. Grounder

9. The Ump (followed by a one-minute cool-down)

Each move is simple, low impact, and easily modified for individuals with limited mobility. The routine is presented in a DVD produced by the Padres in cooperation with UCLA. The DVD features Dr. Yancey and Dave Winfield (a Major League Baseball Hall of Famer and former Padres player, currently executive vice president and senior advisor for the team and an ESPN color commentator) leading youth in the break, with clips of Padres athletes demonstrating moves or snippets of in-game footage highlights. The duration is 10 minutes, with each move lasting for about a minute.

The Padres held training sessions at the ballpark to instruct teachers and other community partners to lead IR in various settings. The location served as an incentive for participation, especially for PE teachers, who were often former athletes themselves. At the training sessions, the rationale for the activity breaks and implementation methods was presented, along with data demonstrating the impact that activity breaks can have on student health and classroom performance. The DVDs were originally labeled with player images and stats in order to serve as "trading discs," similar to baseball trading cards, among students. However, rapid and unanticipated player turnover, even of franchise players, led to a more generic branding with the FriarFit logo.

Implementation at the Ballpark

Before the Sunday, family-focused home baseball games and at special events, the FriarFit IR DVD is shown on a large video scoreboard in the "Park at the Park," a general-use area of Petco Park, adjacent to the stadium. The Pad Squad (fan ambassadors and promotion team) helps to gather children and lead them in the break activities.

IR is advertised on all television monitors throughout the park, along with a countdown, and occurs approximately one hour before the start of the game, which gets spectators to the park early, an added benefit for the team. The Park in the Park area, a joint use venue with San Diego County Parks and Recreation, is popular with families, as it features reduced admission and serves as a place to meet Padres athletes and obtain their autographs in advance of the game. As soon as the athletes depart, the Pad Squad staff and the Friar mascot perform the IR with children and their families.

School and Youth Program Outreach

The Padres Foundation for Children hosted a launch press event to publicize FriarFit in April 2008, at the start of the baseball season. Schools and youth groups were invited, and free transportation was provided. Free tickets are regularly offered to youth-serving organizations throughout the season, providing additional opportunities to expose children and program staff to IR. Media coverage (traditional and social) helped to increase both the popularity and draw of the pregame breaks as well as to drive enthusiasm and interest in participating in IR in other venues. The breaks became a regular feature during player visits to schools and other public service appearances.

In schools and after-school programs, FriarFit leaders encourage teachers to play the IR CD or DVD in the classroom between subjects, during transitions such as settling children down after lunch, and during homeroom or recess periods. For example, the San Francisco Boys and Girls Clubs incorporated IR as a lead-in to its Power Hour study period.

Public and Private Sector Partners of FriarFit

The San Diego Padres organization was one of the first professional sports teams to embrace obesity prevention as a philanthropic goal. Integral to the Padres' interest in partnering with the California Endowment (TCE) was a management decision that a focus on obesity prevention would better align the team's community benefit efforts with its identity as an organization grounded in healthy living (The Sarah Samuels

Center for Public Research & Evaluation 2009). Team leadership also recognized the opportunity to enhance the fan experience and to profit by "doing good" (Elder and Yancey 2009). TCE recognized the natural alignment of pro sports and kids' fitness, and it funded and staffed an exploration of the feasibility of increasing physical activity and access to healthy foods within the stadium. This study contributed to the pool of evidence linking environmental and policy approaches to active living and healthy eating outcomes (The Sarah Samuels Center for Public Research & Evaluation 2010). The foundation took an active role in convening and leveraging support from public health experts to ensure that FriarFit used the most effective educational, policy, and environmental strategies to promote fitness among ballpark patrons and the San Diego community (The Sarah Samuels Center for Public Research & Evaluation 2009). TCE identified and hired an expert consultant (Toni Yancey) to assist the Padres in developing the initiative. TCE provided funding that proved vital to expanding the reach of the initiative. The UCLA School of Public Health created and choreographed the FriarFit IR break, incorporating evidence-based practices into the programmatic approach. The state health department's Network for a Healthy California and California Project LEAN worked with schools and community programs to disseminate IR and encourage participation in the FriarFit initiative. The network also incorporated distribution of the CD and DVD as part of the Children's Power Play! campaign.

The FriarFit consultant, TCE staff, and Padres executives worked with SportsService, Petco Park's concessionaire, to identify and introduce 10 nutrient-rich food options, including sweet pepper hummus with baked pita chips, grilled veggie dogs and burgers on whole wheat buns, salads, yogurt parfaits, and fresh fruit cups.

At the time of this writing, in September 2011, the FriarFit initiative was completing its fourth season. The Pad Squad staff continues to conduct IR prior to each Sunday home game. Throughout the school year, the Pad Squad, and occasionally Padres players or executives, visit local schools to lead the breaks and distribute incentives that encourage youth to be more active. The Padres Foundation for Children hosts special events featuring IR: for example, the launch of the national Let's Move campaign in May 2011. The DVD is updated periodically to replace retired or traded players with talent on the active roster as video subjects.

Program Evaluation

The California Endowment provided funding for an outside organization to evaluate FriarFit's accomplishments, challenges, lessons learned, and best practices. The evaluation provided an opportunity to demonstrate the unique impact of FriarFit as well as to assess the influence of its environmental and policy approach on activity and eating behaviors. The evaluation used a multimethod design to measure FriarFit's influence on outcomes such as changes to the Petco Park menu, integration of physical activity into ballpark routine, and the effect of these changes on park patrons' food purchases and activity levels. The evaluation also covered the Padres' organizational engagement and business approach for promoting fitness and the impact on school and community settings. Qualitative and quantitative methods were used to capture FriarFit's challenges and value-added results. The evaluation focused on three specific components of the initiative that were implemented during the first phase of the FriarFit rollout in the 2008 season:

- Engaging patrons (adults and children) in 10-minute physical activity sessions (IR) in the open area at the ballpark (Park in the Park), using the FriarFit theme, with players and fan ambassadors as role models
- Working with SportService (Petco Park concessionaire) to offer a line of healthy foods and beverages at the ballpark
- Training local school staff and teachers to offer IR breaks to children using FriarFit IR DVDs, to reach school children outside of the ballpark

Process: Qualitative Assessment

According to a survey conducted with Padres professionals and other key stakeholders, fan participation in physical activity breaks was not consistent, as fans were sometimes distracted by other ballpark offerings while IR was taking place. However, IR was well received overall and helped to call attention to the Park in the Park activity space while providing the Padres organization with the unique opportunity to engage fans in fun and exciting activities during games. One of the survey respondents stated,

> It is really unique that [ball park patrons] can be a part of IR before the game and interact with people around them. This is what the ball park experience is all about.

Another stakeholder was especially proud of the increase in children's awareness and interest in IR:

> Kids now realize what's going on and are able to have fun with it. The day we had the YMCA groups out there was great too. It was good to see the whole workout done on a large scale.

Although instituting IR at the ballpark was considered a significant accomplishment, full implementation of FriarFit's environmental changes, particularly those related to marketing and advertising in promoting the breaks and

the initiative's community engagement activities, were not fully developed when the evaluation was conducted. Stakeholders believed that promotion of FriarFit and IR needed to be coordinated across multiple departments within the Padres organization to maximize visibility and recognition. Stakeholders recommended that IR be implemented and more aggressively marketed throughout the stadium.

Outcome: Quantitative Assessment

A modified System for Observing Fitness Instruction Time (SOFIT) tool was used to assess activity levels of individuals before, during, and after IR breaks that occurred before Sunday games in 2008 and 2009. The levels of physical activity during IR did not differ significantly from the baseline to endpoint observation, but there were differences in activity levels at baseline and endpoint before, during, and after IR and for those who were actively engaged in IR. For example, at endpoint the study found that activity equivalent to brisk walking occurred more during IR than before or after. The study also observed less sitting and lying down during IR than after (figure 22.1). Additionally, individuals engaged in IR (actively paying attention and participating in

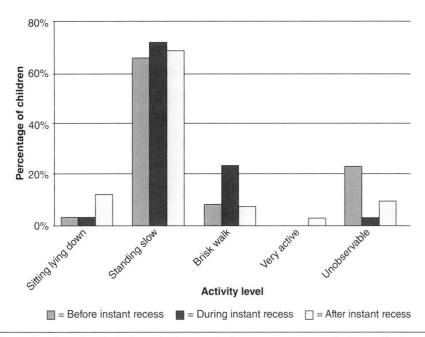

Figure 22.1   Physical activity levels before, during, and after Instant Recess during endpoint observation.

Reprinted, by permission, from Sarah Samuels Center for Public Health Research and Evaluation.

the activities) were significantly more active than those not engaged in IR. On scale of 1 to 4 (1 = sitting, 4 = running), activity levels were 2.22 for those who were engaged in IR versus 1.82 for those who were not engaged. At endpoint, 80 percent of those who were engaged in IR reached levels 3 or 4 (moderate to vigorous physical activity), whereas only 17 percent of those who were not engaged reached the same level of activity. These findings indicate that the activities during IR encouraged more individuals in the Park in the Park area to be physically active while the IR was occurring.

Linkage to National Physical Activity Plan

This approach addresses the following strategies and tactics of the Parks, Recreation, Fitness, and Sport Sector of the National Physical Activity Plan.

Strategy 1: Promote programs and facilities where people work, learn, live, play and worship (i.e., workplace, public, private, and nonprofit recreational sites) to provide easy access to safe and affordable physical activity opportunities.

Tactic: Provide programs in parks, recreation, fitness, and sports that are appropriate for individuals of both genders, diverse cultures, abilities, developmental stages and needs and that have demonstrated positive physical activity outcomes.

Strategy 3: Use existing professional, amateur (Amateur Athletics Union, Olympics), and college (National Collegiate Athletics Association) athletics and sports infrastructures and programs to enhance physical activity opportunities in communities.

Tactic: Train athletes and sports management staff to deliver environmental and policy interventions in addition to individual change interventions.

- Use sporting event venues as opportunities for delivering messages and creating opportunities for active participation.
- Use social marketing approaches to change spectator sports culture and use it as a lever to increase physical activity.

Evidence Base Used During Program Development

IR breaks are scientifically designed to maximize energy expenditure while minimizing injury risk and perceived exertion, permitting individuals of differing levels of fitness and agility to participate together (Yancey et al. 2004). Bouts of physical activity as short as 10 minutes have been found to be more predictive of overweight or obesity status independent of the accumulated volume of minutes engaged in exercise, which can have a substantial impact on largely sedentary populations (Troiano et al. 2008). Elementary school students in classrooms that engaged in Instant Recess for 10 minutes a day were found to have higher levels of light to moderate physical activity than their peers who did not participate (Whitt-Glover et al. 2011). Given that 38 percent of students report that they do not take physical education classes at school, it is important to find alternative ways for youth to be active (Diamant et al. 2011).

By having team athletes demonstrate baseball moves on the DVD, FriarFit leverages the influential capacity of role models to motivate youth to engage in healthy behaviors. A study found that adolescents who listed an athlete as a role model were twice as likely to report engaging in moderate to vigorous physical activity as were their peers who did not report having a role model (Yancey et al. 2011). Finally, FriarFit worked with a nutritionist from the Network for a Healthy California as well as with SportsService to provide fans with the option of purchasing foods that meet recommended standards for fat, saturated fat, and daily caloric intake, in addition to traditional ballpark fare (Patringenaru 2010).

Populations Best Served by the Program

IR initiatives could occur in a variety of communities beyond the Major League Baseball markets. Minor League Baseball, for example, includes 227 teams across the United States.

These Minor League games attract not only the core baseball enthusiasts but also families. Parents bring their children to these venues to enjoy the atmosphere of excitement and anticipation and to participate in promotional activities offered during the games. Although FriarFit IR was implemented at a Major League venue (and in a large urban area), similar programs could serve the 49 million people who attend Minor League baseball games each year.

Lessons Learned

Leadership from senior management helps to ensure the success of a program. Franchise leaders established the initiative as a priority and promoted it with the foundation, concessionaire, and other partners. Dave Winfield's hands-on involvement was pivotal to the substance and success of FriarFit, and the decision to house the initiative under the umbrella of the Padres Foundation for Children protected FriarFit when the team changed ownership.

Academic and public health partners worked with the Padres to guide the development and implementation of the initiative in the ballpark and other settings. As FriarFit unfolded, partners worked to increase the player-featured advertising and the variety of FriarFit foods in the ballpark and to market and position IR in a way that increased fan participation. When production of the DVD was delayed, this slowed program uptake in settings outside of the ballpark, demonstrating that the DVD was a crucial element of intervention exportability.

From the FriarFit experience, the Padres learned that a family-friendly physical activity break program is a good business practice that enriches fans' overall ballpark experience. Teams and sports venues considering a similar Instant Recess initiative should follow these tactics:

- Clarify goals and objectives first.
- Embrace a long-term comprehensive approach that builds on early success.
- Encourage collaboration between public and private organizations to leverage resources.

- Gain top management and executive leadership buy-in.

Tips for Working Across Sectors

Initiatives involving public health entities and professional sports organizations are, in essence, a form of community-based participatory research with a much more powerful community partner (The California Endowment 2008; Yancey et al. 2009). True partnering between these disparate sectors requires strategic realignment of assets and strengths to realize the potential of this collaboration. Public health offers the content expertise or "game plan," while the business of sports provides the dissemination skills to get the message out and to engage the audience. This capitalizes on corporate nimbleness and ability to speak to people's desires and aspirations versus their needs, as defined by health experts and often rejected by the intended audience.

Public health aims must be addressed in a way that is financially viable and fiscally sustainable (presumably an amalgam of product sales and other revenue, public and community relations value, and brand marketing). For example, the profitability of FriarFit product sales versus distribution of materials via the Padres Foundation for Children as giveaways had to be assessed strategically, given the associated overhead (the portion of revenues required by players' agents, contractors that provided services within the stadium, and others). Consequently, FriarFit IR DVDs and CDs must be mass produced through mostly corporate donations to the Padres Foundation for Children, disseminated locally through the regular activities of the foundation, and distributed to partners for dissemination beyond the team's catchment area.

Ideally, the success of the public health effort would increase the corporate bottom line. Near-term seed money (e.g., grant funding through foundations or health care organization community benefit funds) ultimately should be supplanted by public relations value-added and long-term private sector support—corporate sponsorship, sales, and other revenues.

Summary

FriarFit provides a local model for collaboration between professional sports and public health agencies to advance population physical activity. However, to achieve broad-based success in arresting the epidemic of childhood obesity, this model must be scaled up on a national level, with the support and active participation of athletes, sports leagues, foundations, corporations, and elected and appointed government officials. Youth, families, and communities are ready. Bring it on!

Additional Reading and Resources

Barr-Anderson, D.J., M. AuYoung, M.C. Whitt-Glover, B.A. Glenn, and A.K. Yancey. 2011. Integration of short bouts of physical activity into organizational routine: A systematic review of the literature. *Am. J. Prev. Med.* 40(1):76-93.

Brownson, R.C., T.K. Boehmer, and D.A. Luke. 2005. Declining rates of physical activity in the United States: What are the contributors? *Ann. Rev. Public Health* 26(1):421-43.

Donnelly, J.E., J.L. Greene, C.A. Gibson, B.K. Smith, R.A. Washburn, D.K. Sullivan, et al. 2009. Physical Activity Across the Curriculum (PAAC): A randomized controlled trial to promote physical activity and diminish overweight and obesity in elementary school children. *Prev. Med.* 49(4):336-41.

Honas, J., R. Washburn, B. Smith, J. Greene, and J. Donnelly. 2008. Energy expenditure of the Physical Activity across the Curriculum intervention. *Med. Sci. Sports Exerc.* 40(8):1501-5.

Instant Recess: www.toniyancey.com/IR_Book.html

Keen's Recess Is Back campaign to launch a Recess Revolution: http://recess.keenfootwear.com

Knuth, A., and P. Hallal. 2009. Temporal trends in physical activity: A systematic review. *J. Phys. Act. Health* 6(5):548-59.

Mahar, M., S. Murphy, D. Rowe, J. Golden, A. Shields, and T. Raedek. 2006. Effects of a classroom-based program on physical activity and on-task behavior. *Med. Sci. Sports Exerc.* 38(12):2086-94.

Matthews, C.E., K.Y. Chen, P.S. Freedson, M.S. Buchowski, B.M. Beech, R.R. Pate, et al. 2008. Amount of time spent in sedentary behaviors in the United States, 2003-2004. *Am. J. Epidemiol.* 167(7):875-81.

Minor League Baseball Teams by Affiliation: http://web.minorleaguebaseball.com/milb/info/affiliations.jsp

Minor League Attendance Analysis (2012): www.numbertamer.com/files/2012_Minor_League_Analysis.pdf

Padres FriarFit initiative: http://sandiego.padres.mlb.com/sd/community/friarfit.jsp

Sibley, B., R. Ward, T. Yazvac, K. Zullig, and J. Potteiger. 2008. Making the grade with diet and exercise. *Journal of Scholarship and Practice* 5(2):38-45.

The African American Collaborative Obesity Research Network (AACORN): www.aacorn.org

The FriarFit Instant Recess® video: www.youtube.com/watch?v = aEvF3brYvb4

White House Childhood Obesity Task Force Report. 2010. Washington, DC: USDHHS.

World Stadiums. 2011. Stadiums in the United States. www.worldstadiums.com/north_america/countries/united_states.shtml

Yancey, A., N. Pronk, and B. Cole. 2007. Workplace approaches to obesity prevention. In: *Handbook of Obesity Prevention* (pp. 317-47). S. Kumanyika and R.C. Brownson, Eds. New York: Springer.

Yancey, A., J. Siegel, and K. McDaniel. 2002. Role models, ethnic identity, and health-risk behaviors in urban adolescents. *Arch. Pediatr. Adolesc. Med.* 156(1):55-61.

References

Diamant, A., S. Babey, and J. Wolstein. 2011. *Adolescent Physical Education and Physical Activity in California.* Los Angeles: UCLA Center for Health Policy Research.

Elder, S., and A. Yancey. 2009. San Diego Padres' FriarFit: Lessons learned. Partnering with business to prevent obesity break-out session. Presented at the Grantmakers in Health Annual Conference, Long Beach, CA, April 1, 2009.

Institute of Medicine. 2004. Weight management: State of the science and opportunities for military programs. Subcommittee on Military Weight Management, Committee on Military Nutrition Research. www.nap.edu/catalog/10783.html

Institute of Medicine. 2006. *Food Marketing to Children and Youth: Threat or Opportunity?* Washington, DC: National Academies Press.

Institute of Medicine. 2009. *Local Government Actions to Prevent Childhood Obesity*. Washington, DC: National Academies of Sciences.

Mittelmark, M.B. 1999. The psychology of social influence and healthy public policy. *Prev Med. 29*(6 Pt. 2):S24-9.

Patringenaru, I. 2010. Healthy meals a home run for San Diego Padres: Baseball club and UC San Diego team up to offer FriarFit menu at PETCO Park. *This Week @ UCSD: Your Campus Connection*. http://ucsd-news.ucsd.edu/thisweek/2010/06/07_Padres.asp

The Sarah Samuels Center for Public Research & Evaluation. 2009. Findings from the FriarVision Fitness Fanatics Initiative (FriarFit) stakeholder interviews. 1222 Preservation Park Way, Oakland, CA 94612.

The Sarah Samuels Center for Public Research & Evaluation. 2010. Findings from the evaluation of the FriarVision Fitness Fanatics Initiative (FriarFit). 1222 Preservation Park Way, Oakland, CA 94612.

The California Endowment. 2008. The San Diego Padres' FriarFit Initiative: Lessons learned and unlearned in developing strategic alliances between professional sports and public health. 1000 N Alameda St, Los Angeles, CA 90012.

Troiano, R., D. Berrigan, K. Dodd, L. Masse, T. Tilert, and M. McDowell. 2008. Physical activity in the United States measured by accelerometer. *Med. Sci. Sports Exerc.* 40(1):181-8.

Whitt-Glover, M., S. Ham, and A. Yancey. 2011. Instant Recess®: A practical tool for increasing physical activity during the school Day. *Prog. Community Health Partnersh. 5*(3):298-7.

Yancey, A., D. Grant, S. Kurosky, N. Kravitz-Wirtz, and R. Mistry. 2011. Role modeling, risk, and resilience in California adolescents. *J. Adolesc. Health* 48(1):36-43.

Yancey, A., D. Winfield, J. Larsen, M. Anderson, P. Jackson, J. Overton, et al. 2009. "Live, Learn and Play": building strategic alliances between professional sports and public health. *Prev. Med. 49*(4):322-5.

Yancey, A.K. 2006. Changing the sociocultural environment to promote physical activity: capitalizing on cultural assets. Paper presented at the Society of Behavioral Medicine Annual Meeting, San Francisco, CA, March 24, 2006.

Yancey, A.K. 2009. The meta-volition model: Organizational leadership is the key ingredient in getting society moving, literally! *Prev. Med.* 49(4):342-51.

Yancey, A. 2010. *Instant Recess: Building a Fit Nation -- 10 Minutes at a Time*. Berkeley, CA: University of California Press.

Yancey Antronette K, McCarthy William J, Taylor Wendell C, Merlo Angela, Gewa Constance, Weber Mark D, Fielding Jonathan E. 2004. The Los Angeles Lift Off: a sociocultural environmental change intervention to integrate physical activity into the workplace. *Preventive medicine, 38*(6): 848-56.

Business and Industry

Nicolaas P. Pronk, PhD

HealthPartners and Harvard School of Public Health

Overall occupational physical activity in the United States has declined over the past 50 years. In today's workplace, many job tasks are characterized by prolonged periods of sitting and other sedentary activities. Such prolonged periods of low-intensity physical activity, often accompanied by static tension of large muscle groups, predispose workers to musculoskeletal problems, upper-back and neck pain, absenteeism, short-term disability, reduced quality and quantity of work, overall work impairment, and excess health care costs. For these reasons, it behooves employers to implement programs that improve the level of physical activity among workers.

However, for physical activity programs to be adopted and sustained, they need to be designed to fit into the overall context of the workplace. They need to be sensitive to the culture of the organization, be accessible and relevant to the participants, fit effortlessly into the daily workflow, address the psychological and physiological concerns of the workforce, and generate positive impact in both the short and long term. As such, physical activity programs need to be an integral part of a company's business strategy and the overall efforts to promote health and well-being at the work site.

This section of the book presents six case studies that provide important insight into successful implementation efforts for health improvement at the work site. The programs represent a wide variety of industries—from truck drivers to school systems to energy companies and health care organizations. Some programs are newly designed; others celebrate decades of successful implementation and con-

tinuous improvement. Despite their uniqueness, they all share a set of common principles. As you read the case studies, you will undoubtedly notice that each organization paid close attention to its program design. Common design principles include the importance of organizational culture, leadership support, a set of comprehensive program options, multilevel interventions (from individual behavior change efforts to environmental and policy solutions), program communications, programmatic aspects relevant to the employees as well as the company, and evaluation that allows for reporting of program impact and continuous improvement.

Resources that provide high-quality information on work-site-based studies and research are highly accessible. Examples include the Community Preventive Services Task Force, which regularly generates recommendations on what works to promote physical activity and health at the work site and presents these findings as part of the Community Guide (see www.communityguide.org). Other organizations, such as the Cochrane Collaboration and the National Institute for Health and Clinical Excellence, provide similar reviews and reports. Additional support for practitioners in promoting physical activity and health at the work site exists in such organizations as the International Association for Worksite Health Promotion (see www.iawhp.org), an organizational affiliate of the National Physical Activity Plan. Although a lot of information is available on what may effectively promote physical activity in the work site, most of such information is based on generalized knowledge, not necessarily company-specific experiences. The goal of this section is to provide field-based examples, practical advice, and deeper insight into successful programs. The collection of stories presented here more than delivers on that goal.

It is my sincere hope that you will enjoy reading these stellar efforts conducted by organizations that so graciously shared their experiences in order to promote physical activity in our companies and communities across the country.

CHAPTER 23

Fit to Drive
Integrated Injury Prevention, Health, and Wellness for Truck Drivers

Delia Roberts, PhD, FACSM
Selkirk College

NPAP Tactics and Strategies Used in This Program

Business and Industry Sector

STRATEGY 1: Identify, summarize, and disseminate best practices, models, and evidence-based physical activity interventions in the workplace.

STRATEGY 3: Educate business and industry leaders regarding their role as positive agents of change to promote physical activity and healthy lifestyles within the workplace and throughout society, giving particular consideration to efforts targeting low-resource populations.

The purpose of the Fit to Drive program is to improve the health of drivers who haul logs from harvesting sites to the log yard; the intent is to decrease injury claims and increase the safety of their driving.

Program Description

Weyerhaeuser, a multinational corporation headquartered in Federal Way, Washington, was founded in 1900 and currently operates in 10 countries. In recent years the company has begun to implement employee health and wellness programs, and it has been interested for some time in developing an additional program for drivers and heavy equipment operators in Canada and the United States. In 2009, the year preceding development of the Fit to Drive program, two drivers suffered coronary events while driving. In both cases the trucks left the road, resulting in fatalities. Following those tragedies, Weyerhaeuser approached a science researcher who had helped the company develop other health and wellness programs. The company asked the researcher to develop an integrated health and safety program specifically for log haulers, based on a sport science approach. The researcher conducted a study, funded by the company, to evaluate the workplace demands, physiology, and lifestyle of the target population. After the study was initiated, the British Columbia Forest Safety Council joined Weyerhaeuser in funding the program.

First, company executives and the researcher presented the program proposal to company health and safety committees in two geographical regions. In both regions, employees, the union, and management supported the program. However, the union required that multiple test sites be included to ensure that all subregions of the company were engaged in the process. Although expanding the project throughout the company allowed a much greater level of engagement, it also increased the logistical complexity of the project.

The company then recruited 40 participants using a multistep process. Union and occupational health and safety committee representatives reported to their constituent drivers and encouraged them to consider enrolling in the project. Approximately half of the volunteers came forward with this first call. The researcher then conducted short information sessions in an effort to recruit additional participants. The remaining spaces were filled at those sessions.

Hauling volumes for sites in Canada peak during months when the road surfaces are frozen and are more resistant to damage by the very heavy loads on road beds. As a result, data collection at the Canadian test sites was carried out in January 2011. Data were collected in Washington and Oregon in April 2011.

The participant orientation and demographic data collection session began with a step-by-step review of the informed consent form with each participant. This was of particular importance because most participants had not gained a good understanding of the details of the project from the recruitment process. Several participants were very concerned about confidentiality, and many were initially suspicious of the project. Although improving health is ultimately of great benefit to the individual, developing trust with the drivers was critical; without this trust, the project team could not implement changes designed to promote health and wellness. However, enforcement of regulatory requirements by the employer may create a relationship that lacks trust. Addressing risk issues (e.g., financial, medical), ethical concerns, and other culture-specific considerations was considered an absolute necessity in order to engage the group, especially considering the relatively poor level of health in the population. For this reason, the program developers did not measure and record blood pressure as part of the program evaluation.

Each participant completed height, body mass, body mass index, and estimated body composition measures (Omron Model HBF-306CAN, Scarborough, Ontario). The project team interviewed drivers regarding injury and activity history, lifestyle preferences, and dietary habits and helped each participant complete a familiarization session of three to five trials of a reaction time and cognitive testing tool (Brain Checkers software, version 3.01, Behavioral Neuroscience Systems LLC, Springfield, Missouri), run on Palm Tungsten E2, Palm Inc., Milpitas, California). The reaction time and cognition testing consisted of a battery of tests, including a simple stimulus response time as well as more complex tasks that involved executive function, including interpretation of visual input, memory, and decision making. The test output consisted of reaction time, anticipatory events, null events, number of correct scores, and a calculated compilation score that includes both accuracy and speed, called *throughput* (TPut).

Reaction time and cognition (RTC) data, symptom inventory, and blood glucose levels were measured on two successive workdays with similar driving conditions. When drivers reported to the testing site following an eight-hour fast, project staff weighed them, attached a heart rate and activity monitor (Actiheart, Minimitter, Bend, Oregon), and conducted the first glucose and RTC testing session (fasting). On the first day, drivers were instructed to follow their normal eating pattern, including breakfast. On the second day, drivers received a series of small snacks that were prepared according to their food preferences but were designed to provide approximately 200 calories every two hours (60-65 percent carbohydrate, 15-20 percent protein, 15-25 percent fat). On both trial days, drivers reported for RTC evaluation, symptom inventory, and blood glucose testing every time they returned to the log yard, approximately every three hours for the duration of the workday (three times per day). Each time the drivers visited the testing site they spent approximately half an hour with the researcher discussing their lifestyles, goals, concerns, and potential strategies for making positive changes by increasing physical activity and improving diet. At the final testing session the heart rate and activity monitors were removed and subjects were weighed. The difference between morning and afternoon weights was considered to be a measure of hydration status. Drivers also underwent an exit interview to determine their perceptions of what they had learned by participating in the data collection phase.

As a group, the drivers were in very poor health. Although the mean ± standard deviation (SD) age was 45 ± 8 years, 95 percent of the drivers were overweight, including the 85 percent who were obese (based on estimated percentage body fat levels). The mean ± SD estimated body fat was 30 ± 6 percent and the mean calculated body mass index was 34 ± 5. Twenty-five percent of participants were smokers. The mean ± SD fasting blood glucose was 128 ± 49 milligrams per deciliter, with 45 percent of the values exceeding the upper limit of normal. Ten percent of the drivers had fasting levels on both test days that were indicative of undiagnosed diabetes (participants with known diabetes were excluded from participation). Blood glucose levels on the diet intervention day were significantly lower (mean ± SD for the day = 104 ± 29 milligrams per deciliter) than on the day when drivers ate their normal diets (mean ± SD for the day = 116 ± 45 milligrams per deciliter) ($p < .0004$).

The RTC data are unitless calculated values that normalize speed for accuracy; a higher score indicates a better performance. In all cases, performance was better ($p < .02$) on the intervention diet day than on the day when drivers consumed their normal food choices.

The average level of dehydration from a day of driving was 1.8 ± 0.6 percent. Only 12 percent of drivers reported engaging in any physical activity on a regular basis. Ninety-five percent of drivers experienced chronic pain; 65 percent had back pain, 50 percent had knee pain, 45 percent had shoulder pain, 20 percent had ankle pain, 20 percent had upper extremity pain, and 10 percent had neck pain. The mean heart rate for 9.5 hours of driving was 89 ± 13 beats per minute. Drivers spent an average of only 16 ± 14 minutes between a heart rate of 110 and 119 beats per minute, 8 ± 8 minutes between a heart rate of 120 and 129 beats per

minute, 5 ± 6 minutes between a heart rate of 130 and 139 beats per minute, and only 4 ± 5 minutes at a heart rate over 140 beats per minute, confirming the very low physical work output during a day of driving.

Two to four weeks following completion of the data collection for each group, a report of the findings was sent to participating drivers, along with information about how the next phase of the program would be delivered. This communication was intended primarily to maintain the drivers' focus on the lifestyle changes initiated during the data collection phase. No formal counseling was provided to drivers to make any changes at that point; however, drivers were encouraged to try some of the changes and to stay in communication with the research team. One month later, the research team conducted an additional follow-up by e-mail and phone. Although weight loss was not a targeted outcome of the project, 7 of the 40 drivers had lost weight (an average of 20 ± 4 pounds) within two months by implementing what they had learned about improving diet and increasing activity during this early informational phase.

The next phase of the program produced a set of training materials for the drivers that fit with their work culture and the unique situation of their job. These materials included a pocket-sized booklet titled *Top Ten Tips* to present key physical activity and nutrition concepts simply and clearly; a manual titled *Power Driving*, which included more in-depth information on how to increase physical activity levels and make positive diet and lifestyle changes; and a series of double-sided laminated cards that focused on specific topics (Increasing Physical Activity, Choosing a Healthy Diet, and Saving Your Back).

These materials were introduced to the participating drivers during safety meetings at each site; attendance by spouses was optional. Each driver received a package with the training materials and a customized report of his individual results. Program staff then conducted one-on-one coaching sessions with the drivers to set long- and short-term goals and create a specific action plan to achieve the first set of short-term goals by the follow-up visit. During the goal-setting process, drivers were directed toward specific focus areas such as losing weight, lowering blood pressure, decreasing blood glucose, and decreasing specific joint pain and were provided with information to help them achieve their goals. Drivers learned how to use the booklets to access more information on each topic, including step-by-step instructions for making the changes and motivational tips to support behavior change.

As with the preliminary follow-up, the findings at the time of the program launch were surprisingly positive. Drivers who had begun to make lifestyle changes following the testing had been able to maintain their focus over the intervening six months, and other drivers were able to begin the process.

The final results of this program will not be available until after the publication date of this book; however, these preliminary findings show that investigative, intervention-based work-site health and wellness programs can be extremely effective at overcoming barriers to workers' making positive dietary and physical activity changes. Over the next year, the researcher and company management will monitor compliance, injury, and illness rates and compare them to rates in similar operations within the forestry sector that did not implement the program.

Program Evaluation

The Fit to Drive program is being implemented currently, but early results appear very promising. Driver engagement is excellent, with a 94 percent fully committed participation rate. Early results for weight loss, behavior changes, and risk reduction indicators are all very strong. The program will be assessed by comparing injury and illness rates in the sites that receive the Fit to Drive program compared with similar-sized operations that have not received the program.

The concept behind the Fit to Drive program is similar to that of the Fit to Plant program. Eleven years ago, Weyerhaeuser and the same researcher developed the Fit to Plant program, which was based on a similar field study with manual tree planters. That program also

included a *Top Ten Tips* and parent manuals for the nutrition and training programs, which were placed in the public domain (www.selkirk. ca/treeplanting). Weyerhaeuser offered a fee-waived program delivery to all of its tree planting contractors, and after four years the injury rates were reduced by an order of magnitude in the operations that participated in the program. The recordable incidents were so much lower in these operations that the program was instituted across Canada. In August 2011, the company announced that it had achieved zero recordable incidents for the first time in Canadian history.

Linkage to National Physical Activity Plan

Fit to Drive supports these strategies of the Business and Industry Sector of the National Physical Activity Plan:

Strategy 1: Identify, summarize, and disseminate best practices, models, and evidence-based physical activity interventions in the workplace. Data were collected on a representative group of drivers and analyzed with sound scientific principles, and the findings were used to describe the health and lifestyle deficits of this population. The research findings then were used to develop a lifestyle program, designed to promote changes in diet and physical activity. The program is based on sport science and medical research findings and is focused on the interests and needs of the target population. The program will be placed in the public domain, where it can be accessed by business and industry.

Strategy 3: Educate business and industry leaders regarding their role as positive agents of change to promote physical activity and healthy lifestyles within the workplace and throughout society, giving particular consideration to efforts targeting low-resource populations. Industry and government groups have put into place a route for delivery of the program. The program will be announced through various industry publications and presented at a series of important industry and government conferences, seminars and workshops.

Evidence Base Used During Program Development

The incidence of occupational injuries and illness in the transportation sector has been reported to be 8.2 claims per 100 person-years, well in excess of the all-industry average of 3.5 claims per 100 person-years for 1999-2008 (WorkSafe BC 2009). In the United States, injuries in truck drivers account for nearly $900 million and 15 percent of workplace fatalities every year. Furthermore, when drivers are piloting heavy loads on public highways, the human and financial cost of an accident can be greatly exacerbated. These statistics clearly show that truck drivers in the logging industry are in great need of techniques that can help to reduce costly accidents and injuries as well as promote increased vigilance and good health.

The link between vigilance and injury occurrence has been established for other populations. The nervous system requires blood glucose for optimal performance, and when blood glucose levels are variable or drop too low, attentiveness and decision-making capability can decline (Lemaire et al. 2010). Reaction time in response to an unexpected stimulus also is impaired (Lieberman et al. 2005; Stevens et al. 1989; Strachan et al. 2001). Hypoglycemia has been shown previously to be a factor in motor vehicle accidents (Cox et al. 2000) and may contribute to the human error that has been implicated in 80 percent of all aviation accidents (Li et al. 2002). Optimized nutrition can be used to sustain work output and concentration over extended periods of high physical and mental stress with great success, and these techniques can be used to improve occupational health and wellness (Roberts 2005). For example, a nutrition and fitness program in the forestry (silviculture) industry resulted in a reduction of injuries from 20 percent to less than 2 percent and an increase in productivity of 12.5 percent. (Roberts 2003, 2008, 2009). Similar projects with mountain guides (Roberts, 2007), tree fallers and buckers (Roberts and Donnelly 2007), helicopter pilots (Roberts and Dinsmore 2008), and physicians (Lemaire et al. 2010) have shown that improving eating patterns can stabilize blood glucose levels and enhance reaction time and decision making.

Another approach to injury prevention is to reestablish joint and muscle reflexes that protect against changes in loading of these tissues. Sport science techniques have been used with excellent results to reduce back pain and protect against back, knee, and shoulder injuries (Roberts 2006, 2007, 2008, 2009). Sensory motor programs have been shown to increase joint stability in sport injury rehabilitation (Caraffa et al. 1996; Hoffman and Payne 1995) and to decrease work-related injuries in tree planters (Roberts 2003, 2008, 2009) and heli-ski guides (Roberts 2007). Proprioceptive receptors in muscle, tendon, and joint capsules are responsible for coordinating muscular contraction such that a joint is stabilized as the forces applied to it increase. In a healthy system, muscle will contract within 10 milliseconds of the beginning of an applied force, whereas it requires approximately 50 milliseconds for the forces to reach peak levels. Unfortunately, these small proprioceptive nerve endings are easily damaged, which slows the stabilization response or even leads to inappropriate muscle recruitment patterns. Fatigue, vibrations, minor injury, edema, inflammation, dehydration, and low blood glucose will reduce the speed of response such that the pattern of muscle recruitment is slowed and is less likely to result in stabilization of a joint prior to the development of peak force in the joint. This leaves the joint very susceptible to injury. Fortunately, it is also relatively easy to reset the proprioceptive reflexes; simple exercises can be used to relearn the correct movement pattern and speed up the reflex contractions that will stabilize the joint, irrespective of the other contributing factors (Roberts 2007, 2008, 2009).

The current study with log haulers has documented eating patterns, blood glucose and vigilance levels, and physiological responses in drivers during typical workdays. It repeated the measures on days when blood glucose levels were stabilized through an eating regimen. Preliminary findings of the study have shown that performance on a complex visual task improves when blood glucose levels are stable. In addition, the study improved movements and reflexes related to driving tasks. These findings should encourage both companies and drivers to implement diet and physical activity programs designed to improve driving performance.

Populations Best Served by Program

This program is suitable for all types of commercial drivers, including long- and short-haul truck drivers, bus and taxi drivers and couriers, and heavy equipment operators. Many of these occupations require long periods of time in the sitting posture with little opportunity to move and stretch. They also all require a high degree of concentration in the face of repetition and monotony. Many of these occupations are not highly paid.

Tips for Working Across Sectors

In business and industry, the outcomes of a program for increased physical activity are placed into a very clear framework of profit versus loss. Profit and loss are easily reported and are of great interest to the media and educational sectors. Thus, when the outcomes of an industry-sponsored project are communicated with the media and educational sectors, the project gains a much larger audience than would otherwise be possible.

For example, presenting at industry conferences provides an opportunity to describe the program to the target audience. Typically these conferences are attended by the editors of industry-specific publications who can then be approached to include articles about the program in their newsletters and magazines. Because the program is taking a very different approach to a costly and difficult problem for industry, it becomes newsworthy. Likewise, local media are interested in the health of local

business, and because the program combines financial gain (less cost associated with workers' compensation) with social gain (improved health and wellness), it may attract national or even international attention.

The scientific aspect of the data can be presented in the educational sector by describing programs in books and peer-reviewed publications and linking the program to an educational site. For example, a previous study with forestry (silviculture) workers called Fit to Plant established a resource webpage that is hosted on the website of a postsecondary institution (Selkirk College), where it receives well over 15,000 hits annually. The program is used as a case study by instructors in the forestry program, the health and human services programs, and the business programs of the college.

Lessons Learned

For a program to be successful, it must become part of the culture of the organization. Workers will not give the program credence unless all levels within the organization, including unions and management, endorse it. Management must actively demonstrate that it is behind the program in a meaningful way, proving support in the form of time, money, and other aspects. Furthermore, the organization must repeat its endorsement consistently for at least four years before a program becomes incorporated into the culture of the organization.

Workers must feel respected throughout program implementation. Their concerns must be validated or they will not be willing to consider lifestyle changes. Part of this comes from recognition by management regarding the effort each worker makes to do his or her job well, and part of it comes from the value that managers and peers place on the program. The program implementation team must be very aware of this culture of respect and must foster it at all levels. The program must be contextually and culturally specific, and each worker should believe that the program has been customized to meet his needs. Once workers are engaged in the program, the program staff must work to maintain focus and momentum throughout the course of the program.

Each participant, supervisor, and manager must receive an intrinsic reward from the program. The reward will be different for different levels and individuals within the organization, but it should be clearly identified, recognized, and encouraged at every opportunity.

Additional Reading and Resources

The program materials can be viewed at www.selkirk.ca/research/faculty/trucking/.

The tree planting program is available at www.selkirk.ca/treeplanting/

Dinsmore, K., B. MacIntosh, and D. Roberts. Quantifying physiological workload of employees in a plywood processing mill. *Appl. Physiol. Nutr. Met.* Submitted.

Lemaire, J., J. Wallace, K. Dinsmore, and D. Roberts. 2011. Food for thought: An exploratory study of how physicians experience poor workplace nutrition. *Nutr. J.* 10:18.

Roberts, D., and S. Donnelly. 2006. The fluid balance and sweat rates during manual timber harvesting [abstract]. *Med. Sci. Sports Exerc.* 38:S173.

References

Caraffa, A., G. Cerulli, M. Proietti M, et al. 1996. Prevention of anterior cruciate ligament injuries in soccer. *Knee Surg. Sports Traumatol. Arthrosc.* 4:19-21.

Cox, D.J., L.A. Gonder-Frederick, B.P. Kovatchev, D.M. Julian, and W.L. Clarke. 2000. Progressive hypoglycemia's impact on driving simulation performance: Occurrence, awareness and correction. *Diabetes Care* 23:163-70.

Hoffman, M., and G.V. Payne. 1995. The effects of proprioceptive ankle disk training on healthy subjects. *J. Orthop. Sports Phys. Ther.* 21:90-3.

Lemaire, J., J. Wallace, K. Dinsmore, A. Lewin, W. Ghali, and D. Roberts. 2010. Physician nutrition and cognition during work hours: Effect of a nutrition based intervention. *BMC Health Serv. Res.* 10:241.

Li, G., L.P. Baker, M.W. Lamb, J.G. Grabowski, and G.W. Rebok. 2002. Human factors in aviation crashes involving older pilots. *Aviat. Space Environ. Med.* 73:134-8.

Lieberman, H., G. Bathalon, C. Falco, M. Kramer, C. Moran, and P. Niro. 2005. Severe decrements in cognition function and mood induced by sleep loss, heat, dehydration, and undernutrition during simulated combat. *Biol. Psychiatry* 57:422-9.

Roberts, D. 2003. Effects of physiological status of tree-planters on occupational injury and planting productivity and quality (pp. 1-29). Federal Way, WA: Weyerhaeuser Company, North American Forestlands Division.

Roberts, D. 2005. The occupational athlete: Fitness nutrition and hydration. *Med. Sci. Sports Exerc.* Mini-symposium, Nashville TN.

Roberts, D. 2007. Fitness levels, dietary intake and injury rates in heli-ski guides [abstract]. *Med. Sci. Sports Exerc.* 39:S217.

Roberts, D. 2008a. Case studies: a) biochemical evaluation of physical and mental stress in the workplace, b) characterization of workload in the workplace, and c) assessment of workload during manual timber harvesting. In: *Hard Work: Physically Demanding Occupations, Tests and Performance.* B. Sharkey and P. Davis, Eds. Champaign, IL: Human Kinetics.

Roberts, D. 2008b. Efficacy of carbohydrate feeding on occupational injury rate and productivity in reforestation workers in energy deficit [abstract]. *Med. Sci. Sports Exerc.* 40(5 Suppl. 1):S160.

Roberts, D. 2009a. Efficacy effects of chronic consumption of electrolyte beverages by mill workers on markers of metabolic syndrome [abstract]. *Med. Sci. Sports Exerc.* Suppl.

Roberts, D. 2009b. The occupational athlete: Injury reduction and productivity enhancement in reforestation workers. In: *ACSM's Worksite Health Handbook: A Guide to Building Healthy Companies* (pp. 309-16). 2nd ed. N.P. Pronk, Ed. Champaign, IL: Human Kinetics.

Roberts, D., and K. Dinsmore. 2008. Physiological profile and work load assessment of helicopter pilots and ground crews working at Heli-ski lodges [abstract]. *Appl. Physiol. Nutr. Metab.* 33(Suppl. 1).

Stevens, A.B., W.R. McKane, P.M. Bell, P. Bell, D.J. King, and J.R. Hayes. 1989. Psychomotor performance and counterregulatory responses during mild hypoglycemia in healthy volunteers. *Diabetes Care.* 12(1):12-7.

Strachan, M.W., I.F. Deary, F.M. Ewing, S.S. Ferguson, M.J. Young, and B.M. Frier. 2001. Acute hypoglycemia impairs the functioning of the central but not peripheral nervous system. *Physiol. Behav.* 72(1-2):83-92.

CHAPTER 24

Instant Recess

Integrating Physical Activity Into the Workday at Kaiser Permanente South Bay Health Center

Antronette (Toni) K. Yancey, MD, MPH
UCLA School of Public Health

Alison K. Herrmann, PhD
UCLA School of Public Health

Tiffany Creighton, MPH
Kaiser Permanente South Bay Health Center

NPAP Tactics and Strategies Used in This Program

Business and Industry Sector

STRATEGY 1: Identify, summarize, and disseminate best practices, models, and evidence-based physical activity interventions in the workplace.

Health Care Sector

STRATEGY 3: Use a health care systems approach to promote physical activity and to prevent and treat physical inactivity.

Kaiser Permanente (KP) invests in promoting physical activity at both the population level, through its community benefit initiatives, and the individual level, through its clinical prevention services for patients and its work-site wellness program. One KP facility, South Bay Health Center, seeking to augment and complement its existing work-site wellness program, adopted Instant Recess (IR), an evidence-based strategy that integrates brief group activity breaks into the everyday routine of the workday during nondiscretionary time. IR breaks are scientifically designed to maximize engagement, enjoyment, and energy expenditure while minimizing injury risk and perceived exertion among the typical sedentary overweight employee.

Program Description

KP South Bay Health Center is a large urban medical center located in Southern Los Angeles County. One of 12 medical centers in the KP Southern California Medical Group, the KP South Bay facility employs 3,150 staff and 428 physicians throughout its 65 departments. During the first eight months of 2011, South Bay launched IR in 12 departments. In a staggered rollout, the center's wellness coordinator introduces IR and implements it in collaboration with unit-based teams (UBTs) that consist of departmental employees and managers charged with working to achieve department goals and objectives. All departments that have adopted

IR to date have adapted the activity to suit the nature of their work environment and schedule as well as the preferences of their employees. Examples of the different types of departments in which IR has been integrated successfully include the call center, the laboratory and pathology department, and an inpatient unit. Implementation in these departments is detailed next.

The call center was the first department to launch IR at KP. The 85 agents employed in this department work four- to eight-hour shifts, during which nearly all time is spent seated, with little opportunity for physical activity. In late 2010, prior to the launch of IR, the department established as priorities lowering the high rates of reported injuries and sick leave, issues commonly experienced in call centers.

IR was formally introduced to the call center UBT at its November 2010 meeting. At that time, team members were uncertain about the feasibility of implementing IR in their department, where the nature of the work dictates that staff do not take breaks together as a group (i.e., agents need to be available to accept incoming calls). Additionally, middle managers expressed concern regarding potential adverse consequences of IR for performance numbers and hold times. Staff members were concerned about who would lead IR and whether other employees would voluntarily participate. Ultimately, the UBT agreed to consider ways to implement IR prior to its next monthly meeting. Two months following the wellness coordinator's introduction of the IR concept, in large part attributable to strong support from upper management, IR was launched in the call center. To minimize the impact on performance and hold times, the UBT decided to implement a rolling IR, staggered such that each of the department's eight teams conducted the breaks one at a time, beginning at 10:30 a.m. and 3:30 p.m. each day. Team leaders worked with the wellness coordinator to create a shortened IR (4-5 minutes vs. 10 minutes), allowing call agents to stand up, move, and stretch, with the goal of reducing ergonomic strain, since ergonomic injuries were the leading source of injury in the call

center in 2010. Team leaders gained increased confidence and comfort in leading IR by practicing with new agents, who were training in a separate location, prior to leading IR breaks among existing call center staff.

The UBT decided to launch IR in a fashion similar to that of a movie premiere. Announcements, "Recess is coming January 20, 2011," were posted throughout the call center. On the launch date, staff members were permitted to wear workout clothes and were provided with "goodie bags" containing healthy living resources (e.g., pedometers, water bottles, and fitness logs). The wellness coordinator and several members of upper management were present for the IR launch, visibly and verbally signaling their enthusiastic and unqualified support.

The call center UBT has developed creative solutions to issues that arose following the implementation of IR, including an increase in hold times. The duration of IR was further shortened from four to two minutes, and team groupings were made more flexible so that employees on a call when their team began IR could complete that call and join another team for IR after the call had ended.

Following the successful launch of IR in the call center, upper management requested that the wellness coordinator launch IR in the laboratory, a department that had recently experienced multiple significant changes, including a need for employees to reapply for their job positions, a move to a temporary space, shift changes, new processes, new equipment, and a new computer system. Employee morale had suffered, and workplace injury reports had soared.

Lab managers were initially skeptical of IR and did not think that it would work for their large and busy department. Upper-management executives intervened, however, relaying positive changes experienced following adoption of IR in the call center—a department with more employees and less flexible work schedules than the lab. The wellness coordinator again chose to implement IR with the help of the UBT, whose members were enthusiastic about IR after she

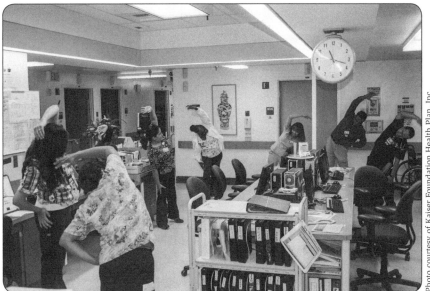

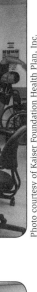

Photo courtesy of Kaiser Foundation Health Plan, Inc.

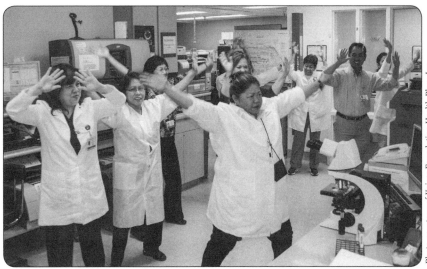

Photo courtesy of Kaiser Foundation Health Plan, Inc.

led them through a break. Staff reported that their department was already set up for IR since the breaks could be incorporated at the end of two daily department huddles, during which all areas of the lab stop work and provide an update on their work status. Additionally, UBT members were optimistic about the potential for IR to improve group cohesiveness in the lab.

Since the entire lab was able to do IR together, energy and excitement levels surrounding implementation of IR were even greater in this department than in the call center. Several lab staff requested to take turns leading IR and adapted the breaks to correspond to their personal and cultural preferences. Employees did the chicken dance, incorporated meringue dance moves, and choreographed moves to Michael Jackson's "Beat It" (by far the most popular break). In addition to taking part in the two regularly scheduled daily IR breaks held at the conclusion of staff huddles, lab staff reported using IR at other times to lower their stress levels. For example, a clinical lab scientist commented that running a certain series of tests is time-sensitive and very stressful for her. Since IR implementation, she often announces to her team that an IR is needed after finishing the test series to provide a fresh start before moving on to the next task.

After launching IR in several additional and smaller outpatient departments, the wellness coordinator decided to explore the feasibility of IR in an inpatient setting. Managers of Unit 3000, an inpatient medical-surgical floor that had employee attendance issues, were approached to gauge their interest in IR. They were very supportive and passed the idea along to the UBT. Although initially skeptical, after participating in an IR break the UBT enthusiastically agreed to adopt IR and nominated two charge nurses to lead the department activity.

Once again, the wellness coordinator worked with the UBT to fit IR into the departmental work schedule, ultimately settling on the end of peak times (e.g., medication passing, change of shift) to avoid compromising patient care. Unit 3000 decided to implement IR three times per day, so that staff on each of the three shifts (day, evening, and night) would have an opportunity to participate. During the day and evening IR, available staff members gather around the nurses' station, inform the patients and visitors that IR is about to begin, and invite them to join in—which often occurs. The department has made IR its own by starting breaks with standard stretches and movements led by the charge nurse and then asking each employee to lead the group through free-style movements of his or her choice. Recently, a patient being discharged joined IR and commented that she had heard the music all week and was happy that she could finally participate, even while seated in her wheelchair!

Program Evaluation

The impact of IR at the KP South Bay Health Center was evaluated with both subjective and objective measures. Subjective measures were used to capture changes in staff morale and the working environment associated with IR as reported by departmental managers and staff. Objective measures were used to assess changes in absenteeism and injury rates in relation to IR implementation.

Subjective Measures

Since launching IR in the call center, managers have observed improvements in the department's morale. On days that the leads forget to start IR, the staff request it, and many staff members have reported that it helps them to manage their stress. During a recent Employee Assistance Program event at the call center, several staff members reported lower levels of stress since the launch of IR.

Management also has observed a change in morale and collaboration within the lab. Line staff report that doing IR with their managers has made them feel more connected and that the managers seem more approachable. As noted earlier, the laboratory was under construction and was to move to a new location in fall 2011; a major concern of the staff when they met with construction planners was that they wanted their new space to allow them enough room to continue IR. As is typical for many scientific personnel, the lab staff tends to be quiet and introverted, which did not foster a collaborative work environment. IR has brought the entire team together, from management to lab assistants, and promoted bonding. This department was recently asked to attend the Torrance Leadership Conference, a training workshop for the city's business leaders. Four employees from the lab attended the conference and led the group in a five-minute IR break to "Staying Alive." It was considered the highlight of the day. Many business leaders said that IR was an easy and low-cost way to give their staff a boost in energy and reduce their sick time and injury rates.

There is ample evidence that Unit 3000 has perceived IR very positively. "I feel that Instant Recess takes you out of the stress of the moment," said one of the RNs, quoted in the monthly KP newsletter. "You come back with a new attitude and have a smile on your face."

Seven large departments at the South Bay Health Center have implemented IR, and four other departments are in the process of training and developing their work plan for IR. Leaders of several regularly scheduled meetings now incorporate IR into those meetings, and the program has earned a slot on the agenda of the monthly meeting of department administrators. At a recent meeting with approximately 100 volunteers for the medical center, staff incorporated IR into the meeting, following a period of extended sitting. The mood in the room changed, and the activity sparked requests from many of the volunteers that IR be incorporated into their day on a regular basis. One older volunteer said that he volunteered in order "to get out of my house and get up on my feet!"

Objective Measures

Each of the three large departments implementing IR for at least two months has documented improvements in injury rates, absenteeism, or both. Data retrieval and analyses were conducted jointly by each department director and the wellness coordinator.

Decreases in sick time and injuries have been observed in the eight months since the call center implemented IR. An evaluation of sick leave in 2010 compared with 2011, for the same pay periods, revealed that the call center experienced a decrease of 1.8 days per full-time employee (FTE) (from 7.5 to 5.7). Injuries, as reflected in accepted claims (those deemed legitimate by KP's workers' compensation department), have decreased from 3 in 2010 to 0 during the same time period in 2011 among the department's 85 employees, with no ergonomic injuries reported since IR's launch.

The laboratory-pathology department has seen substantive changes. This department did not previously have high absenteeism rates, having met its goals in this area, and no change was apparent. However, a comparison of 2010 and 2011 data showed that the department

recorded a 35 percent decrease in injury reports among its 86 employees. Accepted claims have decreased from 18 to 12, again with no ergonomic injuries reported since IR began.

Unit 3000 has experienced a significant reduction in sick leave of 1.9 days per FTE (from 6.2 to 4.3) compared with the same time period in 2010, and the unit has not had a workplace injury in the two months since implementing IR.

Linkage to the National Physical Activity Plan

KP's approach bridges two of the NPAP's sectors: the Business and Industry Sector and the Health Care Sector.

Strategy 1: Identify, summarize, and disseminate best practices, models, and evidence-based physical activity interventions in the workplace. Implementation of Instant Recess falls within Strategy 1 of the Business and Industry Sector. Specifically, IR aligns with the tactics recommending that specific approaches be developed that appeal to work sites with large numbers of lower-income and ethnic minority workers and that key business and industry leaders play central roles in influencing their peers (Pronk & Kottke 2009). IR provides unique opportunities to model physical activity promotion by "walking the talk" for patients, partners, grantees, and competitors (Boyle, et al. 2009).

Strategy 3: Use a health care systems approach to promote physical activity and to prevent and treat physical inactivity. IR implementation resides in Strategy 3 of the Health Care Sector. The tactic most consistent with this KP approach is the identification and evaluation of best practices for physical activity in health care, particularly those effective in population segments at high risk of physical inactivity. However, KP also builds on successful programs already in place to create a central role for physical activity, in this case adopting an evidence-based model that influences sociocultural norms and grants high visibility and priority to physical activity.

Evidence Base Used During Program Development

A growing body of evidence suggests that interrupting prolonged periods of sitting and other sedentary behaviors, and increasing engagement in moderate to vigorous physical activity, are necessary to promote well-being and prevent chronic disease (Danaei et al., 2009; Owen et al., 2009; Bankoski et al., 2011; Thorp et al., 2011). Workdays are associated with nearly one hour more of sitting than are nonwork days (McCrady & Levine 2009). In fact, the 50-year decline in occupational energy expenditure was recently equated to the caloric imbalance associated with the obesity epidemic (Church, et al. 2011).

Physical activity programs have typically been regarded as the "easiest sell" in worksite wellness (Batt 2009). However, even mature and comprehensive work-site health promotion programs have typically been less successful in influencing physical activity than other risk indicators, such as tobacco use, dietary fat, and blood pressure (Soler et al., 2010; Henke et al., 2011). In part, this may be attributable to dismally low participation rates, particularly among workers at higher risk of chronic disease, and to approaches that use organizations as staging venues for individually targeted education and counseling rather than address the organizational infrastructure (Dishman et al., 1998; Mattson-Koffman et al., 2005; Beresford et al., 2007; Yancey, Pronk, & Cole 2007; Robroek et al, 2009). According to the National Business Group on Health, the typical corporate "pull" strategies that rely on individual motivation (e.g., onsite fitness centers and classes, gym membership subsidies) are being abandoned by many corporations, which consider these strategies to be costly and ineffective (Yancey 2010).

Emerging models of policy and environmental intervention enhance regularity and sustainability of participation by making short bouts of activity the default option. The viability of these models is predicated on (1) the very low average adult physical activity levels (eight minutes per day) documented by objective monitoring (Troiano et al. 2008); (2) the modest amount of physical activity delivered by most workplace interventions—slightly more than 600 steps per day (Conn, et al. 2009); (3) the association of monitored activity and compulsory participation with higher levels of adherence and greater effectiveness, particularly among the sedentary (Seymour, et al. 2004; PAGAC 2008); (4) emerging evidence of a link between moderate to vigorous physical activity that is accumulated in bouts of 10 minutes or more and body mass index and waist circumference (Strath, et al. 2008); and (5) the potential of these models to deliver both individual and organizational benefits.

Populations Best Served by the Program

Workers lower in the organizational hierarchy usually derive greater benefits from "active by default" practices and policies than do managers and executives (Yancey, Bastani, & Glenn 2007). Lower-level workers are at higher risk for inactivity and associated chronic illnesses and injuries, and thus small incremental changes are more likely to produce health and economic benefits. These workers also have less private space and greater exposure to others, increasing the influence of the social interaction sparked by IR. Typical workplace culture dictates that good employees are those who are work-focused, that is, "chained to their desks"; they arrive early, leave late, and remain tethered to their smartphones or tablet computers and laptops when traveling. Consequently, structured group activity breaks tend to be more appealing to blue and pink collar or lower-level administrative staff whose hours are closely supervised and controlled (e.g., workers who punch a time clock) than to "knowledge economy" workers who are paid to accomplish certain outcomes and have flexible schedules and decisional latitude. In addition, IR builds on such cultural assets as dance, music and sports traditions, and collectivist versus individualist community values.

Workplace physical activity promotion is particularly critical among less affluent workers, given the obstacles of lack of discretionary time (e.g., longer workdays and commutes), less decisional latitude, less flexible time schedules, more pressing basic priorities, and fewer resources for active leisure (Wolin, et al. 2008; Yancey 2010; Day 2006; Marcus, et al. 2006). In 2008, 23 percent of whites in the United States reported no leisure activity, compared with 32 percent of blacks and 35 percent of Hispanics, respectively (CDC 2008). Thus, lowering the "cost" of physical activity participation for workers by intervening on paid time is critical. Diffusion of active living practices in socioeconomically and ethnically diverse populations is more likely to occur at work than in other settings (Sorenson, et al. 2005). Spillover of activity breaks from work and school to outside life has been documented (Yancey, et al. 2006; Donnelly, et al. 2009).

Lessons Learned

KP South Bay Health Center provides an excellent example of important issues associated with successfully implementing and maintaining IR. As the intervention spread throughout the medical center, the importance of factors such as involvement of individuals at multiple levels of the organization (i.e., upper management, middle management, supervisors and line staff), clear and unwavering leadership support and engagement, tailoring of the program to suit the needs of the organization and preferences of employees, and the presence of readily identifiable and committed program champions ("sparkplugs," in IR parlance) became increasingly evident. Each of these factors has been demonstrated in prior research to be critical to the success of IR and similar innovations (Barr-Anderson, et al. 2011; Hopkins, et al. 2012).

KP South Bay Health Center represents a "perfect storm" of the key elements needed to make IR work. The wellness coordinator, a well-connected and public health–trained employee, selected IR as a possible solution to her organization's challenges, and implementation and evaluation of the program became a part of her job responsibilities and accountability. Individuals across the organizational hierarchy were involved and actively demonstrated their support for IR as it was being launched at departments throughout the health center. When managers or leaders who were hesitant to begin IR in their departments presented roadblocks, these roadblocks were easily managed when upper management communicated support for IR to middle management.

As in many large organizations, each department within the Health Center has a unique climate, workflow, and schedule. With this in mind, the wellness coordinator engaged each department UBT and provided technical assistance and troubleshooting to encourage the team to take ownership of IR and select the best method by which to implement it. This collaboration has allowed for ongoing modifications in IR that keep pace with changing departmental needs and staff preferences, such as shortening the breaks in the call center and sharing responsibility for choosing and leading activity among participants in the breaks on Unit 3000.

The importance of an energetic leader, or sparkplug, within each department was also apparent. Having someone available, energetic, and motivated to gather the staff, encourage participation, and lead other staff members through movements proved to be a critical component of IR's success in a department. However, having only one sparkplug could jeopardize the sustainability of IR within that department. Momentum may be difficult to maintain if that person is out of the office (on sick leave or vacation), transfers out of the department, or leaves the organization. Having a higher ratio of sparkplugs to staff members improves IR's sustainability (Maxwell, et al. 2011).

Finally, throughout the implementation process, leaders at the health center have noted a synergistic energy created by IR. As more departments successfully launched IR and demonstrated positive results, more managers and staff have requested that IR be brought to their departments. Initial levels of resistance to IR expressed by departmental managers and staff have lessened significantly. In fact, a recent feature on IR in the KP Southern California employee newsletter and website resulted in five new requests from other departments for the wellness coordinator's assistance in bringing IR to their employees.

Tips for Working Across Sectors

"Minimal intensity" intervention strategies may be particularly appealing to the vast majority of employers who, unlike KP, do not have the will, resources, or capacity to implement comprehensive work-site wellness programs. Documented return on investment in economic and health benefits is frequently cited by employers as a critical factor in their willingness to adopt brief group activity breaks, and this chapter illustrates the organizational benefits of IR to KP. This approach to increasing physical activity is especially relevant to the health care sector, as KP is both an employer and a health care delivery system.

Additional Reading and Resources

Instant Recess Products and Resources are available at www.toniyancey.com.

Toolkits for implementation of Instant Recess are available at www.keenfootwear.com/recess.

Details about the development and rationale of Instant Recess are available in Yancey, T. 2010. *Instant Recess: Building a Fit Nation 10 Minutes at a Time*. Berkeley, CA: University of California Press. This book is available from the publisher, in many Barnes & Noble and BooksAMillion stores, or online at www.amazon.com or www.bn.com.

References

Bankoski, A., T. Harris, J. McClain, R. Brychta, P. Caserotti, K. Chen, D. Berrigan, R. Troiano, and A. Koster. 2011. Sedentary activity associated with metabolic syndrome independent of physical activity. *Diabetes Care* 34:497-503.

Barr-Anderson, D., M. AuYoung, M. Whitt-Glover, B. Glenn, and A. Yancey. 2011. Structural integration of brief bouts of physical activity into organizational routine: A systematic review of the literature. *Am. J. Prev. Med.* 40:76-93.

Batt, M.E. 2009. Physical activity interventions in the workplace: The rationale and future direction for workplace wellness. *Br. J. Sports Med.* 43:47-8.

Beresford, S.A, E. Locke, S. Bishop, et al. Worksite study promoting activity and changes in eating (PACE): Design and baseline results. Obesity (Silver Spring). 2007;15 Suppl 1:4S-15S.

Boyle, M., S. Lawrence, L. Schwarte, L. Samuels, and W. McCarthy. 2009. Health care providers' perceived role in changing environments to promote healthy eating and physical activity: Baseline findings from health care providers participating in the healthy eating, active communities program. *Pediatrics* 123(Suppl. 5):S293-300.

Centers for Disease Control and Prevention. 2008. *US Physical Activity Statistics: State Comparisons*. Division of Nutrition, Physical Activity, and Obesity, National Center for Chronic Disease Prevention and Health Promotion. Centers for Disease Control and Prevention. Atlanta, GA.

Church, T.S., D.M. Thomas, C. Tudor-Locke, P.T. Katzmarzyk, C.P Earnest, et al. 2011. Trends over 5 decades in U.S. occupation-related physical activity and their associations with obesity. *PLoS One* 6:e19657.

Conn, V., A. Hafdahl, P. Cooper, L. Brown, and S. Lusk. 2009. Meta-analysis of workplace physical activity interventions. *Am. J. Prev. Med.* 37:330-9.

Danaei, G., E.L. Ding, D. Mozaffarian, B. Taylor, J. Rehm, C.J. Murray, et al. 2009. The preventable causes of death in the U.S.: Comparative risk assessment of dietary, lifestyle, and metabolic risk factors. *PLoS Med.* 6:e1000058.

Day, K. 2006. Active living and social justice: Planning for physical activity in low-income, black, and Latino communities. *J. Am. Plann. Assoc.* 72:88-99.

Dishman, R.K., B. Oldenburg, H. O'Neal, and R.J. Shephard. 1998. Worksite physical activity interventions. *Am. J. Prev. Med.* 15(4):344-61.

Donnelly, J.E., J.L. Greene, C.A. Gibson, et al. 2009. Physical Activity Across the Curriculum (PAAC): A randomized, controlled trial to promote physical activity and diminish overweight and obesity in elementary school children. *Prev. Med.* 49:336-41.

Henke R.M., R.Z. Goetzel, J. McHugh, and F. Isaac. Recent experience in health promotion at Johnson & Johnson: Lower health spending, strong return on investment. Health Aff (Millwood). 2011;30(3):490-499.

Hopkins, J.M,, B.A. Glenn, B.L. Cole, W. McCarthy, and A. Yancey. 2012. Implementing organizational physical activity and healthy eating strategies on paid time: Process evaluation of the UCLA WORKING pilot study. *Health Educ Res.* 27(3):385-398.

Marcus, B., D. Williams, P.M. Dubbert, J.F. Sallis, A.C. King, A.K. Yancey, et al. 2006. Physical activity interventions: What we know and what we need to know. A statement from the American Heart Association. *Circulation* 114:2739-52.

Matson-Koffman, D.M., J.N. Brownstein, J.A. Neiner, and M.L. Greaney. 2005. A site-specific literature review of policy and environmental interventions that promote physical activity and nutrition for cardiovascular health: What works? *Am. J. Health Promot.* 19:167-93.

Maxwell, A.E., A.K. Yancey, M. AuYoung, J.J. Guinyard, W.J. McCarthy, and R. Bastani. 2011. Dissemination of organizational wellness practice and policy change: A mid-point evaluation of the L.A. basin REACH US Center of Excellence in Eliminating Disparities. *Prev. Chronic Dis.* 8(5) [serial online].

McCrady, S.K., and J.A. Levine. 2009. Sedentariness at work: How much do we really sit? *Obesity* 17(11):2103-5.

Owen, N., A. Bauman, and W. Brown. 2009. Too much sitting: A novel and important predictor of chronic disease risk? *Br. J. Sports Med.* 43(2):81-3.

Physical Activity Guidelines Advisory Committee (PAGAC). Physical Activity Guidelines Advisory Committee Report. 2008. Washington, DC: U.S. Department of Health and Human Services. www.health.gov/paguidelines/committeereport.aspx.

Pronk, N.P., and T.E. Kottke. 2009. Physical activity promotion as a strategic corporate priority to improve worker health and business performance. *Prev. Med.* 49:316-21.

Robroek, S., F.J. van Lenthe, P. van Empelen, and A. Burdorf. 2009. Determinants of participation in worksite health promotion programs: A systematic review. *Int. J. Behav. Nutr. Phys. Act.* 6:26.

Seymour, J.D., A.L. Yaroch, M. Serdula, H.M. Blanck, and L.K. Khan. 2004. Impact of nutrition environmental interventions on point-of-purchase behavior in adults: A review. *Prev. Med.* 39(Suppl. 2):S108-36.

Soler, R., K. Leeks, S. Razi, et al. 2010. A systematic review of selected interventions for worksite health promotion. *Am. J. Prev. Med.* 38(2S):S237-62.

Sorensen, G., E. Barbeau, A.M. Stoddard, M.K. Hunt, K. Kaphingst, and L. Wallace. 2005. Promoting behavior change among working-class, multiethnic workers: Results of the healthy directions—small business study. *Am. J. Public Health* 95(8):1389-95.

Strath, S.J., R.G. Holleman, D.L. Ronis, A.M. Swartz, and C.R. Richardson. 2008. Objective physical activity accumulation in bouts and nonbouts and relation to markers of obesity in US adults. *Prev. Chronic Dis.* 5:A131.

Thorp, A., N. Owen, M. Neuhaus, and D. Dunstan. 2011. Sedentary behaviors and subsequent health outcomes in adults. *Am. J. Prev. Med.* 41:207-15.

Troiano, R., D. Berrigan, K. Dodd, L. Masse, T. Tilertand, and M. McDowell. 2008. Physical activity in the United States measured by accelerometer. *Med. Sci. Sports Exerc.* 40:181-8.

Wolin, K.Y., G.G. Bennett, L.H. McNeill, G. Sorensen, and K.M. Emmons. 2008. Low discretionary time as a barrier to physical activity and intervention uptake. *Am. J. Health Behav.* 32:563-9.

Yancey, A. K. (2010). *Instant recess: Building a fit nation 10 minutes at a time.* Berkeley: University of California Press.

Yancey, A.K., R. Bastani, and B. Glenn. 2007. Racial/ethnic disparities in health status. In: *Changing the U.S. Health Care System: Key Issues in Health Services, Policy, and Management.* 3rd ed. R. Andersen, T.H. Rice, and G.F. Kominski, Eds. San Francisco: Jossey-Bass.

Yancey, A.K., L.B. Lewis, J.J. Guinyard, D.C. Sloan, L.M. Nascimento, L. Galloway-Gilliam, A. Diamant, and W.J. McCarthy. 2006. Putting promotion into practice: The African Americans Building a Legacy of Health organizational wellness program. *Health Promot. Pract.* 7:233S-46S.

Yancey, A., N. Pronk, and B. Cole. 2007. Environmental and policy approaches to obesity prevention in the workplace. In: *Handbook of obesity prevention : a resource for health professionals.* S. Kumanyika and R. Brownson, Eds. New York: Springer; 2007.

CHAPTER 25

ChooseWell LiveWell

An Employee Health Promotion Partnership Between Saint Paul Public Schools and HealthPartners

Abigail S. Katz, PhD
HealthPartners and HealthPartners Institute for Education and Research

Terri Bopp, MPA
Saint Paul Public Schools

Richard O. Burmeister, III, BAS
HealthPartners and Saint Paul Public Schools

Suzanne P. Kelly, MS
Saint Paul Public Schools

Nicolaas P. Pronk, PhD
HealthPartners, HealthPartners Institute for Education and Research, and Harvard University

NPAP Tactics and Strategies Used in This Program

Business and Industry Sector

STRATEGY 1: Identify, summarize, and disseminate best practices, models, and evidence-based physical activity interventions in the workplace.

STRATEGY 2: Encourage business and industry to interact with all other sectors to identify opportunities to promote physical activity within the workplace and throughout society.

STRATEGY 3: Educate business and industry leaders regarding their role as positive agents of change to promote physical activity and healthy lifestyles within the workplace and throughout society, giving particular consideration to efforts targeting low-resource populations.

STRATEGY 4: Develop legislation and policy agendas that promote employer-sponsored physical activity programs while protecting individual employees' and dependents' rights.

STRATEGY 5: Develop a plan for monitoring and evaluating worksite health promotion programs.

This chapter describes a multiyear community partnership aimed at improving the health and well-being of employees of the Saint Paul Public Schools (SPPS) system in Minnesota. In partnership with HealthPartners, a not-for-profit, member-governed integrated health system, SPPS implemented a worksite health promotion program that focused on creating a culture of wellness among employees. The partnership, which began in 2005 with a pilot program at 9 sites and expanded to 80 sites by 2011, includes a variety of physical activity interventions. The program, titled ChooseWell LiveWell, has resulted in sustained health improvements among the more than 5,800 employees in the school district.

Program Description

The ChooseWell LiveWell program was developed in partnership with HealthPartners in an effort to improve employee health and address the affordability of health care for the SPPS district. The goal of the program is to cultivate a wellness culture within the school system for the purpose of improving employee health and to model positive lifestyle behaviors for students in the district.

Saint Paul Public School System

As Minnesota's second-largest school district, SPPS consists of 64 schools with a total of 80 sites, more than 5,800 employees, and a diverse student body. The district is committed to the health and well-being of both employees and students.

Employee Wellness Programs

Effective health promotion programs include multiple components, most notably an individual health risk assessment and programs to support employee health. In each year of ChooseWell LiveWell, the program has offered employees an online self-reported health assessment as well as a variety of wellness program options of varying lengths, ranging from eight weeks to a full calendar year (table 25.1). Many of the programs have been well received and are repeated annually; additional program offerings vary each school year. More than one third of all program offerings have focused specifically on physical activity. Other activities, such as those related to stress management, often include a physical activity component.

Beginning as a pilot program and developing into a comprehensive wellness program, ChooseWell LiveWell worked to create a strong culture of health at SPPS. Program volunteers and staff promoted available programs, distributed communications, and worked in conjunction with student wellness programs and administration on policy and program development. The program offered incentives to encourage employee participation in ChooseWell LiveWell. The value of the incentives increased over each program year, and all involved some form of preferred health plan benefit—that is, a lower co-pay or deductible for participants. In the first years of the program, employees who participated were given the choice of a $10 medical plan co-pay reduction or a $100 lower deductible. Over time, the incentive evolved to a $20 medical plan co-pay reduction or $200 deductible and a $1,000 difference of the out-of-pocket minimum between participants and nonparticipants.

In the initial two years of the program, employees, retirees, and their covered spouses could participate in ChooseWell LiveWell. Beginning in the third year, and in subsequent years of the program, COBRA members also could participate.

Implementation

The ChooseWell LiveWell program was first implemented in 2005 across different segments of the school system. District schools and offices were invited to participate through an application process. Requirements for a site to participate included a staff member designated as a wellness champion, a functioning wellness committee, and a dedicated wellness bulletin board. In the first year, nine sites were selected: three elementary schools, two middle schools, two high schools, and two administrative buildings.

The program made an effort to connect and partner with other wellness programs within the school district, including one related to the Steps to a HealthierUS grant (Steps), which focused on physical activity at the student level. By leveraging the existing Steps network, ChooseWell LiveWell was able to reach beyond the initial sites selected for the program.

The initial nine sites continued into September 2006. Later that fall, the district launched the employee wellness website. Since that time, the wellness website has served as the hub of the ChooseWell LiveWell program, enabling staff to access wellness information, including program registration, program materials, and related resources. SPPS also enacted a school district-wide wellness policy in year 2.

The wellness policy requires physical activity and nutrition to be addressed for students within the district. Section IX of the wellness policy specifically addresses the valued role of district staff in affecting student wellness:

Table 25.1 SPPS ChooseWell LiveWell Physical Activity Programs by Year

Program year	School year	Program title	Program description
1	2005-2006	10,000 Steps Walk to Key West Hydrate and Head-out	Online walking program Group walking challenge Individual activity program
2	2006-2007	10,000 Steps Get Moving, Get Fit Walkabout Wellness Walking Tour of Italy GetFit Twin Cities Tour de SPPS cycling club	Online walking program 1:1 telephonic coaching Individual activity program Group walking challenge Group walking challenge Individual cycling program
3	2007-2008	10,000 Steps Get Moving, Get Fit Walkabout Wellness Tour de SPPS cycling club Walking Tour of Australia	Online walking program 1:1 telephonic coaching Individual activity program Individual cycling program Group walking challenge
4	2008-2009	10,000 Steps Get Moving, Get Fit Tour de SPPS cycling club Walking Tour of America	Online walking program 1:1 telephonic coaching Individual cycling program Group walking challenge
5	2009-2010	10,000 Steps Get Moving, Get Fit Tour de SPPS cycling club Start to Finish 5K training Exercise Your Right 5K event	Online walking program 1:1 telephonic coaching Individual cycling program Individual training program Group run-walk event
6	2010-2011	10,000 Steps Get Moving, Get Fit Tour de SPPS cycling club Start to Finish 5K training Exercise Your Right 5K event Tri It	Online walking program 1:1 telephonic coaching Individual cycling program Individual training program Group run-walk event Triathlon training online program

"School staff serves as role models for students and are the key to successful implementation of student wellness programs. Therefore, the district and schools should offer staff wellness programs. This may include workshops, and presentations on health promotion, education, and resources that will enhance morale, encourage healthy lifestyles, prevent injury, reduce chronic diseases and foster exceptional role modeling."

The program expanded in year 3 with the addition of 15 sites, for a total of 24 pilot sites out of 80 total sites districtwide. The district strengthened its commitment to wellness in year 3 with the introduction of the employee wellness DVD. This DVD was shown at each new employee orientation, distributed to leaders throughout the district, and posted on the district's wellness website. The video sought to demonstrate to new staff that the district understands and recognizes the key role staff play in facilitating and modeling wellness throughout the district.

By year 4 of the program, 43 of 80 sites were participating. Although the program had implemented several successful short-term walking challenges in previous years, year 4 included the first year-long physical activity challenge, the Walking Tour of America. Participants in the walking tour received pedometers to track daily steps in a virtual tour of the globe.

By September 2009, the beginning of year 5, all 80 sites were participating, which provided the potential to reach all 5,800 employees. The program increased access in year 5 by removing cost barriers and providing programs to employees at no cost. These included health coaching and online health improvement programs.

The 2010-2011 school year marked the sixth year of the ChooseWell LiveWell program. Programs were up and running at all district sites and provided at no cost to employees. Many popular programs from previous years continued, such as the fifth annual Tour de SPPS cycling club. ChooseWell LiveWell added new activities, including the Tri It triathlon training program, a six-week online program that consists of two levels of training to accommodate both beginner and experienced triathletes (table 25.2).

Staffing

At the start of the ChooseWell LiveWell program in 2005, employee wellness in the district was organized through a network of wellness champions. The champions network consisted of SPPS staff serving in a volunteer capacity. The district then created a wellness program manager position. The paid full-time professional who fills this position is dedicated to coordinating employee wellness within the district, including collaborating with the network of volunteer wellness champions. The responsibilities of the wellness program manager include drafting and disseminating wellness communications, creating and delivering health promotion campaigns, distributing monthly wellness newsletters, facilitating group-based health coaching, and serving as the main point of contact for wellness within the district.

The existing network of wellness champions has continued to develop. In a survey of the wellness champions conducted in fall 2009, this group of leaders reported noticeable changes in both employee and student health attributable to the program. Among these changes, champions reported an increased sense of community, a shared goal among employees to make healthy choices, a visible difference in physical activity during work time, and modeling of positive behaviors for the student body (e.g., walking breaks, healthy food choices).

Evidence Base Used During Program Development

The ChooseWell LiveWell program was designed to build progressively toward a full-scale, comprehensive, multicomponent, and multilevel work-site health promotion program that

Table 25.2 SPPS ChooseWell LiveWell Program Expansion

Program year	School year	Number of ChooseWell LiveWell program sites
1	2005-2006	9
2	2006-2007	9
3	2007-2008	24
4	2008-2009	43
5	2009-2010	Districtwide (80+)
6	2010-2011	Districtwide (80+)

resulted in measurable outcomes in employee health and health care costs. Physical activity is often at the heart of health and wellness programming because of its wide-ranging health benefits, and such has been the case with ChooseWell LiveWell. Inactivity is a modifiable risk factor for many chronic conditions, including diabetes, heart disease, back pain, and certain cancers. Low levels of physical activity have been associated with negative consequences in the workplace, including absenteeism, reduced quality and quantity of work, excess health care costs, short-term disability, and overall work impairment. For SPPS, a goal of the wellness program included improving the ability of staff to tackle the challenges of working in a busy urban school system by building a comprehensive program with a focus on physical activity.

The ChooseWell LiveWell program is grounded in the Transtheoretical Model of Behavior Change. Because all individuals vary in their readiness to make changes regarding their health, the program offers a variety of program options, program lengths, and modalities.

Tracking one's own behavior, or self-monitoring, is a key feature of many of the ChooseWell LiveWell program options (tables 25.3 and 25.4). Self-monitoring is most commonly associated with weight loss interventions and also has been applied to physical activity interventions. All of the physical activity programs offered as part of ChooseWell LiveWell include a log for tracking physical activity or a pedometer for participants to track their daily steps. When applied to physical activity interventions, the process of documenting behavior (e.g., pedometer steps) involves purposeful attention to the behavior. To change behaviors, individuals need to pay close attention to their own actions, the conditions under which those actions occur, and the short- and long-term effects of those actions.

Linkage to National Physical Activity Plan

The ChooseWell LiveWell program addresses all five of the strategies included in the Business and Industry Sector of the National Physical Activity Plan (NPAP).

Strategy 1: Identify, summarize, and disseminate best practices, models, and evidence-based physical activity interventions in the workplace. Working in partnership with HealthPartners, the ChooseWell LiveWell program has offered participants new evidence-based physical activity interventions each year of the program. These have included the use of pedometers or logs for tracking physical activity, the use of social support for health behavior change, and interactive online health interventions. America's Health Insurance Plan has summarized and shared the program as an employer–health plan partnership model of best practices in the area of intersectoral collaborations around health and wellness.

Strategy 2: Encourage business and industry to interact with all other sectors to identify opportunities to promote physical activity within the workplace and throughout society. The ChooseWell LiveWell program is a partnership between HealthPartners and SPPS, an urban school district. HealthPartners' mission is to improve the health of its members, its patients, and the community. Through disseminating lessons learned from this six-year partnership, HealthPartners and SPPS set an example for the broader community, representing an effective intersectoral health promotion partnership.

Strategy 3: Educate business and industry leaders regarding their role as positive agents of change to promote physical activity and healthy lifestyles within the workplace and throughout society, giving particular consideration to efforts targeting low-resource populations. Although the ChooseWell LiveWell program has been aimed at employees of SPPS, it was designed to complement and reinforce existing student-focused health promotion efforts in the district. The district serves a diverse urban population, where nearly half of the student body (45 percent) come from a home where English is not the primary language and more than 70 percent are eligible for free and reduce priced lunches.

Strategy 4: Develop legislation and policy agendas that promote employer-sponsored

Table 25.3 Baseline Characteristics of the Sample (*N* = 1,942)

Average age (years)	47
Gender (% female)	72
Average body mass index (kg/m²)	27.4
Race American Indian or Alaska Native Asian or Pacific Islander African American or Black Caucasian Other race Unknown	 1% 3% 5% 80% 2% 9%
Ethnicity (% Hispanic or Latino)	3%

Table 25.4 Physical Activity Indicators Over Time

School year	2005-2006	2006-2007	2007-2008	2008-2009	2009-2010
% Below 2008 DHHS Physical Activity Guideline*	21.1%	14.7%	13.7%	13.9%	13.1%
% Low muscle strengthening	64.5%	58.4%	53.9%	53.6%	52.6%
% Low muscle stretching (flexibility)	41.3%	31.7%	30.7%	31.2%	29.5%
% Sedentary	2.1%	1.0%	1.4%	1.2%	1.4%
Vigorous activity (days/week)	3.01	3.50	3.54	3.54	3.59
Vigorous activity (minutes)	38.39	40.28	39.61	38.40	39.38
Moderate activity (days/week)	4.27	4.59	4.61	4.62	4.58
Moderate activity (minutes)	41.10	41.28	41.73	41.80	42.23
Muscle strengthening (days/week)	1.27	1.45	1.60	1.65	1.69
Flexibility (days/week)	2.48	2.89	3.00	2.93	3.07

Data pertain to the cohort of the Saint Paul Public Schools employees (*N* = 1,942) who participated in all 5 program years. Data from year 6 were not available at the time of publication.

*2008 U.S. Department of Health and Human Services. Guidelines available at www.health.gov/paguidelines/

physical activity programs while protecting individual employees' and dependents' rights. The ChooseWell LiveWell program has evolved to a stage where policy solutions have been implemented to effectively scale the program to reach all employees. A districtwide wellness policy was designed and implemented and now may be used as an example to other school districts to show what is possible.

Strategy 5: Develop a plan for monitoring and evaluating worksite health promotion programs. ChooseWell LiveWell includes an ongoing evaluation component, enabling the program to demonstrate marked changes in employee health. Annually, representatives from the school district and HealthPartners meet to review population-level results obtained through the annual health assessment, as well as outcomes specific to each of the programs offered. Estimated cost savings and return on investment based on changes in the summary health scores are reviewed periodically, and changes in the program are based on a combination of these data and input and feedback from participants.

Lessons Learned

Program leaders identified three major lessons that will assist with future implementation of similar programming: (1) use technology to automate administrative components of the program; (2) cultivate community partnerships and leverage existing partnerships to enhance program success; and (3) introduce gradually and progress mindfully.

The first year of ChooseWell LiveWell was entirely "paper-based." The wellness program manager and SPPS wellness champions administered program registration, materials, and communications manually. The administrative burden placed on these individuals detracted from their ability to focus on motivating and coaching employees and limited the scope of the program's reach. The development and launch of the district wellness website enabled program staff and volunteers to focus their roles on health promotion. The website helped broaden the reach of the program by facilitating 24/7 access to program information, registration, and materials.

Another key lesson was to form partnerships whenever possible. By design, ChooseWell LiveWell was created as a partnership between a local health services organization and a community school district. Annual meetings among leaders from both institutions have helped to facilitate communication and ensure that programming is informed by the latest evidence and industry knowledge and meets the needs of the population. The success of the program also can be attributed to partnerships within the school district. In the first three years of the program, ChooseWell LiveWell staff partnered with staff who worked on student-focused wellness efforts. The program leveraged the existing network of wellness champions from the Steps grant, as well as Minnesota's Statewide Health Improvement Program, to partner and promote program options available to employees throughout the district.

ChooseWell LiveWell was developed at a gradual pace, and monitoring and evaluation were used to inform program changes from year to year. Program expansion was mindful and deliberate, taking into account the needs of the employee population and the latest evidence-based interventions.

Program Evaluation

An advisory group consisting of program staff and leaders from both the school district and HealthPartners convenes annually to evaluate and assess the effectiveness of the program. The group's meetings include a program overview and discussions about the number of sites involved, available program options, and population-level health indicators from the health assessment. The discussions have informed annual program planning and staffing and provide an opportunity for leaders within the school district and HealthPartners to share ideas and discuss planning for the coming year and strategy going forward.

Central to evaluation of the ChooseWell LiveWell program is the employee health assessment offered each fall. Developed by HealthPartners, the health assessment contains a cross section of scientifically validated questions and medically approved algorithms that can accurately predict a person's likelihood of developing diabetes or heart disease in the next two to three years. It includes a series of questions in several areas: personal demographics and health history, self-care, women's health, nutrition, physical activity, alcohol and tobacco, safety, and readiness to change. The health assessment is predictive of health care costs and worker productivity indicators and has been a key instrument for the documentation of the program's impact on health and costs over time.

Annual reports are generated based on health assessment information, including summary health scores. The summary health scores allow for tracking of population health over time and are used to estimate the impact of the program on cost-related outcomes, such as estimated health care cost savings over time. In general, these indicators have shown a progressive improvement in overall population health, resulting in cost savings. In year 5 of the program, HealthPartners estimated cumulative four-year (2005-2006 through 2008-2009) health care cost savings of $632 per participant (or $158 per participant per year), based on the improvements in summary health scores. Additionally, a group of 1,942 unique individuals who participated in the program for all 5 program years, from 2005 to 2010, experienced statistically significant improvements in physical activity.

Tables 25.3 and 25.4 display the descriptive characteristics, key physical activity indicators, and aggregate improvement over time among a unique cohort of 1,942 participants who participated in the first five years of the ChooseWell LiveWell program.

Populations Best Served by the Program

The ChooseWell LiveWell program could be replicated in a variety of employer settings. The wellness website enabled easy communication and access to employees across the many sites in the school district. This program feature would serve employer populations in all sectors well, including small and medium-sized employers, and especially those with offices in many different locations.

Tips for Working Across Sectors

The core ChooseWell LiveWell program components—annual employee health assessment with personalized feedback, a variety of program options, incentives for participation and effective communications—have been demonstrated to be effective in other industries. Key to the success of this program was the leadership support from both major program partners as

well as the focus on building and optimizing a culture of health within the organization. Future programs should consider the specifics of organizational culture and potential impacts on program implementation. The role of the wellness website, for example, may be less impactful in sectors in which computer access is limited.

Additional Reading and Resources

Bandura, A. Health promotion from the perspective of social cognitive theory. *Psychol. Health* 13:623-49.

Burke, L.E., J. Wang, and M.S. Sevick. 2010. Self-monitoring in weight loss: A systematic review of the literature. *J. Am. Diet. Assoc.* 111:92-102.

Helsel, D.L., J.M. Jakicic, and A.D. Otto. 2007. Comparison of techniques for self monitoring, eating and exercise behaviors on weight loss in a correspondence-based intervention. *J. Am. Diet. Assoc.* 107:1807-10.

Hogan, B.E., W. Linden, and B. Najarian. 2002. Social support interventions: Do they work? *Clin. Psychol. Rev.* 22(3):381.

Lindberg, R. 2000. Active living: On the road with the 10,000 steps program. *J. Am. Diet. Assoc.* 100(8):878-9.

Prochaska, J.O., and W.G. Velicer. 1997. The transtheoretical model of health behavior change. *Am. J. Health Promot.* 12(1):38-48.

N.P. Pronk. 2008. Designing a multisector approach to health and wellness. In: America's Health Insurance Plans (AHIP). AHIP innovations in prevention, wellness and risk reduction (pp. 18-21). www.ahip.org/redirect/AHIP_Innovations_Prevention.pdf.

Pronk, N.P., Ed. 2009. *ACSM's Worksite Health Handbook, Second Edition. A Guide to Building Healthy and Productive Companies*. Champaign, IL: Human Kinetics.

Pronk, N.P. 2009. Physical activity promotion in business and industry: Evidence, context, and recommendations for a national plan. *Journal of Physical Activity and Health* 6(Suppl. 2):S220-35.

Pronk, N.P., M. Lowry, M. Maciosek, and J. Gallagher. 2011. The association between health assessment-derived summary health scores and health care costs. *J. Occup. Environ. Med.* 53(8):872-8.

Thygeson, M.N., J.M. Gallagher, K.K. Cross, and N.P. Pronk. 2009. Employee health at BAE Systems: An employer-health plan partnership approach. In: *ACSM's Worksite Health Handbook: A Guide to Building Healthy and Productive Companies* (pp. 318-326). N.P. Pronk, Ed. Champaign, IL: Human Kinetics.

Wantland, D.J., C.J. Portillo, W. Holzemer, R. Slaughter, and E.M. McGhee. 2004. The effectiveness of web-based vs. non-web-based interventions: A meta-analysis of behavioral change outcomes. *J. Med. Internet Res.* 6(4).

CHAPTER 26

What's Next? Keeping NextEra Energy's Health & Well-Being Program Active for 20 Years

Andrew Scibelli, MBA, MA
NextEra Energy

NPAP Tactics and Strategies Used in This Program

Business and Industry Sector

STRATEGY 1: Identify, summarize, and disseminate best practices for physical interventions in the workplace.

STRATEGY 2: Encourage business and industry to interact with all other sectors to identify opportunities to promote physical activity within the workplace and throughout society.

STRATEGY 3: Educate business and industry leaders regarding their role as positive agents of change to promote physical activity and healthy lifestyles within the workplace and throughout society, giving particular consideration to efforts targeting low-resource populations.

STRATEGY 5: Develop a plan for monitoring and evaluating worksite health promotion programs.

The NextEra Energy Health & Well-Being program began in 1991 as FPL-WELL, a wellness program designed for Florida Power & Light Company (FPL) employees. For the next 20 years, the program flourished as it grew and changed in tandem with the company. In January 2009, when FPL changed its name into NextEra Energy, Inc., the FPL-WELL program transitioned into the NextEra Health & Well-Being program. NextEra Energy, which operates in 26 U.S. states and Canada, is one of the leading clean energy companies in the United States and employs nearly 15,000 employees globally. Although the program's offerings have evolved to better target its audience of 33,000 employees, dependents, and retirees, the program has continued to focus primarily on employee health and well-being.

Program Description

The NextEra Health & Well-Being program was implemented 20 years ago at the direction of the CEO of FPL as an employee wellness pro-gram for FPL employees and their families. The program was created primarily as a benefit for employees to help improve their overall health and well-being. A secondary motivation for investing in employee health was the belief that encouraging employees to take charge of their health could help the company control health care costs. The initial program included on-site fitness centers and exercise program-ming, health promotion programming, and an employee assistance program (EAP).

During the program's early years, a network of volunteer wellness coordinators supported the small staff at the corporate headquarters. Together, they worked to engage FPL employees by delivering wellness programs and services to the company's many sites throughout Florida.

Leadership has been fundamental to the program's success. Since its inception in 1991, the program has enjoyed strong support from senior leaders. In fact, leadership constitutes three of the five pillars that support NextEra Energy's corporate culture of health:

1. Senior leadership demonstrates its support by incorporating employee health into the company culture and including health as a potential core competency for senior management, operational leaders, and employees.

2. Operational leaders add further support by encouraging employee participation in wellness programs and being flexible with employees who want to participate in programs during work hours.

3. Management encourages employees to practice self-leadership in health matters by assuming responsibility for their own health and the health of their families.

4. The company reinforces employees' self-leadership and positive health behaviors through well-placed program incentives.

5. Measurement across all aspects of the program—risk status changes, costs, engagement, participation, vendor performance, health claims data, and performance indicators—drives future program growth and direction.

With senior leadership support, NextEra Energy has ingrained wellness into all aspects of the work environment. The company has tobacco-free policies in all facilities, and cafeterias offer subsidized wellness meals. On-site exercise opportunities thrive even in moderate-sized work sites, and signage and coworker watchfulness reinforce safety policies.

Basic health and wellness programming is structured along five focus areas:

1. Fitness centers offer exercise prescriptions, group classes, specialty classes, personal training, fitness assessments, team challenges, and independent exercise opportunities.

2. Health promotion includes office and field ergonomic assessments, health screenings, flu shots, tobacco cessation options, massage therapy, and wellness challenges.

3. Health centers include annual physicals, preventive screenings, primary care, disease management, body composition analysis, allergy shots, physical therapy, dietary counseling, and immunizations.

4. Nutrition and weight management offers personal nutrition counseling, group nutrition presentations, dietary consultation for company cafeterias, catering services, and healthy options for on-site vending machines.

5. EAP and mental health programming includes personal consultation, triage, and referral and group presentations and workshops on behavioral health issues.

The NextEra Health & Well-Being program consists of many programs and activities:

- Steps to Success is a personalized, long-term weight management program that pairs individuals who are obese or overweight and have multiple risk factors with a health team, including a dietitian, fitness center staff member, and EAP counselor, who help them lose weight and sustain weight loss.

- Healthy Back/Healthy Neck is an exercise and lecture series designed to prevent musculoskeletal injury and discomfort by strengthening the back, core, and neck and teaching proper body mechanics.

- Active Parenting Now is a video-based parent education program led by an EAP specialist who uses video vignettes to demonstrate parenting skills and lead a discussion on positive discipline and communication techniques.

- NextEra Health & Well-Being staff and safety group teamed up to create the Back Reinjury Prevention Program, which includes specialized materials on stretching, lifting, and body mechanics for employees who have experienced a loss-time back injury.

- The Cigna Personal Health Team delivers an integrated approach to health and well-being in the form of confidential, one-on-one support for employees and family members with multiple risk factors or maternity or chronic health needs. A team of 12 health professionals, staffed by the company's contracted health insurer (Cigna), coach participants to achieve optimal health through education, intervention programs, and assistance working with the health care delivery system.

Short-term or seasonal programs complement the ongoing programs and keep the offerings fresh and employees engaged. The 20-20-20 Challenge, which motivates employees to exercise at least 20 minutes each day for a month, is an example of a seasonal program. Employees earn tokens for each workout and increase their chances to win a raffle with each additional token they earn. In another seasonal program, Spring Into Fitness!, fitness center members are encouraged to engage in physical activity and exercise routines with weekly challenges and prizes, including a prize for referring a new member to one of the fitness centers.

Company and program managers continuously measure the success of the NextEra Health & Well-Being program in terms of participant health maintenance and improvement. Although health for any large population is distributed along points of a continuum, the program's founder holds a core belief that success depends on some key items:

- Keeping risk low for healthy people
- Encouraging behavior change to reduce risk for marginally healthy people
- Providing effective programs for people with chronic conditions or catastrophic health events

The program's success starts with strong participation from employees and their family members:

- Ninety percent of employees participated in at least one on-site program in 2010, a 7 percent increase over 2009.
- Forty-five percent of employees reported they had participated in the program continuously for three years in 2010, a 10 percent increase since 2008.
- In 2010, 80 percent of employees eligible to receive incentives had taken the annual

health assessment, and 49 percent had participated in a health screening.

- Participation in the on-site health centers increased by 10 percent from 2009 to 2010, with a total of more than 20,000 visits in 2010. The average return on investment (ROI) for the company's three health centers was $2.29 for every dollar spent in 2010.
- Flu shots were administered to 41 percent of employees in 2010, an increase of 11 percent over the previous year.
- In the company cafeterias, 27 percent of employees chose the healthy food option in 2010, an increase of 4 percent since 2008. These healthy options represented 39 percent of the total cafeteria sales in 2010.
- With 62 fitness centers across the company, ample opportunity exists to use an on-site facility; 60 percent of eligible employees are enrolled in their on-site fitness center. In 2010, the total number of fitness center visits increased by 5 percent compared with 2009.
- The internal EAP staff counseled 1,952 employees and family members in 2010.

Strong employee participation is an important component of the company's multiyear health benefits strategy. In 2009, the program encouraged employees to participate in health assessments and screenings to "know their numbers" and to reduce their risks by participating in behavior change programs. The company reinforced these behavior changes by offering health incentives to employees who participated in the assessments and took action to reduce identified risks.

Linkage to National Physical Activity Plan

This approach addresses the following strategies and tactics of the National Physical Activity Plan Business and Industry Sector.

Strategy 1: Identify, summarize, and disseminate best practices for physical interventions in the workplace. NextEra Energy was one of only 22 employers to be awarded platinum-level recognition as the Best Employer for Healthy Lifestyles for Employees by the National Business Group on Health. NextEra Energy participates in several regional and national health care forums to share ideas with other companies and agencies. Andrew Scibelli, manager of Employee Health & Well-Being at NextEra Energy, is a founding board member of the Institute on the Cost and Health Effects of Obesity and, as a national subject matter expert, has addressed the Florida Health Coalition and published numerous articles in health journals.

Strategy 2: Encourage business and industry to interact with all other sectors to identify opportunities to promote physical activity within the workplace and throughout society. Although primarily geared toward employees and their families, NextEra Health & Well-Being recognizes its responsibility to reach out within its communities. NextEra Energy has been the local sponsor of Race for the Cure in West Palm Beach, Florida, an event held by Susan G. Komen for the Cure, and consistently recruits more than 900 employees to participate in the race. Employee teams also participate in the American Heart Association's annual Heart Walk. Each year on Take Your Child to Work Day, physical activities are conducted throughout the company for children of employees. Most recently, staff members consulted with the Palm Beach County School District regarding additional ways to promote fitness in county schools.

Strategy 3: Educate business and industry leaders regarding their role as positive agents of change to promote physical activity and healthy lifestyles within the workplace and throughout society, giving particular consideration to efforts targeting low-resource populations. The program takes special care to target underserved populations and those with the highest-risk behaviors. The underserved employee population includes those working outside of the corporate offices who have limited access to health centers and larger fitness centers located at central facilities. When space is available at a remote location, on-site exercise rooms or outdoor recreational areas, such as sand volleyball courts, are created using staff expertise and local financial resources. Community resources are used to offer on-site health fairs and screenings, and sometimes local management pays to bring wellness staff members on site to offer ergonomic assessment of job tasks. For example, at one wind energy site, workers were experiencing some muscular stress from carrying tools up the stairs to the top of the wind turbines. The wellness staff created a series of stretching and strengthening exercises to help alleviate potential strains.

Members of the Cigna Personal Health Team identify and confidentially contact high-risk individuals, who receive one-on-one coaching and are directed to tailored health improvement programs.

Strategy 5: Develop a plan for monitoring and evaluating worksite health promotion programs. Twenty years ago, as the NextEra Health & Well-Being program was under development, a nationwide assessment in the United States was conducted to help define what the program would include. Program leaders interviewed senior managers, studied medical claims, and evaluated the corporate culture to determine which health promotion services employees needed and which offerings would be successful. The company has conducted similar evaluations on a biannual basis to ensure that the services remain relevant and useful to employees.

Lessons Learned

The most important lesson that company and program managers learned was to understand how the organization operates before designing programs. A successful health promotion program must have a champion who is willing to visibly and vocally influence the rest of the organization in favor of the program. A mistake many new health promotion programs make is to roll out initiatives without identifying and engaging such a champion or without understanding the organization and culture. Even if employees support healthy lifestyles and would choose health promotion benefits over other forms of indirect compensation, if the corporate culture is not one that supports wellness, employees will be reluctant to participate. Once managers begin to serve as role models for wellness, programming will naturally follow.

Once established, a successful program must continue to re-create itself before its life cycle ends. In the case of the NextEra Health & Well-Being program, integrating services—such as traditional wellness services with safety and employee benefits—keeps offerings meaningful to employees and simplifies their personal health improvement efforts. Integrating wellness with safety means that health promotion has both a personal improvement component and tangible work significance. Similarly, integrating wellness with health care benefits expands awareness of health promotion to family members who previously would have shown interest only in benefits.

Finally, program managers need to stay on top of current trends. With the proliferation of social media and near-universal online access, the program is placing greater emphasis on reaching people online. The internal health and well-being website was redesigned to make it easier to use and accessible from almost anywhere. The web-based programs offered and housed on this website make achieving health and wellness more convenient for employees and their families.

Populations Best Served by the Program

Employees at highly populated sites are the easiest to reach for programming given economies of scale. NextEra Energy staffs fitness centers and health centers at the company's most highly populated sites, making services more readily accessible and allowing staff to increase employee awareness of additional program services.

Because NextEra Energy operates in so many locations, it is important to offer programming that can be implemented at remote sites. Locations willing to pay for staff travel costs can bring wellness staff members on site to offer a series of lectures, fitness testing, nutrition counseling, and other programming. These staff members also work with the on-site wellness champion and local community resources to arrange for on-site services such as flu shots, health fairs, and biometric testing. Whenever possible and within security limitations, these programs also are available to covered spouses and dependents.

Because unionized employees generally work in the field during the day, special arrangements must be made to include them in any on-site programming. With local management approval, work hours can be adjusted and program times altered so that wellness services are available to all employees. When feasible, wellness programming can be incorporated into monthly safety meetings for unionized employees.

Tips for Working Across Sectors

Strong leadership support has helped the NextEra Health & Well-Being program operate successfully for 20 years. Because of this support, the program has been able to circumvent the challenges that a geographically diverse company often faces.

Support from senior leaders opens the door to working with management at remote company sites. When NextEra Energy senior leaders made "fostering a culture of health" a performance indicator, they motivated general managers of remote sites to seek out health and wellness programs to bring to their locations. Local support is further demonstrated when managers and supervisors identify a wellness coordinator or champion who distributes monthly wellness materials sent by corporate staff, schedules health fairs, and promotes fitness challenges and other events among site employees. Local management support is needed to give the wellness coordinator time each month to devote to these activities and allow employees to participate in the scheduled events during work hours.

Because some employees at remote sites are part of a bargaining group, support of union leadership is necessary. Meeting with union representatives regularly and giving them advance notice of upcoming events and promotions are critical to garnering full employee participation among the unionized workforce. Since benefits differ between union and nonunion employees, and because wellness is closely integrated with health benefits, clear communications about which programs are available to union employees encourages greater involvement.

Program Evaluation

Since winning the prestigious Deming Award for quality improvement in 1989, NextEra Energy has made it standard practice to base actions on research findings. The health and well-being program is no exception.

The company has conducted several studies of the program throughout its 20-year history, and in 2010, OptumInsight, a health care analytics vendor, evaluated the effectiveness of the on-site health centers. The study set out to test the hypothesis that employees who use the health centers have lower health care costs and better compliance with nationally recognized medical guidelines. Episode risk groups and evidence-based medicine were used to evaluate current and future health risks and compliance. The episode risk groups used medical claims and demographic data to predict an individual's need for health services and costs. Evidence-based medicine is a quality-of-care assessment tool that evaluates compliance with the predicted need for services. The treatment cost of an off-site health care provider versus an on-site health center was collected and incorporated into the ROI analysis. The population size of 2,630 was based on unique employee visits to one of NextEra Energy's three on-site health centers during two years; the average number of visits per patient ranged between 3.9 and 5.7 at the different locations.

Findings from the study demonstrated that on a risk-adjusted basis, employees who use the on-site health centers have annual costs that are $706 lower than employees who do not use the health centers. Employees who use the on-site health centers also showed a compliance rate with nationally recognized medical guidelines of 81 percent, compared with a compliance rate of 74 percent for employees who did not use the

health center. Last, the average ROI for all three health centers was $2.13 per dollar invested in 2009 and $2.29 per dollar invested in 2010. Higher compliance with medical guidelines and a larger ROI provide a strong business case for offering on-site health centers.

Recognizing that outcomes drive strategy, NextEra Energy tracks and assesses metrics relative to health improvement, engagement, participation, employee satisfaction, vendor performance, program integration, health claims data, and leadership engagement.

In 2011, NextEra Energy began matching incentives with healthy outcomes. Employees who meet certain biometric indicators are eligible to receive a credit to their health reimbursement account. This approach was incorporated into the employee benefit plan for 2012.

NextEra Energy regularly publishes metrics that reflect program objectives and track effectiveness. These metrics include a 16-risk health assessment, which surveys active employees regarding self-reported conditions and willingness to change. The health assessment also includes a productivity review that monitors changes in both presenteeism (productivity loss while at work) and absenteeism (productivity loss due to absence from work) and compares them with a national norm.

The program consistently seeks and benefits from employee feedback, collecting pre-to-post measurements on all programs. A vendor conducts a survey every two years to assess employee perceptions of the health and well-being program and offer suggestions for improvement. The last survey was conducted in 2010 and demonstrated an 89 percent satisfaction rate with the health and well-being program, compared with an 84 percent satisfaction rate in 2008. These results show that even a progressive, evolving program like the NextEra Health & Well-Being program has room to improve.

Additional Reading and Resources

NextEra Health & Well-Being (formerly known as FPL-WELL) was featured on ABC World News

Tonight on March 22, 2007. This two-minute video shows the fitness center, health center, and cafeteria in the corporate headquarters in Juno Beach, Florida. http://video.google.com/videoplay?docid = -348372692272836281#

FPL group wins award for health program. 2007, November 27. *South Florida Business Journal.*

FPL successful with on-site clinics, fitness centers. 2008, September 22. *Disease Management News.*

"Value-based" health plan designs focus on health, not merely dollars: Successes found in upfront spending that avoids long-term, higher costs. 2007, October 29. *Business Insurance.*

Working at change: executive lifestyles, workplace wellness. 2008, January 1. *Florida Trend.*

How FPL's approach to weight management helped improve its company wellness. 2004, October 1. *Managing Benefit Plans.*

CHAPTER 27

Johnson & Johnson

Bringing Physical Activity, Fitness, and Movement to the Workplace

Fik Isaac, MD, MPH, FACOEM
Johnson & Johnson

Melinda Vertin, MSN, NP
Johnson & Johnson

NPAP Tactics and Strategies Used in This Program

Business and Industry Sector

STRATEGY 1: Identify, summarize, and disseminate best practices, models, and evidence-based physical activity interventions in the workplace.

STRATEGY 2: Encourage business and industry to interact with all other sectors to identify opportunities to promote physical activity within the workplace and throughout society.

STRATEGY 3: Educate business and industry leaders regarding their role as positive agents of change to promote physical activity and healthy lifestyles within the workplace and throughout society, giving particular consideration to efforts targeting low-resource populations.

STRATEGY 4: Develop legislation and policy agendas that promote employer-sponsored physical activity programs while protecting individual employees' and dependents' rights.

STRATEGY 5: Develop a plan for monitoring and evaluating worksite health promotion programs.

This chapter tells the story of how Johnson and Johnson (J&J) created and then sustained a culture of health for its employees. Although physical activity and movement play important roles in the story, good nutrition, mental well-being, and other health-related components contribute to the global culture of health. Programs that encompass all of these health components have made significant contributions to the overall health and well-being of J&J employees for the past 125 years.

J&J has longstanding dedication to the health of its employees. This commitment is based in its credo, which drives decisions and actions at all levels of the corporation. The credo includes a pledge to the health and welfare of all J&J employees and retirees. Even before General Robert Wood Johnson created the credo in 1943, this dedication was understood and valued. As far back as 100 years ago, J&J provided medical centers, health education and lectures, and physical activity resources for all company employees.

Program Description

Given this commitment and history, in 1979, the company created a successful health and wellness initiative: Live for Life. At that time, J&J's company group chairman, Jim Burke, believed that unhealthy behaviors, such as smoking, overeating, alcohol abuse, emotional stress, hypertension, and unsafe driving, were responsible for a large share of the company's health care costs in the United States.

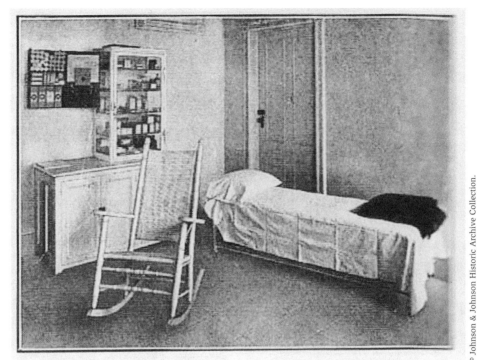

Program success required understanding the workplace culture and setting goals and targets that drove the program and led to sustained improvements in health outcomes. Such goals garnered the support of management at all levels, which was essential if the program was to achieve goals and sustain results year after year.

Employee health promotion goals have evolved over time at J&J, expanding the program's reach and targets. For example, program goals have been aligned with external goals (such as Healthy People 2010 or the National Physical Activity Plan), which allow the company to standardize and validate its efforts. Additionally, initial program efforts focused on four key risk factors; current efforts focus on 11, including physical inactivity.

Programs that were initially based in the United States have now moved to company locations across the globe. For example, in 2012, 95 percent of all sites worldwide (379) offered some form of physical activity opportunities to their employees. More than 84 percent of sites (335) offered comprehensive programs. These outcomes resulted from goals and targets that sought to expand physical activity and other

health offerings. Prior to expanding these goals, the company had only offered these programs in a few sites outside of the United States.

In 2010, the company set corporate sustainability goals called Healthy Future 2015. These goals are centered on the philosophy of sustainability and managing for the long term. Goals in the area of employee health challenge all employees to "know their health numbers" and reduce their health risk factors. The aim is to encourage sites to actively choose and use available health programs to assist employees in lowering their health risks.

Established health and wellness policies and standards support Healthy Future 2015 goals as well as define minimum program expectations. The company conducts assessments to monitor these standards (as well as other environmental health and safety standards) at least annually. For example, operating companies are required to provide access to and improve physical activity initiatives. Management action plans address these expectations to ensure that senior managers are aware of and support the initiatives. The Office of the Chairman and members of the Executive committee support these programs,

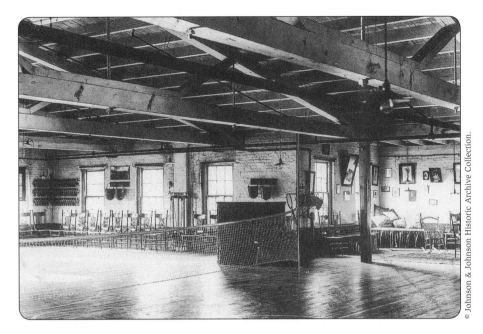

© Johnson & Johnson Historic Archive Collection.

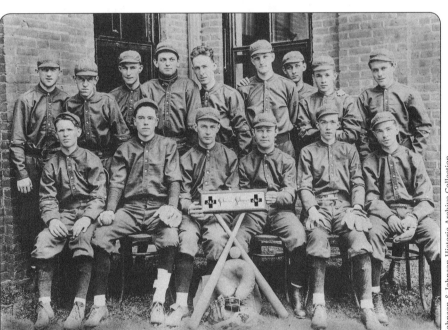

© Johnson & Johnson Historic Archive Collection.

policies, and practices related to the health and safety of employees. This high level of corporate commitment ensures that employee health programs remain a priority of the company.

J&J has a long history of understanding the value of physical activity and providing physical activity opportunities for employees. As early as 1895, the company fielded a men's baseball team. In the early 1900s, it built outdoor and indoor tennis and badminton courts and a swimming pool for employees. Female employees were offered dancing and callisthenic classes, and the male employees formed the J&J Athletic Association. Many employees joined sports clubs for basketball, tennis, or bowling. Today, of the 11 population health risks that J&J has targeted to track and reduce over time, physical inactivity remains one of the most important. The company recognizes the well-documented positive effects of physical activity on other health risk factors (e.g., obesity, high glucose, hypertension, stress) and the role physical activity can play as a positive alternative to negative health habits (smoking, alcohol use).

Despite the well-known positive effects of physical activity, inactivity is increasing in the workplace. A recent study found that up to 80 percent of jobs in today's workforce are predominantly sedentary. This has been an issue for J&J as well, and physical inactivity continues to be one of the top three health risks for our employees (along with obesity and unhealthy eating).

Table 27.1 illustrates that compared with national norms (with trends moving in the wrong direction), J&J has made steady progress in addressing the issue. The success J&J has achieved in reducing physical inactivity and improving employee health behaviors is built on the success of the following programs:

• On-site fitness centers: On-site employee fitness centers are located at 210 company sites worldwide. These centers are fully equipped and staffed with fitness professionals who provide personal coaching and advice. Exercise classes are offered based on the site's needs and requests. Fitness professionals tailor fitness offerings specifically to the employee population at each site. Access to the fitness centers is free of charge for all employees and retirees.

• Exercise reimbursement: For employees who cannot access on-site fitness centers, J&J provides reimbursement of $200 per year so that employees can purchase gym memberships, enroll in exercise classes close to home, or buy exercise-related equipment.

• Walking trails: Most locations strive to offer safe pathways around the facility for walkers as a means to promote activity throughout the day. A checklist is used to ensure the trails are walkable, allowing for adequate distance and safety.

• Million Step Challenge: This program encourages movement by providing free pedometers and sponsoring competitions that motivate employees to increase their daily steps (with the goal of 10,000 steps a day). In 2012, 7,307 unique employees participated in the Million Step Challenge (22.3 percent of the U.S. J&J population) compared with 7,268 in 2011. Of these participants, 1,562 employees walked at least one million steps by year-end, whereas 1,725 employees walked two million or more steps. A 2012 survey of participants found that 60 percent reported more energy, 40 percent lost weight, 15 percent lowered blood pressure, 14 percent lowered cholesterol, and 27 percent were less troubled by stress.

• Job Fit: This program is designed to improve health and productivity by preventing and reducing musculoskeletal injuries. The program focuses on ergonomic demands of the job as well as the employee's overall fitness.

• Community health activities: Each site works to align with community and recreational events and may coordinate with fundraising events like Race for the Cure, American Heart Association Heart Walk, and Relay for Life. For example, LifeScan (a J&J company) has been involved in the rider recruitment, fund-raising,

Table 27.1 Percentages of Physically Inactive Employees Over Time

	1995-1999 average	2007-2008*	2009	2010	2011
Johnson & Johnson	39%	31.5%	20.4%	20.8%	20.9%
CDC Comparison		52.7%			

*Questions addressing physical inactivity were altered in 2008 to better align with the new physical activity guidelines and accurately capture employees' moderate- and vigorous-intensity activity. This update may have affected the risk percentage for physical inactivity when compared with previous years since those numbers were calculated differently.

and marketing of the Silicon Valley Tour de Cure. This is an annual benefit ride supporting the American Diabetes Association. In 2010, the LifeScan team played an integral role in recruiting more than 100 riders and helping to raise $103,000. Over the last two years, the team has raised nearly $200,000 for the American Diabetes Association. The on-site staff has partnered with other wellness professionals to promote the Tour de Cure at other J&J operating companies. These efforts have drawn more than 1,000 riders, and more than $540,000 is raised nationally.

• Family activity challenge: This 12-month program is built on the concept that becoming active as a family and focusing on good health habits are rewarding ways to improve the health of loved ones while teaching children healthy habits that will last a lifetime. Included are monthly activity calendars encompassing healthy eating, physical activity, hydration, the importance of sleep, and reducing screen time. Principles from Energy for Performance in Life and healthy eating are incorporated in the calendar activities. A pedometer challenge incorporates e-mails, raffle prizes, and incentives.

• Move (from HealthMedia): Move is a virtual training program that provides unique and tailored online assistance and digital coaching to J&J employees. The program devises a customized activity plan specific for each employee and works with the employee to track progress and goals.

Program Evaluation

Evaluations of the Live for Life program have proven Jim Burke to be right and have demonstrated that good health is good business. An independent study evaluated the program's results from 1979 through 1983 and found that hospitalization costs at J&J locations that implemented the program were a third of those at other company locations. Absenteeism rates were 18 percent lower, and improvements in weight, blood pressure, cholesterol, and smoking cessation contributed to an estimated 3 to 5 percent reduction in overall health care costs. (Bly et al. 1986)

More recent evaluations revealed similar findings. Figure 27.1 shows the overall decrease in employees considered to be "high risk" (five or more lifestyle risk factors) over the past five years, and figure 27.2 shows the decline of specific risks since 1995.

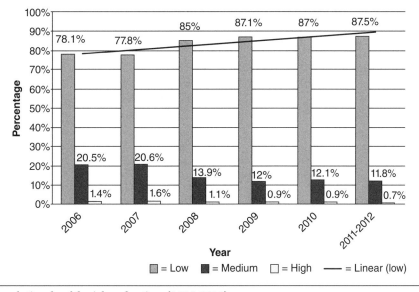

Figure 27.1 Population health risk reduction (2006-2012).

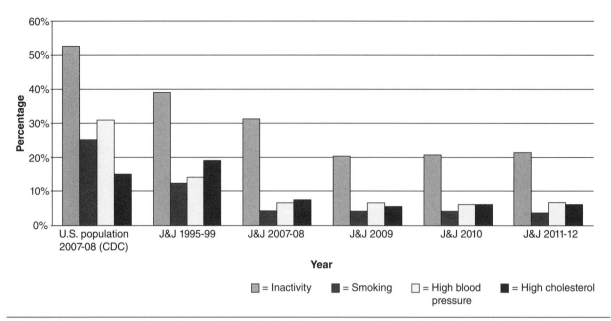

Figure 27.2   Johnson & Johnson decline in four major health risks (1995-2012).

Following are key findings from recent studies of the Live for Life program:

- Johnson & Johnson had significantly fewer employees at risk for high blood pressure, unhealthy eating, obesity, and tobacco use compared with benchmarked companies.

- Johnson & Johnson's program produced a $565 savings per employee per year.

- With an average annual program cost ranging from $144 to $300 per person, the return on investment for Johnson & Johnson's program ranged from $1.88 to $3.92 saved for every dollar spent.

Linkage to the National Activity Plan

The J&J programs have a natural synergy with the efforts described for the Business and Industry Sector of the U.S. National Physical Activity Plan:

Strategy 1: Identify, summarize, and disseminate best practices, models, and evidence-based physical activity interventions in the workplace. By providing a consistent approach to delivering known best practices (to a decentralized organization), J&J is able to leverage resources and gather data in a consistent, quality-driven fashion. Data are reported to the highest levels of the company to bring attention to population health risk status and progress; the data are also used at the site level to develop customized interventions that address population health risk needs. Strong incentives drive participation in the Health Profile (J&J's health risk assessment), which highlights an individual's unique risks and follows through with specific interventions (such as physical activity) to address them.

Strategy 2: Encourage business and industry to interact with all other sectors to identify opportunities to promote physical activity within the workplace and throughout society. J&J recognizes the importance of affecting change in the external community as a strategy for maintaining change within the organization. In a recent article, Jack Groppel, cofounder of the Human Performance Institute, a J&J company, explored the possibility of achieving effective community behavior change through the application of sport science. According to Groppel, helping people understand their missions and the reason for movement and wellness is where community leaders must step in. He implores leaders in the fields of health, physical education, recreation, and dance to lead the charge by improving awareness, making movement matter on an individual level, and helping individual communities rewrite their stories. Starting the conversation across sectors is the first step. (Groppel 2011)

Strategy 3: Educate business and industry leaders regarding their role as positive agents of change to promote physical activity and healthy lifestyles within the workplace and throughout society, giving particular consideration to efforts targeting low-resource populations. The J&J Global Health leadership team sets an annual goal to participate with and give back to external organizations (other employers, government and nongovernment organizations, academics, and professional organizations) through speaking engagements, benchmarking and sharing of best practices, and participation on relevant boards. Beyond J&J Global Health, the executive business leadership within J&J has helped develop and implement initiatives such as the CEO Cancer Gold Standard, a series of cancer-related recommendations developed by the CEO Roundtable on Cancer, to fight cancer in workplaces in the United States.

In 2008, J&J acquired the Human Performance Institute (HPI) and is continuing the legacy that the institute has brought to the field of human energy management. The institute's 30-plus year history is deeply rooted in the arena of high performance in the face of enormous stress, and it continues to reach business leaders. In 2009, 24 of the Fortune 100 companies participated in the Corporate Athlete, HPI's premier training program.

Strategy 4: Develop legislation and policy agendas that promote employer-sponsored physical activity programs while protecting individual employees' and dependents' rights. J&J is a leader in the field of employee health and well-being. As a result, other companies and organizations often ask J&J to share opinions or advice on best practices. During the most recent health care reform activities, J&J was asked by the White House to share its best practices and observations in regard to what works in health and wellness programs. These programs are respected because they continue to be completely voluntary, observe all privacy regulations and recommendations, and remain accessible to present and past employees and their families.

Strategy 5: Develop a plan for monitoring and evaluating worksite health promotion programs. The real success of these programs is often seen in the personal stories of employees: *No longer required to take cholesterol medication; lost 30+ pounds; lowered blood pressure; lost 5 inches off waistline; quit smoking!* These are real results attained by real Johnson & Johnson employees. However, although such anecdotes help tell the story, it is also critical to rigorously measure and analyze results. Two studies have done this. The first, published in *Health Affairs* (Henke et al. 2011), measured the long-term effectiveness of the workplace health and wellness programs to contain costs and reduce health risks among employees compared with 16 other large employers (detailed results are mentioned in the Commitment to Health section of the article). A second study, published in the *Journal of Occupational and Environmental Medicine* (Carls et al. 2011), found that Johnson & Johnson employees who maintain a healthy weight have average annual medical costs of $285 per year, whereas those who gain weight and are at risk for obesity have average annual medical costs of $1,267. Combined, these studies are a testament to the effectiveness of the Johnson and Johnson workplace wellness programs.

Evidence Base Used During Development

Although the company has achieved some success in this area, physical activity remains a key focus area for J&J given ongoing employee risk assessments, the increasing number of predominantly sedentary jobs within the company (and the associated risks), and current literature indicating ever-increasing inactivity within employee and general populations. Most recently, the principles of "energy management" have been incorporated into the program.

Energy management uses a holistic approach to incorporate personal wellness goals as part of a deeper personal mission to improve health. This mission provides a long-term goal and purpose that drives short-term aspirations and lifestyle changes. (For example, "I am purposefully making healthier choices so that I can be fully present and active with my children as they grow up.") Part of this energy management approach shifts the emphasis from program goals and corporate objectives to individualized stories and motivation that drive behavior.

Employees are now taught that movement and physical activity are linked to their energy levels. There are three key principles of energy management:

- Manage your energy through strategic movement, deep breathing, and sleep.
- Expand your energy capacity through strategic exercise.
- Incorporate strategic movement into your daily routine.

The company uses communication and marketing campaigns to remind and motivate employees to remain active. Some of the campaigns provide video links and training. Some are tailored to the employee (such as those from the Move program), whereas others are site-specific and related to activity campaigns and competitions for that location.

J&J recently implemented the concept of the health champion as a strategy designed to sustain positive changes and ensure that senior managers, who serve as health champions, are visible and engaged in health promotion programs in their regions. This approach combines top-down encouragement and regional solutions and encourages employees at all levels to get involved. The company's vice president of human resources, who is an Executive committee board member, leads this effort.

Populations Best Served by the Program

Many of the J&J physical activity programs encourage involvement of family and the community. Building this connection helps employ-ees make changes and sustain them over the long haul. Annual marathons, bikathons, and other team events to raise money for charity are popular—employees train for and participate in these events year after year. Leveraging social media has allowed for a virtual community among remote and global employees in order to encourage and reinforce healthy practices. J&J also develops or supports health programs that encourage community residents to take charge of their health. The Five Steps for Your Health initiative, for example, trained health care workers to help diabetes patients stay active, eat well, monitor body weight, and increase other positive health behaviors. As an established global leader in the field of employee wellness, J&J supports many of its leaders to serve on national and international committees and forums in order to promote growth and development of the field. Therefore, the populations served by the program are widespread and varied.

Lessons Learned

The essence of J&J is that it is the "caring" health care company. As such, it continues to commit to the health and well-being of its employees. Its employee health programs build on the legacy and foundation of the past 125 years while evolving to meet the challenges of the 21st century. An important piece of this journey has been to recognize and understand key lessons along the way:

- A focus on health risk factors can yield strong results.
- To sustain health and well-being within an organization, leadership is critical, including that of middle management.
- Engaging employees in the program is a critical success factor.
- Increased productivity and engagement can generate significant cost savings and improved performance.
- Start small, and build on simple gains to increase program engagement.
- A seamless and holistic approach at the organizational and individual level will drive participation and behavior change.

- Increasing rates of chronic disease, rising health care costs, economic downturns, a stretched work force, and health care reform present the opportunity to improve employees' health and wellness.

- Partnering with policy makers can be an effective strategy to improve labor productivity and economic competitiveness. Successful U.S. strategies and tactics can be leveraged in other regions across the world.

These lessons highlight the notion that from a business and industry perspective, employee health can be positioned as a strategic and competitive advantage. Physical activity, fitness, and human movement are important factors in the adoption and long-term maintenance of employee health.

Tips for Working Across Sectors

A successful global program depends on the following minimal criteria:

- Ensure that upper and middle management personnel provide committed leadership and lead by example. Executive and senior leaders who have taken the lead in creating a sustainable global culture of health have been essential drivers in the alignment of health and business priorities. This leadership commitment, coupled with challenging goals, has been pivotal in making health and wellness programs sustainable at Johnson & Johnson.

- Recognize the importance of setting goals, establishing a baseline, and assessing progress. In 2009, J&J began to look back at its progress toward the healthiest employee population while considering the next five-year goals. What emerged is Healthy Future 2015, which presents the five-year goals for corporate citizenship and sustainability commitments across key strategic priorities. Each business sector worldwide has embedded these goals into its business imperatives and performance, and the progress of those goals (related to employee health) is tracked annually through a global health assessment tool.

- Identify site-specific population risk factors and develop culturally appropriate programs to address these risk factors. Because J&J operates within a diverse range of countries and operating environments, it introduced "culture of health" toolkits that assist companies in developing a local culture of health strategy. Each operating company may be at a different stage of its health promotion strategy, so the toolkits help each site either enhance an existing strategy or start from step 1 and develop a fully comprehensive strategy.

- Partner with external resources, community leaders, and policy makers to create an environment that focuses on health education and health promotion; this highlights the importance of effecting change in the external community as a strategy for maintaining change within the organization.

- Strive for continuous improvement by evaluating and re-evaluating programs and by creating, revising, and resetting goals based on emerging trends within employee and general populations.

Summary

Johnson & Johnson has not written "the end" to the story of bringing physical activity, fitness, and movement to the workplace but rather has written "to be continued". J&J will continue to build on its successes and progress toward having the healthiest, most engaged workforce possible, allowing for full and productive lives, and providing sustainable and effective services to improve the health of its employees worldwide.

Additional Reading and Resources

Arnst, C. 2009, November 23. 10 ways to cut health-care costs now. *Business Week*. www.businessweek.com/magazine/content/09_47/b4156034717852.htm.

Carls, G.S., R.Z. Goetzel, R.M. Henke, et al. 2011. The impact of weight gain or loss on health care costs for employees at the Johnson & Johnson family of companies. *J. Occcup. Environ. Med.* 53(1):8-16.

Isaac, F., & P. Flynn. 2001. Johnson & Johnson Live for Life® program: Now and then. *Am. J. Health Promot.* 15(5):365-67.

Isaac, F. 2010, August. A legacy of health and wellness. *Benefits & Compensation Digest.* 47(8):1-15.

Ozminkowski, R., D. Ling, R. Goetzel, et. al. 2002. Long-term impact of Johnson & Johnson's health & wellness program on health care utilization and expenditures. *J. Occcup. Environ. Med.* 44(1):21-9.

Robertson, I., and C. Cooper, Eds. 2011. *Well-Being—Productivity and Happiness at Work.* Great Britain, London: Palgrave McMillan.

Weldon, B. 2011, January/February. Fix the health care crisis, one employee at a time. *Harvard Business Review.* http://hbr.org/2011/01/web-exclusive-fix-the-health-care-crisis-one-employee-at-a-time/ar/1

References

Bly, J., R.C. Jones, and J.E. Richardson. Impact of worksite health promotion on health care costs and utilization: evaluation of Johnson & Johnson's LIVE FOR LIFE programs. JAMA. 1986; 256: 235-240.

Goetzel, R., R. Ozminkowski, J. Bruno, et.al. 2002. The long-term impact of Johnson & Johnson's health and wellness program on employee health risks. *J. Occcup. Environ. Med.* 44(5):417-24.

Groppel, J. 2011. Thinking beyond the playing field. *Journal of Physical Education, Recreation and Dance.* 82(6):35-40.

Henke, R., R. Goetzel, J. McHugh, and F. Isaac. 2011. Recent experience in health promotion at Johnson & Johnson: Lower health spending, strong return on investment. *Health Aff.* 30(3):490-9.

CHAPTER 28

Building Vitality at IBM

Physical Activity and Fitness as One Component of a Comprehensive Strategy for Employee Well-Being

Nicolaas P. Pronk, PhD
*HealthPartners and HealthPartners Institute
for Education and Research, and Harvard University*

Megan Benedict, BS
IBM Corporation

Joyce Young, MD, MPH
IBM Corporation

Stewart Sill, MS
IBM Corporation

NPAP Tactics and Strategies Used in This Program

Business and Industry Sector

STRATEGY 1: Identify, summarize, and disseminate best practices, models, and evidence-based physical activity interventions in the workplace.

STRATEGY 2: Encourage business and industry to interact with all other sectors to identify opportunities to promote physical activity within the workplace and throughout society.

STRATEGY 3: Educate business and industry leaders regarding their role as positive agents of change to promote physical activity and healthy lifestyles within the workplace and throughout society, giving particular consideration to efforts targeting low-resource populations.

STRATEGY 4: Develop legislation and policy agendas that promote employer-sponsored physical activity programs while protecting individual employees' and dependents' rights.

STRATEGY 5: Develop a plan for monitoring and evaluating worksite health promotion programs.

The IBM Corporation is redefining wellness, moving from focusing on health risk reduction to building the capacity to flourish. The goal is to better meet the emerging needs of employees and the company by using multiple approaches to build employees' capacity to flourish in business settings that feature fast pace, constant change, and demand for creative solutions. Building capacity to flourish and thrive offers new and exciting opportunities for employees to experience higher levels of energy and vitality. This approach positions IBM employees to be healthy, optimistic, energetic, and resilient.

Physical activity promotion remains an important component of the overall Vitality Strategy for IBM. Physical activity and fitness are integral parts of all dimensions of vitality, including the physical, mental, emotional, and values dimensions. As such, the company implements a variety of physical activity programs. The program highlighted in this chapter,

Acknowledgments: The support in this project from the following Medifit Corporate Services employees is greatly appreciated: Paul Couzelis, PhD, Linda Raymond, Aymii Couzelis, and Debi Kelly.

the Virtual Fitness Center (VFC), has reached tens of thousands of IBM employees and families over the past decade, improved employees' health status, and reduced health care costs. The VFC program is only one component of the overall Vitality Strategy of IBM but deploys all five strategies included in the Business and Industry Sector of the National Physical Activity Plan.

The VFC was introduced by IBM as an online resource for promoting physical activity after many years of using approaches such as onsite fitness centers, campaigns, and other programs (figure 28.1). Although the VFC continues to be an important tool in the IBM toolbox for physical activity behavior change, it represents only one part of the overall Vitality Strategy that is designed to improve and optimize the health and well-being of IBM employees across the corporation.

To build the capacity for employees to flourish and thrive, the IBM program needs to encompass strategies beyond health risk reduction. Additional programmatic approaches need to be included in the overall program options and choices that move into the area of well-being, a strategy that IBM refers to as its Vitality Strategy. The Vitality Strategy considers four dimensions that collectively refer to an employee's overall vitality level:

1. Physical dimension—the ability to respond physically to everyday situations. Physical activity remains an integral part of this dimension, which also includes functional movement, nutrition, hydration, and sleep.

2. Mental dimension—the capacity to sustain focus and attention. It prepares the mind for challenging situations, reframes negative thoughts, and identifies achievements. Research shows that physical activity is directly relevant to mental health. Other components include daily recovery, energized thinking, and meeting preparation.

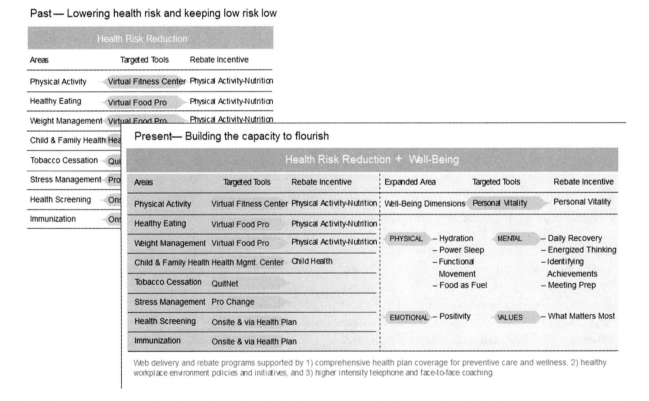

Figure 28.1 Redefining wellness at IBM.

Reprinted, by permission, from IBM Integrated Health Services.

3. Emotional dimension—the capacity to manage positive and negative emotions. Higher levels of physical activity are associated with fewer emotional concerns, even when physical activity is only one of a cluster of modifiable health behaviors. Positive thinking and optimism are key components of the emotional dimension.

4. Values dimension—the capacity of a person to connect with his or her purpose and understand the value of good health. By identifying and prioritizing personal values (i.e., figuring out what matters most), employees enhance overall vitality.

The Vitality Strategy ensures that physical activity is part of a larger set of programmatic options from which employees can choose in order to personalize their own and their families' health goals. The strategy recognizes that physical activity programs are most successful when they are implemented as part of a larger health and wellness strategy. This observation was also noted in the National Physical Activity Plan white paper for business and industry. Although individual physical activity programs may result in successful outcomes, the net benefit of comprehensive, multicomponent, multilevel worksite health programs (that include physical activity options) appears to be larger than the sum of all individual physical activity programs combined.

Program Description

This chapter focuses on the VFC, a program that targets adoption and maintenance of physical activity and fitness within the larger set of employee health initiatives that IBM offers to its employees. The VFC is an Internet-based resource that employees can use to participate in an online physical activity program. IBM worked with Medifit Corporate Services to develop the program and launched it in 1999. Originally, it adapted the Centers for Disease Control and Prevention's March Into May physical activity campaign into an online application. However, the VFC evolved over time into a state-of-the-art, online interactive behavior change tool that provides access to information and resources to support year-round physical activity programming.

IBM has provided access to on-site fitness centers and other physical activity programs for many years. However, not all of the approximately 300 sites across the United States are large enough to house a fitness center, and a large number of employees work remotely.

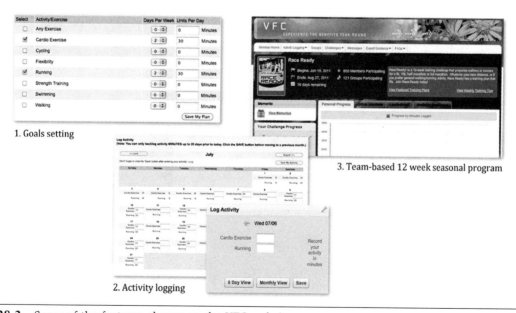

1. Goals setting

2. Activity logging

3. Team-based 12 week seasonal program

Figure 28.2   Some of the features shown on the VFC website.
Reprinted, by permission, from IBM Integrated Health Services.

Hence, creating an online resource for promoting physical activity improved access significantly.

The VFC program includes several key features that are fundamental to supporting behavior change (see figure 28.2):

• Goal setting—Employees can establish and monitor customized physical activity goals across a variety of aerobic (e.g., walking, running, cycling) and nonaerobic (e.g., strength training, flexibility) activities.

• Activity logging—The VFC provides physical activity logs to keep track of activities performed. Employees can use month-by-month calendar views to monitor their progress.

• Team-based 12-week seasonal program campaigns throughout the year—Workout campaigns offered during the winter, summer, and fall provide opportunities for teams to engage in friendly competition while moving toward achieving physical activity goals. The program provides weekly motivational messages via e-mail, and the campaigns often offer small incentives such as pedometers, books, or other token items.

• Progress reports—Participants can monitor their progress in the program by viewing activity graphs in the VFC, including graphs of the physical activity trend over time and progress by specific exercise categories (figure 28.3).

• Ask Our Pros online Q&A—Participants can submit questions via an online portal and receive answers from professionally trained and certified staff. Fitness staff members use the most common questions to develop e-mail messages for all program participants.

• Incentives—In 2004, IBM enhanced its commitment to physical activity promotion by adding the Healthy Living Rebate, a $150 cash incentive for employees who participate in the VFC program. Employees are eligible to receive the incentive if they elect to participate during the annual fall benefits enrollment, join the VFC program, log their minutes of physical activity online, and engage in at least 20 minutes of physical activity, three days per week, for 10 of 12 consecutive weeks.

Linkage to National Physical Activity Plan

IBM's efforts meet all five strategies of the Business and Industry Sector of the National Physical Activity Plan.

Strategy 1: Identify, summarize, and disseminate best practices, models, and evidence-based

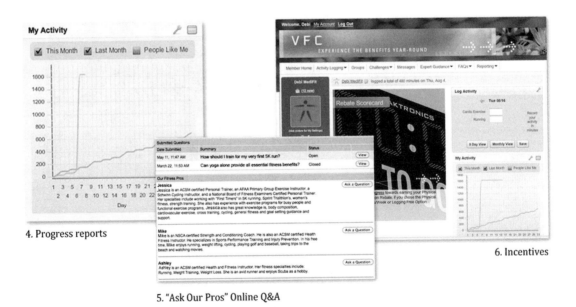

4. Progress reports

5. "Ask Our Pros" Online Q&A

6. Incentives

Figure 28.3   Progress report, Q&A, and incentives features of the VFC website.
Reprinted, by permission, from IBM Integrated Health Services.

physical activity interventions in the workplace. Through the VFC program and the broader Vitality Strategy, IBM has become a best practice organization for promoting physical activity and fitness. The web-based delivery of the VFC is supported by comprehensive health plan coverage for preventive care and wellness and healthy workplace environment policies and initiatives. The VFC program is highly scalable and can be applied to all types of worksites and workforces.

Strategy 2: Encourage business and industry to interact with all other sectors to identify opportunities to promote physical activity within the workplace and throughout society. IBM is a well-recognized leader with a strong track record of working across sectors to encourage physical activity within the workplace and throughout society. The company plays key leadership roles in organizations and initiatives such as the National Business Group on Health, the Institute of Medicine, efforts to address childhood obesity, and efforts to establish the patient-centered medical home, among others. Within each of these examples, physical activity plays a central role related to preventing disease or optimizing health.

Strategy 3: Educate business and industry leaders regarding their role as positive agents of change to promote physical activity and healthy lifestyles within the workplace and throughout society, giving particular consideration to efforts targeting low-resource populations. Strong leadership within IBM continues to promote an agenda that focuses on promoting health and well-being, reducing risk, and creating the capacity to flourish. This agenda applies to all employees regardless of income, race, gender, or health risk status. The company's integrated approach brings together components of occupational medicine, industrial hygiene, safety, health benefits, and wellness and implements programs that are proactive, relevant, and effective in managing the highly complex, diverse, and ever-changing health and safety needs of the employees.

Strategy 4: Develop legislation and policy agendas that promote employer-sponsored physical activity programs while protecting individual employees' and dependents' rights. The IBM global strategy for improving the health of employees includes investing in prevention and primary care, developing programs for healthy lifestyles among employees and their families, and scaling programs and services through web-based health care tools in ways that enable employees to be informed, activated, and engaged in their health care. This strategy entails developing supportive policies at the workplace and playing an active role in collaborations with other employers through coalitions such as the National Business Group on Health.

Strategy 5: Develop a plan for monitoring and evaluating worksite health promotion programs. Monitoring and evaluation of worksite health promotion programs are integral parts of IBM's process for managing employee health programs. Independent researchers have conducted formal evaluations of the VFC program, and the results are published and shared in the public domain so that the field can learn from the IBM experiences.

Program Evaluation

IBM implemented the VFC in 1999, and initially it generated approximately 16,000 users per year. However, when the company added the Healthy Living Rebate incentive program in 2004, participation increased significantly, to an average of more than 80,000 participants per year. Although participation statistics are important, the company wanted more information and a more extensive evaluation. Formal research conducted by independent researchers was designed to answer two questions:

1. Is a financial incentive for participation in an online physical activity program associated with increased employee participation and improved health status among participants compared with nonparticipants?

2. Is participation in an incentive-based online physical activity program for employees associated with moderation of health care costs?

Research on question 1 was conducted among VFC participants and nonparticipants during 2004 and was based on responses to a health risk appraisal. Among the 126,372 eligible employees, 78,952 (62.5 percent) enrolled in the VFC and 67,324 (53.3 percent) were considered active participants. This 53 percent active participation rate represents an increase over the prior year of almost 400 percent (16,777 participants of 129,628 eligible employees). On average, health risks related to low physical activity were reduced by −8.2 percentage points (a 52 percent relative reduction) among VFC participants. In addition, participants experienced significant improvements in life satisfaction, perception of health, risk status, smoking, and body weight. Although improvements were greatest among VFC participants who completed enough physical activity to earn the rebate incentive, all VFC participants demonstrated significant improvements.

The study that addressed question 2 considered the trends in health care claims from 2003 to 2005 among a matched sample of participants and nonparticipants. Medical, pharmacy, hospital inpatient, and emergency room costs were examined. Results of this analysis indicated that average annual health care expenditures among VFC participants increased by $291 per year, compared with an increase of $360 per year among nonparticipants ($p = .09$). The study found significant differences between participants and nonparticipants for inpatient hospital costs, heart disease costs, and costs to treat diabetes. In addition, higher levels of participation were associated with smaller increases in health care costs.

In general, the results of formal research studies on the VFC program indicated that a cash incentive can boost participation in an online physical activity program, reduce population health risks, and, as a result, reduce the increase in health care costs among participating employees.

Evidence Base Used During Program Development

A strong evidence base undergirds the design of the VFC and IBM's approach to health and well-being. Epidemiological data clearly show the importance of physical activity in disease prevention, health maintenance, and functional status, including work performance. Senior health managers have been guided by national guidelines for physical activity, the results of major intervention studies, and the Guide to Community Preventive Services. The scientific literature on self-monitoring techniques, stages of change, social support, incentives, and exercise science has played an important role in IBM's program design approach. The company has continuously translated research findings into practical tools and approaches, tested these tools in real-life workplace settings, and revised and improved programs based on the results of this testing. This cycle of continuous improvement is an integral part of the IBM wellness management system and allows for innovations to improve after they are introduced into practice.

Lessons Learned

Several observations are recognized by the program staff as important lessons learned. These lessons relate to the program's reach, the degree of engagement over time, the type and diversity of workers involved, the role of champions and local leaders, and the importance of capturing the program's value.

Maximize Employee Engagement

Worksite health promotion efforts have traditionally been plagued by low participation rates and, therefore, limited impact. Employee engagement relies on creative approaches that maximize visibility and interest. IBM's Healthy Living Rebate programs have provided significant exposure to wellness initiatives and stimulated positive employee response. Increasing intervention penetration in this way is the first step in influencing the population.

Reach a Diverse, Dispersed Employee Population

Facilitating employee access to health and wellness programs is challenging when employees live in many locations and participate in a wide range of work arrangements. IBM's 300-plus U.S. worksites and its increasing population of mobile and remote employees require unique approaches to employee engagement. Variety and flexibility are key program attributes for such a diverse population, which has a wide range of needs, interests, and motivations. IBM has determined that using multiple delivery mechanisms, including online, telephone, onsite, and hard copy materials, leads to maximum population impact.

Health champions provide peer support and encouragement. The volunteer team captains in the VFC programs serve as influential models of healthy behavior and mentors to those needing assistance. Company management support for wellness initiatives has also contributed to consistent delivery and engagement.

Demonstrate the Value of Well-Being as a Personal Benefit

IBM's wellness communications strategy incorporates a key concept of behavior change science, that the benefits of engaging in healthy behaviors must outweigh the barriers in order for people to take action. As many program messages as possible highlight the value of maintaining and improving health status. Leading employees to measure and record their individual results is a key component of this strategy. This focus helps them recognize the personal outcomes they achieve from their healthy living efforts. A Personal Outcomes Assessment feature is included on the VFC to measure fitness, central body fat, and energy balance so that participants can determine the specific impact of their physical activity behaviors. Use of the Personal Outcomes Assessment reinforces the value of well-being to the individual and helps him or her refine actions to better achieve personal targets.

Populations Best Served by the Program

The VFC program was designed for active adult employees, and this chapter reports on its implementation among employees of a single company. It is reasonable, however, to consider this a highly scalable program across participant age (with a range of at least 18-65 years), gender, income level, race, and ethnicity groups. It is also reasonable to consider that this program may be effective among various types of industry (service, manufacturing), business environments (union, nonunion), and company sizes (small, medium, large). Obviously, a limitation is the fact that it is implemented online.

Tips for Working Across Sectors

The following recommendations can facilitate efforts to implement similar programs across various sectors in the community setting:

- Ensure equitable access to online resources.
- Address any disparities in health literacy, web-based training and knowledge, and language.
- Translate implementation processes from the worksite setting into the specifics of the other sectors, for example, a community setting, an education or school setting, or a health care setting.

Additional Reading and Resources

Books

Committee to Assess Worksite Preventive Health Program Needs for NASA Employees, Food and Nutrition Board. 2005. *Integrating Employee Health: A Model Program for NASA*. Institute of Medicine, National Academy of Sciences. Washington, D.C.

Prochaska, J.O., C.A. Redding, and K.E. Evers. 1997. The transtheoretical model and stages of change. In: *Health Behavior and Health Education: Theory, Research, and Practice* (pp. 60-84). 2nd ed. K. Glanz, F.M. Lewis, and B.K. Rimer, Eds. San Francisco: Jossey-Bass.

Seligman, M.P. 2011. *Flourish: A Visionary New Understanding of Happiness and Well-Being*. New York: Free Press.

Articles

Helsel, D.L., J.M. Jakicic, and A.D. Otto. 2007. Comparison of techniques for self monitoring, eating and exercise behaviors on weight loss in a correspondence-based intervention. *J. Am. Diet. Assoc.* 107:1807-10.

Herman, C.W., S. Musich, C. Lu, S. Sill, J.M. Young, and D.E. Edington. 2006. Effectiveness of an incentive-based online physical activity intervention on employee health status. *J. Occup. Environ. Med.* 48(9):889-95.

Keyes, C., and J.G. Grzywacz. 2005. Health as a complete state: The added value in work performance and health care costs. *J. Occup. Environ. Med.* 47(5):523-32.

Lu, C., A.B. Schultz, S. Sill, R. Petersen, J.M. Young, and D.W. Edington. 2008. Effects of an incentive-based online physical activity intervention on health care costs. *J. Occup. Environ. Med.* 50(11):1209-15.

Pronk, N.P. 2009. Physical activity promotion in business and industry: Evidence, context, and recommendations for a national plan. *J. Physical Activity Health.* 6 (Suppl. 2), S220-S235.

Pronk, N.P., M. Lowry, T.E. Kottke, E. Austin, J. Gallagher, and E. Katz. 2010. The association between optimal lifestyle adherence and short-term incidence of chronic conditions among employees. *Popul. Health Manag.* 13(6):289-95.

Pronk, N.P., A.S. Katz, J. Gallagher, E. Austin, D. Mullen, M. Lowry, and T.W. Kottke. 2011. Adherence to optimal lifestyle behaviors is related to emotional health indicators among employees. *Popul. Health Manag.* 14(2):59-67.

Sepúlveda, M-J., C. Lu, S. Sill, J.M. Young, and D.W. Edington. 2010. An observational study of an employer intervention for children's healthy weight behaviors. *Pediatrics* 128(5):1153-60.

Other Materials and Web-Based Resources

The National Physical Activity Plan website: www.physicalactivityplan.org/index.php

The National Physical Activity Plan Business and Industry Sector web pages including the strategies and tactics: www.physicalactivityplan.org/theplan.php and www.physicalactivityplan.org/business.php

Guide to Community Preventive Services and the Task Force on Community Preventive Services: www.thecommunityguide.org/index.html

Public Health

Jackie Epping, MEd

U.S. Centers for Disease Control and Prevention,
Division of Nutrition, Physical Activity and Obesity

The public health sector plays a critical role in promoting physical activity at the population level. Physical activity is fundamental to maintaining health and preventing disease, and public health organizations and professionals are responsible for monitoring, protecting, and promoting the public's health. As the field of physical activity and public health has grown and evolved, particularly over the past decade, several key roles for the public health sector have emerged. One of those roles is developing and maintaining a diverse and competent physical activity and public health (PAPH) workforce, which requires developing professional standards, creating and providing professional development opportunities, connecting PAPH professionals, and developing and providing physical activity resources. Another role is creating, maintaining, and leveraging partnerships and coalitions that can promote physical activity across all sectors of society. Because the public health sector exists at the national, state, and local levels, it is well positioned to convene and connect partners and stakeholders at multiple levels and across many sectors. The public health sector also can engage in PAPH policy development by educating policy makers at all levels, conducting PAPH surveillance, and evaluating programs and policies to promote physical activity. These roles are specifically identified within the five strategies outlined in the Public Health Sector of the National Physical Activity Plan.

The chapters in this section illustrate the ways that public health organizations and professionals promote physical activity in a variety of settings and contexts. The section includes case studies of cross-sectoral collaborations to promote physical activity, including collaborations that use health impact assessments to inform policy decisions about land use. The section also describes programs that are developing the PAPH workforce at both the state and national levels. One chapter discusses the use of surveillance and evaluation to inform physical activity policy, and two chapters describe the process of developing state physical activity plans.

The authors and editors hope that these chapters will provide useful examples of the roles the public health sector can play in advancing the field of physical activity and public health and promoting physical activity at the population level.

CHAPTER 29

State-Based Efforts for Physical Activity Planning

Experience From Texas and West Virginia

Eloise Elliott, PhD
West Virginia University

Emily Jones, PhD
West Virginia University

Donna C. Nichols, MSEd, CHES
University of Texas Health Science Center - Houston

Tinker D. Murray, PhD
Texas State University

Harold W. Kohl, III, PhD
University of Texas Health Science Center – Houston and University of Texas at Austin

NPAP Tactics and Strategies Used in This Program

Public Health Sector

STRATEGY 2: Create, maintain, and leverage cross-sector partnerships and coalitions that implement effective strategies to promote physical activity. Partnerships should include representatives from public health; health care; education; parks, recreation, fitness, and sports; transportation, urban design, and community planning; business and industry; volunteer and non-profit organizations; faith communities; mass media; and organizations serving historically underserved and understudied populations.

OVERARCHING STRATEGY 3: Disseminate best practice physical activity models, programs, and policies to the widest extent practicable to ensure Americans can access strategies that will enable them to meet federal physical activity guidelines.

Planning is an essential function for public health. Strategic public health planning allows agencies and organizations to set priorities for action, ensures access to services and activities across a broad population, and helps develop essential partnerships across and within sectors to identify and achieve common goals. Nations, states, and local governments have established public health plans to address a wide range of health problems (Kohl et al. 2012). Planning is key to addressing public health problems and maximizing the health of populations, because although plans don't ensure success, success is much less likely without a plan.

Historically, state health departments have developed public health plans to reflect state health priorities, which are usually tied to funding sources. U.S. federal and private funding sources often require states that request funding to have a formal plan for using the funding and other resources. State plans often address cardiovascular disease, diabetes, tobacco control, cancer, obesity, and other major areas of public health concern. Some state plans include physical activity in sections or plans that address noncommunicable diseases, but until very recently no state plans have focused specifically on physical activity.

The development of the U.S. National Physical Activity Plan (NPAP) emphasized physical activity as an independent public health priority and focused attention on the importance of physical activity planning (Pate 2009). NPAP provides a key framework for translating and mobilizing efforts at the state and local levels. In this chapter, we describe two state efforts that resulted from the development of NPAP and were designed to make physical activity a state public health priority through public health planning efforts.

Texas Program Description— Active Texas 2020

While the National Physical Activity Plan was being conceptualized and formulated, Texas convened a steering committee in mid-2008 to determine how to make the U.S. national plan relevant to Texas. The committee, consisting of School of Public Health faculty, other academic leaders, and members of the Texas Governor's Advisory Council on Physical Fitness (GCPF), discussed strategies and approaches to making physical activity a health priority in the state. The steering committee decided to back an effort to develop a statewide planning document for physical activity. Active Texas 2020, the Texas physical activity plan, resulted from this effort (Active Texas 2020, 2012).

The partnership between the School of Public Health and the GCPF was advantageous for several reasons. First, the GCPF is a group of state leaders already committed to physical activity. These leaders strongly supported the idea of a state physical activity plan. Second, the School of Public Health was able to provide expertise in public health planning. Third, developing a plan under the auspices of the GCPF provided structure for the plan and created avenues for developing partnerships and involving multiple sectors. This allowed the Texas planners to avoid the limited buy-in that often occurs when one agency develops a state plan (e.g., if the state health department develops a plan, then implementing the plan becomes the sole responsibility of the health department) and positioned physical activity as a multisectoral problem that must be addressed on many fronts. Fourth, housing the plan in the governor's office instead of a specific state agency allowed for flexibility to leverage partnerships across a wide variety of agencies and organizations.

Capacity Building

In January 2009, state planners organized a two-day conference in Austin to gather input on developing a state plan for making physical activity a health priority. Known as the Fit City Summit, the conference attracted community leaders, elected officials, representatives of state and municipal agencies, and other interested stakeholders. The summit was hosted by the mayor of Austin, and several state-level officials participated. Approximately 400 people attended this meeting.

During the summit, breakout sessions addressed several key questions. These sessions, organized by sector (schools, work sites, transportation, health, parks and recreation) were designed to get maximal input from local leaders about how municipalities in the state could make physical activity a health priority. Each session began with a review of evidence-based strategies for promoting physical activity, and moderators were prepared with discussion points to lead the discussion. Extensive notes were obtained from each 90-minute session. These notes and the session summary were used to inform the development of the state plan.

After gathering input from the summit, a writing group began to draft the state plan. This effort was supported by a small development grant from the Directors of Health Promotion and Education, a national nonprofit public health organization. The writing group circulated drafts to various leaders and requested feedback and input. The group then posted a penultimate draft on the internet for public comment. The Texas state plan for promoting physical activity—Active Texas 2020—was finalized in September 2010.

The vision of Active Texas 2020 is that "Texas will succeed in efforts to improve health by making physical activity a health priority across the state." An overarching theme of Active Texas 2020 is to enable and empower local leaders to advance physical activity as a health priority. Active Texas 2020 assumes that state and local leaders across Texas share a sense of priority for improving health and that a key strategy to improve health is to increase physical activity. Guided by that assumption, Active Texas 2020 focuses on informing and supporting community leaders across the state to take action and make changes that will increase physical activity in their communities. The six main sections of the plan highlight ways that local leaders can develop strategies for effectively promoting physical activity.

Plan Development

Eight guiding principles form the foundation for Active Texas 2020 (table 29.1). These principles were established to ensure that efforts to

Table 29.1 Guiding Principles for Active Texas 2020

Principle	Rationale
Physical activity improves health.	Active Texas 2020 relies on recent public health guidelines (U.S. Department of Health and Human Services 2008) and the vast scientific literature on physical activity and health.
Public health approaches to increasing physical activity are needed to improve the health of populations.	Individually based promotion programs are effective for individuals; public health approaches are needed for populations.
Make the healthier choice the easier choice.	Public health approaches can focus on removing barriers and promoting enablers for physical activity where people eat, work, play, and pray.
All health is local.	The emphasis on improving health through increased physical activity must take place at the community level. National and state health officials can and should provide a scientific and policy context and information, tools, and resources for making changes that will improve health. However, local leaders hold the power to make necessary changes.
Health is everyone's business.	In addition to the health benefits of physical activity, substantial economic benefits can be realized with a population that is more physically active.
Prioritize leadership collaboration and partnerships.	Success in changing communities to promote physical activity will require community leaders to create collaborative partnerships with a diverse set of partners, including elected officials, business leaders, faith-based organizations, medical professionals, nonprofits, school districts, neighborhoods, and more.
Work from the evidence base.	Strategies for successful physical activity promotion must be rooted in the scientific evidence. Nothing is gained (and much can be lost) if non-effective or non-recommended strategies are implemented.
Evaluate effectiveness.	Fundamentally, evaluating the effectiveness of any implemented strategy is a core element of public health practice. Evaluation of the strategies used is critical to understanding how the population's health has changed with certain interventions. The evaluation should provide further evidence of which practices are effective for increasing activity and which are not.

increase physical activity to improve health will focus on effective leadership, evidence-based recommendations, and actionable strategies.

Measuring Plan Success

Implementation and evaluation efforts for Active Texas 2020 are ongoing. The emphasis on local actions for physical activity promotion extends to the measurement and evaluation of success. A guiding principle used in developing the plan (table 29.1) addresses effectiveness evaluation. Process and outcome evaluation strategies are ideal for evaluation of Active Texas 2020. Because local actions to promote physical activity will differ, a cookbook approach to evaluation was not supportable; rather, the importance of doing the work and collecting appropriate data relevant to a local community's goals is emphasized.

Currently, the state has not identified resources to evaluate overall dissemination, diffusion, and implementation strategies for Active Texas 2020, although efforts to secure evaluation resources are underway.

The National Physical Activity Plan as the Foundation

The NPAP provided the framework for translating and mobilizing efforts at the state level. The activity at the national level helped to justify attention and commitments at the state level. The evidence-informed strategies within the NPAP were used to develop the strategies and tactics that provide the foundation for Active Texas 2020.

Concluding Comments

Active Texas 2020 is one of the first state-level physical activity plans in the United States. It was designed to make physical activity a health priority in the state by providing specific strategies for local design and implementation of physical activity promotion. The plan can be used to enhance existing planning efforts regarding noncommunicable disease because of the role that physical activity plays in promoting health.

West Virginia Program Description—Active WV 2015

Although West Virginia has a number of health problems and disparities, it also has a population of enthusiastic citizens and leaders who are dedicated to improving the state and, specifically, improving the health of the state's citizens. These citizens and leaders have worked across sectors to address a number of health issues. For example, state government has passed legislation related to health promotion, including improved physical education and nutrition offerings in schools; state agencies have adopted policies and developed plans to include physical activity promotion and practice; nonprofit organizations are spearheading programs that educate children and adults about the need for physical activity and are providing suggestions for community initiatives; and community groups are stepping up to showcase local projects that are working in their communities. These efforts reflect a state ready to make positive changes in the health and well-being of its citizens. However, the missing element among all of these efforts is a strategic vision to unify activities to address increasing health care costs, the need for environmental changes, and the prevalence of chronic diseases.

Based on recommendations from the NPAP, a statewide initiative to develop a physical activity plan for West Virginia was born. Active WV is designed to provide a strategic vision and direction to create a culture that facilitates physically active lifestyles in every societal sector and region of the state, regardless of barriers. Active WV provides the strategic vision and represents the collective voice of West Virginians proclaiming the values and physical activity needs of our state. The following sections provide an overview of the capacity-building efforts, development process, launch, and measures of success of Active WV.

Capacity Building

For Active WV to effectively guide state and local policies and practices, key individuals needed to be involved in every step of the development, implementation, and dissemination.

The target audience of Active WV consists of three main constituency groups: (1) state and local policy leaders, (2) key stakeholders who represent state and local organizations and groups in each sector, and (3) West Virginia citizens. Individuals in each group serve as leaders, contributors, and advocates in the process of creating a physically active West Virginia. Key capacity building efforts involved in creating Active WV are described next.

Establishing Organizational Governance

Following the May 2010 release of the NPAP, a multidisciplinary group of researchers and organizational leaders from across West Virginia convened to discuss the potential of a statewide physical activity plan. Participants concluded that West Virginia needed strategic direction for physical activity promotion, and the Active WV coordinating committee, which would serve as the primary governing body of the statewide initiative, was established. The coordinating committee, whose members represent a variety of social and professional sectors, determined that the goal of Active WV would be "to serve as a blueprint for connecting, supporting, and building upon existing efforts within the state," while focusing on strategies that would require policy, environmental, and systems changes at both the state and local levels. To that end, the committee identified key factors for ensuring the effectiveness of the plan, including (1) input and participation from all sectors, as identified in the NPAP; (2) a unified leadership team of dedicated state and local stakeholders working toward a solution; and (3) policy leaders who see physical activity as a health priority in the state and will advocate for policy and environmental changes to provide more localized physical activity opportunities.

Garnering Support From Policy Leaders and Key Stakeholders

During the early stages of conceptualizing and developing the plan, the chair of the Active WV coordinating committee met with many state government officials and health policy leaders to increase the visibility of Active WV and to seek advice and recommendations. These leaders included the governor's chief of staff, members of a joint Senate and House health committee, funding officers of foundations, directors of state agencies, and health coalition leaders. Many key partnerships transpired from the recommendations that emerged from these meetings, and the leaders provided advice on coordinating strategies to involve government, funding agencies, and local decision makers (e.g., county commissioners). The opportunity to inform these key stakeholders at the beginning of the planning process proved to be significant in moving forward.

Establishing Sector Teams and Organizational Partners

Another Active WV capacity-building strategy used the NPAP's eight-sector framework to identify targeted population groups. Unique to Active WV, a policy group was added to the list of sectors in an attempt to intentionally involve those who may directly influence state, regional, and local policies related to physical activity and health. As a result, the representative sectors included education; public health; business and industry; volunteer and nonprofit; parks, recreation, fitness, and sports; transportation, land use, and community design; health care; mass media; and policy. Participation and leadership of key stakeholders within each sector was formalized through the development of sector teams. The sector teams consist of 70 leaders from organizations such as state government, local health departments, county and city leaders, medical schools, community and worksite wellness programs, and state media outlets. These teams, each of which is led by a team leader, finalized the development of the plan strategies and tactics for their respective sectors. This 70-member group continues to lead efforts to implement the plan statewide and at the community level. The roles of the sector team members and the team leaders were adapted from the NPAP and are outlined in table 29.2.

Hosting a Statewide Event

The first West Virginia Physical Activity Symposium was held in Charleston in June 2010 as the initial step in developing a working plan that could potentially change the state's

Table 29.2   Roles of Sector Leaders and Sector Team Representatives

Sector leaders	Sector team representatives
• Review national strategies from the NPAP and make recommendation for refinement for West Virginia, based on the outcomes of West Virginia systematic analyses	• Review national strategies from the NPAP and make recommendation for refinement for West Virginia, based on the outcomes of West Virginia systematic analyses
• Designate leaders for specific strategies within a sector	• Contribute to the final development of Active WV strategies and tactics
• Lead the final development of Active WV strategies and tactics	• Advocate for changes in policies and practices that will influence physical activity behaviors
• Set forth changes in policies and practices that will influence PA behaviors	• Influence plan implementation on the state and local levels
• Advise and influence plan implementation	• Represent the plan within their respective organizations and throughout the sector
• Support state and local advocacy related to the plan	• Encourage community action
• Represent the plan within their respective organizations and throughout the sector	

physical activity culture. The intent of the two-day symposium was to bring together as many people as possible from all nine sectors and all regions of the state to learn about the NPAP, showcase what is currently happening in West Virginia related to physical activity programs and research, and build awareness and support for a statewide strategic plan for physical activity. More than 250 participants representing all sectors and regions of the state attended the event. Seven nationally recognized speakers, including the chair of the NPAP coordinating committee, shared national and global perspectives on physical activity related to all of the sectors. More than 50 West Virginia programs and research projects presented information in either poster or oral formats. The West Virginia governor and first lady provided support for the event, including an all-conference reception at the governor's mansion. Celebrities who carry the message for increased physical activity participated and truly enhanced the symposium program. Twenty-three organizations and agencies sponsored or contributed to the success of the symposium. During day 2, sector and regional working group sessions began the process of gathering input pertinent to developing the plan. Small group discussions, focused on some of the NPAP strategies in each sector, resulted in sector-specific recommendations for action steps and identification of regional barri-

ers and gaps. Data from these working groups informed the development of the final strategies and tactics for Active WV.

Securing Financial Support

Three organizational partners, including two university-based programs and a statewide nonprofit physical activity advocacy group, provided the primary resources for the development of Active WV. Many businesses, organizations, agencies, and a regional foundation provided support for the statewide symposium. Efforts are underway to secure financial support and resources for implementing, disseminating, and evaluating Active WV.

Plan Development

The coordinating committee used a systematic process to develop the plan and to ensure input from a wide range of audiences, sectors, and regions. Input used in formulating the final written plan came from four sources—the NPAP's strategies and tactics, results of the West Virginia Physical Activity Symposium sector working groups, results of an online concept mapping exercise, and sector team expertise.

National Physical Activity Plan as the Foundation

The NPAP provided the framework for translating and mobilizing efforts at the state level. The evidence-informed strategies and tactics within the NPAP underpinned the Active WV strategies and tactics, although planners considered the contextual variables specific to West Virginia.

Concept Mapping Exercise

In an attempt to gather input from citizens throughout the state regarding the need for physical activity policy and environmental changes, Active WV planners used an integrated, web-based approach called *concept mapping*. Concept mapping is a strategy used to help show connections between ideas and concepts, and it proved to be a valuable tool for gathering and synthesizing strategies for the statewide plan. For the purposes of Active WV, planners implemented a multiphase concept mapping process. The four phases included brainstorming; statement analysis and synthesis; sorting and rating of statements; and data analysis and interpretation. The actions and results of each phase of the concept mapping exercise and plan development are shown in table 29.3.

Face-to-Face Sector Team Meeting

At a face-to-face meeting, sector team participants ($N = 72$) wrote sector-specific strategies for each of the five priority areas identified by the concept mapping process. For each priority area, each sector team generated one specific strategy that best represented its sector. Tactics, or action steps, for each strategy were then considered from all data sources. Each sector team selected five top tactics that team members believed could be achieved in the next five years for inclusion in the final written plan. The Activ eWV plan development subcommittee finalized the written document and, after public review, prepared it for widespread dissemination.

Release of Active WV 2015

Active WV 2015: The West Virginia Physical Activity Plan was officially released on January 19, 2012, at the State Capitol in Charleston (Active WV n.d.). The all-day event at the Capitol included displays, physical activity demonstration groups, state dignitaries and key stakeholders, and two national celebrities who are role models for physical activity. A launch ceremony included the signing of a declaration by the governor to make the day West Virginia Physical Activity Day, a proclamation by the West Virginia Legislative Senate to make physical activity a health priority, and support messages from West Virginia congressional leaders. Across the state, schools and communities supported the launch of Active WV by hosting local

Table 29.3 Phases of the Concept Mapping Process

Phase	Action	Result
Phase 1: brainstorming	Informational Active WV webinar Invitation to respond to a prompt that encouraged submission of ideas	154 participants from all sectors responded to the prompt. 240 ideas generated
Phase 2: statement analysis and synthesis	Review of the 240 ideas Elimination of non–physical activity ideas Synthesis of similar ideas into single-statements	61 single-idea, physical activity-related statements were generated.
Phase 3: sorting and rating of statements	Statements sorted into like groups Statements rated on importance and feasibility scales	Five discrete priority areas for Active WV were determined.
Phase 4: data analysis and interpretation	Informational Active WV webinar Sector team review of priority areas and statements	Sector-specific Active WV strategies and tactics were identified and finalized.

events. A powerful example was the participation of the schools throughout West Virginia. In conjunction with the West Virginia Department of Education's Office of Healthy Schools Let's Move WV initiative, 100,652 students (from 313 schools) did a popular line dance simultaneously at 1:00 p.m. to highlight physical activity in the schools. Also, 44 county commissioners (out of 55) signed resolutions to support increased physical activity in the communities where West Virginia citizens live, learn, work, and play. Key television, radio, and newspaper media outlets participated in both the capitol event as well as many local happenings.

Shortly after the release of the plan, the sector teams were reconvened for another face-to-face meeting to begin formulating the implementation plan and to make recommendations for the next steps in implementation, dissemination, and evaluation of Active WV.

Measuring Plan Success

Although the ultimate goal of the plan is to increase physical activity among all West Virginians, other more immediate measures of effectiveness are whether

- state and local organizations adopt the plan's strategies,
- local communities implement the actionable tactics that are outlined in the plan, and
- West Virginia policy makers and other key stakeholders support and enact change for improved physical activity opportunities.

Process, impact, and outcome evaluation methods were developed at the state and local levels. Process evaluation will review and document the plan development process. Impact evaluation will examine the short-term impact of program interventions and disseminate efforts on the physical activity behaviors; public awareness; and policy, system, and environmental changes within the state. Finally, outcome evaluation methods will monitor the long-term influence on statewide public health goals related to physical activity.

Concluding Comments

With a comprehensive physical activity blueprint now in place, West Virginia is poised to influence the culture of physical activity statewide. Through the organizational partnerships developed as a result of the sector teams, and through positive leadership of policy leaders, West Virginia may now make physical activity a primary health priority. Communication and implementation, however, will drive its success. Lead organizations and groups must step up and assume primary roles in advocacy, implementation, and evaluation. Funding must be secured to support these endeavors as well as to create a state coordinator position to ensure accountability, continuity, and sustainability. Communities must be targeted as the real venues for change. An ongoing social marketing campaign is needed to raise awareness of the importance of physical activity, and community leaders will need action strategies to guide implementation of the plan at the local level. Community groups interested in physical activity promotion will need support, including strategies for assessing local needs, overcoming barriers, planning interventions, and evaluating outcomes. Evaluation of the plan's success must focus on the community. As with the initial plan development process, there must remain a focus on "one vision, one voice." West Virginia still has much work ahead to make a difference in the health and quality of life of its citizens. The West Virginia Physical Activity Plan is a step toward success—toward Active WV 2015.

Linkage to National Physical Activity Plan

Although the physical activity plans in Texas and West Virginia were developed by processes different than that of the NPAP, both plans have elements that include the eight sectors and strategies of the NPAP. The local articulation of the overarching vision of the NPAP is a common thread between the two state plans. Other states can use these models to develop localized plans using the NPAP as a framework that create, maintain, and leverage cross-sectional partnerships and coalitions that can be used for physical activity promotion.

Lessons Learned

State-level planning for physical activity is rare, but the need for such action has never been clearer. When the NPAP was released in 2010, it called for grassroots efforts to mobilize and support strategies and tactics nationally but also provided an evidence-based blueprint to enable states to develop their own physical activity plans. Texas and West Virginia are two of the first states to follow a systematic process to develop such plans. Although these two states followed different development processes, they learned many of the same lessons:

- Involve key stakeholders and partners from many sectors.
- Take steps in the beginning and throughout the process to establish a systematic and ongoing forum for discussion, input, buy-in, and participation.
- Empower local and state leaders to make physical activity a health priority.
- Encourage and enable communities to take responsibility for implementing the plan at the local level.

Once states have developed, disseminated, and implemented statewide physical activity plans, these plans should be integrated into other state plans for which physical activity is a relevant issue (e.g., public health, education, economic development, health care, transportation). As a result, physical activity promotion becomes everyone's responsibility and physical activity becomes a public health priority for the entire population. After all, the goal of the NPAP is to "improve health, prevent disease and disability, and enhance quality of life" (National Physical Activity Plan 2010); this can become a reality when states invest in and take steps to change the environments, systems, and policies that can affect the physical activity behaviors of all citizens where they live, work, learn, and play.

References

Active Texas 2020: Taking action to promote physical activity. 2012. https://sph.uth.tmc.edu/research/centers/dell/active-texas-2020/.

ActiveWV 2015: The West Virginia Physical Activity Plan. n.d. http://wvphysicalactivity.org/.

Kohl, H.W., III, C.L. Craig, E.V. Lambert, S. Inoue, J.R. Alkandari, G. Leetongin, S. Kahlmeier; Lancet Physical Activity Series Working Group. 2012. The pandemic of physical inactivity: global action for public health. *Lancet* 380:294-305.

The National Physical Activity Plan. 2010. www.physicalactivityplan.org.

Pate, R.R. 2009. A national physical activity plan for the United States. *J. Phys. Activ. Health* 6(Suppl. 3):S157-8.

U.S. Department of Health and Human Services. 2008 Physical Activity Guidelines for Americans. www.health.gov/paguidelines.

CHAPTER 30

Health Impact Assessments
A Means to Initiate and Maintain Cross-Sector Partnerships to Promote Physical Activity

Katherine Hebert, MCRP
Davidson Design for Life

Candace Rutt, PhD
Centers for Disease Control and Prevention

NPAP Tactics and Strategies Used in This Program

Public Health Sector

STRATEGY 2: Create, maintain, and leverage cross-sector partnerships and coalitions that implement effective strategies to promote physical activity. Partnerships should include representatives from public health; health care; education; parks, recreation, fitness, and sports; transportation, urban design, and community planning; business and industry; volunteer and nonprofit organizations; faith communities; mass media; and organizations serving historically underserved and understudied populations.

STRATEGY 3: Engage in advocacy and policy development to elevate the priority of physical activity in public health practice, policy, and research.

STRATEGY 4: Disseminate tools and resources important to promoting physical activity, including resources that address the burden of disease due to inactivity, the implementation of evidence-based interventions, and funding opportunities for physical activity initiatives.

Transportation, Land Use, and Community Design Sector

STRATEGY 3: Integrate land-use, transportation, community design, and economic development planning with public health planning to increase active transportation and other physical activity.

D ecisions made outside of the traditional public health and health care sectors can have immense effects on individual and population health. For example, policy and planning decisions that shape the built environment (defined as human-made resources and infrastructure designed to support human activity, including buildings, roads, parks, and other amenities; County Health Rankings & Roadmaps 2013) may determine an individual's ability to be physically active every day. By increasing access to means of active transportation (such as bicycle lanes and sidewalks), places of inexpensive recreation (such as parks and greenways), and safe environments for walking, playing, and learning within neighborhoods and

Acknowledgments: The authors thank Dr. Holly Avey (Fort McPherson HIA), Amanda Thompson (Decatur Transportation Plan HIA), Karen Leone de Nie (Decatur Transportation Plan HIA), and Michelle Marcus (Atlanta BeltLine HIA) for their insight on the collaborations that were necessary to conduct the HIA. The authors also thank Amy Lang with the CDC's Geospatial Research, Analysis, and Services Program (GRASP) for her assistance with the map titled HIA Case Studies in the Greater Atlanta Region.

urban areas, city planners and decision makers can positively influence many aspects of health (figure 30.1).

The social determinants of health (defined as the conditions in which people are born, grow, live, work, and age; World Health Organization 2013) include the options and resources available to people in their neighborhoods; the cleanliness of the air, water, and food they consume; the safety of their neighborhoods and workplaces; their education; and their social ties to friends, family, and neighbors (Healthy People 2020, 2012). These conditions play a vital role in determining health. Health inequities can be attributed largely to differences in social determinants of health. Cross-sectoral collaborations that focus on the potential health impacts of decisions on vulnerable populations, who often lack access to the resources needed to live a healthy and physically active lifestyle, can help to address these disparities. A health impact assessment is one means of addressing health inequities and changing policies and environments by promoting cross-sectoral collaboration and bringing potential public health concerns to the attention of decision makers from various sectors.

Program Description

Health impact assessment (HIA) is "a systematic process that uses an array of data sources and analytic methods and considers input from stakeholders to determine the potential effects of a proposed policy, plan, program, or project on the health of a population and the distribution of those effects within the population. HIA provides recommendations on monitoring and managing those effects" (National Research Council 2011, p. 46).

HIA consists of six steps: screening, scoping, assessment, recommendations, report-

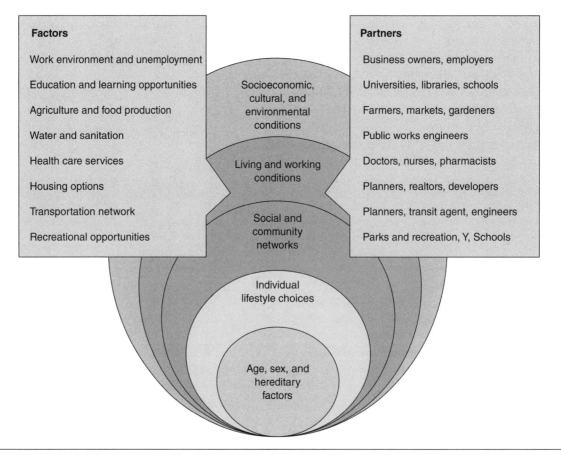

Figure 30.1 Social determinants of health and potential partners.

ing, and monitoring and evaluation (figure 30.2). These steps are fluid and tend to influence each other. HIA uses a combination of sources and methods of analysis, depending on the topic and sector in which the HIA is being conducted. Each sector is unique, and the flexibility of the HIA process to evaluate potential health outcomes of diverse decisions is one of its greatest strengths. Because it is a participatory process, HIA involves gathering stakeholder input and involving the public at every stage. It emphasizes considering the needs of people who may be most adversely affected by a policy decision (such as the placement of a new road or the opening or closing of a park). Perhaps most important, HIA is proactive and offers recommendations to promote positive health impacts and prevent or mitigate negative health impacts. This means that the HIA must be completed

before a decision is made, preferably early enough in the process that the HIA findings can be incorporated into the decision-making process.

The overarching purpose of an HIA is to provide decision makers with accurate and scientifically based information and recommendations concerning the potential health impacts of their decisions. As well as leading to better-informed decisions, HIAs typically result in increased awareness of community health concerns; collaborations across multiple disciplines and a better understanding of each discipline's influence on the social determinants of health; broader spillover effects and support for encompassing policies, such as a Complete Streets policy; and more equitable and community-driven planning and policy making through increased community engagement (NACCHO 2008).

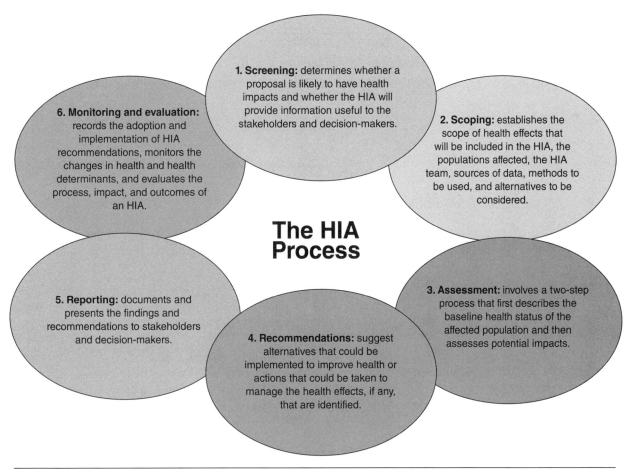

Figure 30.2   HIA process.

The principles guiding the practice of HIA support the use of collaborations in health promotion and disease prevention. These principles include democracy and public participation, equity and equality, ethical and transparent use of evidence, sustainability, a comprehensive approach to health and health promotion, interdisciplinary or collaborative orientation, and an efficient use of time and resources (Hebert et al. 2012).

The type of HIA conducted—rapid, intermediate, or comprehensive—depends on the amount of time available before a decision is made and the resources that can be dedicated to the HIA. Rapid HIAs take days to weeks to finish, use limited resources, and typically provide a broad overview of potential health impacts without collecting new, site-specific data. Intermediate HIAs can take weeks to months to complete, involve a greater degree of community engagement, and provide more detailed information

than a rapid HIA. If a very thorough assessment of the potential health impacts is warranted (usually in the case of major projects or policies that affect a large number of people or are considered politically controversial), then a comprehensive HIA should be done. Comprehensive HIAs commonly involve collecting new quantitative and qualitative data and engaging the community at a high level, and these can take years to complete.

The remainder of this chapter describes partnerships formed to conduct three HIAs that considered the potential impacts of three proposals on physical activity in the greater Atlanta area: the interim zoning policies for the redevelopment of Fort McPherson, Decatur's Community Transportation Plan, and the proposed Atlanta BeltLine (figure 30.3). Each HIA was conducted at a different geography (development site, city, and regional scale) and focused on a different type of decision, and all three resulted in the

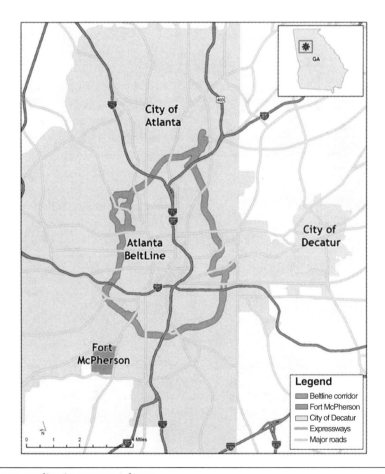

Figure 30.3 HIA case studies in greater Atlanta.

development of partnerships to perform and implement the HIA recommendations.

Fort McPherson

Fort McPherson, an Army installation consisting of 488 acres located between downtown Atlanta and Hartsfield Jackson International Airport, was scheduled to be shut down in 2011 as part of the Department of Defense's Base Realignment and Closure program. A city unto itself, Fort McPherson supports a wide variety of community facilities, including a bank, library, convenience store, gas station, health facilities, office space, and more than 200 acres of outdoor recreational facilities, including historic parade grounds and a golf course.

The closure and redevelopment of Fort McPherson could potentially span decades. Interim use of the property during the first 5 to 10 years of redevelopment could have significant economic and health impacts on the surrounding communities. As a result of a larger Health in All Policies (HiAP) project funded by the Centers for Disease Control and Prevention, the Georgia Health Policy Center conducted an HIA of the proposed redevelopment plan. The scope of the HIA was limited to the 5- to 10-year interim period and focused on the zoning provisions that address permitted uses, available green space, and transportation. The center estimated impacts on physical activity levels (among other impacts) for those living within a half mile of the property. At the beginning of the HIA, the Centers for Disease Control and Prevention brought together all of the stakeholders in the redevelopment process to learn more about HIA and to share their perspectives.

To conduct the Fort McPherson HIA, the Georgia Health Policy Center worked closely with multiple partners, including the City of Atlanta Department of Planning and Community Development, which regulates the zoning and permitting process for the redevelopment; the McPherson Local Redevelopment Authority, which is responsible for planning the redevelopment of the property; and the McPherson Action Community Coalition, which represents interested residents from the surrounding neighborhoods. Through these partnerships, the Health Policy Center's leaders were introduced to other participants and important organizations, including a Department of Defense representative; contractors from the planning and architectural design firm hired to revise the redevelopment plan; Georgia Stand Up, which is a community organizing group affiliated with the McPherson Action Community Coalition; and a professor at the Georgia Institute of Technology who conducted a design studio on the redevelopment project for planning students.

At the conclusion of the HIA, the HIA report recommended zoning actions to the City of Atlanta Department of Planning and Community Development that could improve opportunities for physical activity during the interim period while the property is redeveloped. Recommendations were based on several premises: (1) people are more physically active when they have access to trails and parks; (2) people are more likely to use trails when they can access them from multiple places; and (3) walking trails may increase physical activity in particular for two population subgroups that are less likely to exercise—women and people of limited income. The recommendations included permitting the use of existing outdoor recreational facilities and green space by neighboring communities and maximizing accessibility to existing recreational facilities and green space with ADA-compliant roads or paths at multiple entry points.

City of Decatur's Community Transportation Plan

The City of Decatur's Community Transportation Plan, completed in 2007, is organized around the goal of creating an "active living community," defined in the plan as "a place where residents and visitors can readily participate in everyday physical activity, regardless of physical limitations" (Decatur Community Transportation Plan 2007, appendix F, p. 2). Decatur is a historic town 6 miles (9.6 kilometers) east of downtown Atlanta, spanning 4.2 square miles (10.8 square kilometers) and consisting of approximately 20,000 residents. Founded in 1826 and experiencing a lack of developable land since the 1960s, Decatur has increased development in the core of the city and has redeveloped surface parking lots over the last 10 years to restructure the built environment to include mixed-use midrise buildings featuring residential units on the upper floors and commercial development on the ground floor.

With the task of incorporating an "active living framework" into the transportation plan, the City of Decatur partnered with the Georgia Institute of Technology's Center for Quality Growth and Regional Development, Kimley Horn and Associates, and Sycamore Consulting to conduct an HIA to evaluate the plan's goals from a health perspective. These goals included (1) setting a course for a transportation and land use connection to make Decatur a healthy place to live and work; (2) maintaining a high quality of life in Decatur; and (3) increasing opportunities to use alternative modes of transportation (Decatur Community Transportation Plan 2007).

To help identify potential community health concerns about the plan, the city hosted a one-day workshop and invited local residents and business owners; nonprofit organizations and area churches; and local, regional, and state government officials. During the workshop, experts on the built environment, HIA, and public health from the Centers for Disease Control and Prevention, the Center for Quality Growth and Regional Development, and the DeKalb County Board of Health provided participants with local health information, background information on the relationship between the built environment and health, and group facilitation assistance. At the conclusion of the workshop, participants identified four broad areas within the plan that would have a direct effect on health: (1) intersection improvements, (2) biking facilities, (3) sidewalk improvements, and (4) traffic safety. They also identified particularly vulnerable populations, including youth and the elderly, persons with disabilities, and low-income and minority populations.

After the workshop, each element of the plan was evaluated for its potential impacts on health. There were three major findings of the HIA: (1) the plan could help the city increase physical activity levels and promote other posi-

tive health impacts; (2) concerns over bicyclist and pedestrian safety could be mitigated by the plan; and (3) implementation of the plan should be prioritized to meet the needs of vulnerable populations. Since the adoption of the plan and the completion of the HIA, the city has formed an Active Living Advisory Board, composed of Decatur residents and business owners, and an Active Living Division within the city government to continue to coordinate efforts to promote physical activity and healthy eating within the city.

Atlanta BeltLine

The Atlanta BeltLine, considered one of the largest redevelopment projects in United States history, is expected to convert 22 miles (35.4 kilometers) of abandoned railway into a combination of trails, parks, light rail transit, residential buildings, and commercial development. The oval loop, measuring 2 to 4 miles (3.2-6.4 kilometers) from Atlanta's city center, travels through 45 distinct neighborhoods and each of Atlanta's council districts. The project is expected to improve 700 acres of existing parks and add 1,300 acres (5.3 square kilometers) of new green space, including 33 miles (53 kilometers) of trails. Construction along the BeltLine is expected to produce 12 million square feet (slightly more than 1 million square meters) of office, retail, light industrial, and public or private institutional space and create 29,000 housing units. The tax allocation district established to fund the BeltLine is expected to raise $1.7 billion over the next 25 years, while increasing the overall tax base by $20 billion within the same period.

In 2005, the Georgia Institute of Technology's Center for Quality Growth and Regional Development, with funding from the Robert Wood Johnson Foundation and technical assistance from the Centers for Disease Control and Prevention, embarked on a comprehensive HIA that would take more than a year to complete. The HIA's study area consisted of 30,500 acres (123.4 square kilometers) (35 percent of the city's land area), forming a half-mile (.8-kilometer) buffer around the BeltLine's Tax Allocation District. The HIA considered the following health impacts: (1) access and social equity as they related to parks and trails, transit, housing, and healthy food; (2) physical activity levels, particularly in the southeast, southwest, and west-side areas where mortality rates are higher because of the prevalence of chronic disease; (3) safety from injury and crime; (4) social capital; and (5) environmental factors such as air and water pollution, noise and vibration, and the cleanup of formerly polluted sites.

Because of the vast differences in the social and economic characteristics of the regions through which the BeltLine passes (the southeast, southwest, and west-side populations are primarily nonwhite and, compared with the north-side and northeast populations, are younger and have almost twice the level of poverty and significantly lower levels of car ownership), health equity and the distribution of the associated health impacts were critical components of the HIA. Vulnerable populations identified within the HIA included low-income populations, children, older adults, those who have disabilities, renters, and those who do not have access to a car.

After a series of public workshops and surveys, detailed health data collection, and an intensive literature review, the HIA team reported on more than 50 recommendations for improving health along the BeltLine. Some of the recommendations were specifically tailored to increasing physical activity levels: (1) form a Safe Routes to School program; (2) include bicycle and pedestrian advocates on the BeltLine's advisory committees; (3) create park access equal to 10 acres (40,500 square meters) per 1,000 people and trail access every quarter of a mile (400 meters); (4) develop trail spurs, especially to underserved neighborhoods; (5) set design standards for multiuse trails and offer a variety of park types; and (6) launch an educational campaign for increasing physical activity on the BeltLine.

Because of the complexity of the BeltLine project, the HIA team consisted of numerous partners, including an HIA advisory committee that assisted with "overall project direction, component-specific guidance, and analytical

expertise" (Atlanta BeltLine HIA 2007, p. 38). The larger HIA team was responsible for the scoping and appraisal steps of the HIA and included representatives from Atlanta BeltLine, the Atlanta Development Authority, BeltLine Partnership, the Metropolitan Atlanta Rapid Transit Authority (MARTA), Park Pride, the Path Foundation, the Trust for Public Land, and City of Atlanta departments (planning and community development, public works, watershed management, and parks, recreation and cultural affairs).

Linkage to National Physical Activity Plan

The practice and application of HIA can contribute to accomplishing four of the strategies included within the National Physical Activity Plan: Public Health Sector Strategies 2, 3, and 4 and the Transportation, Land Use, and Community Design Sector Strategy 3.

Strategy 2: Create, maintain, and leverage cross-sector partnerships and coalitions that implement effective strategies to promote physical activity. Partnerships should include representatives from public health; health care; education; parks, recreation, fitness, and sports; transportation, urban design, and community planning; business and industry; volunteer and nonprofit organizations; faith communities; mass media; and organizations serving historically underserved and understudied populations. HIAs often are led by public health professionals, who make a concerted effort to involve professionals from many sectors, community residents, and other stakeholders.

Strategy 3: Engage in advocacy and policy development to elevate the priority of physical activity in public health practice, policy, and research. The findings of an HIA can be used in advocacy efforts and for promoting physical activity in all policy decisions.

Strategy 4: Disseminate tools and resources important to promoting physical activity, including resources that address the burden of disease due to inactivity, the implementation of evidence-based interventions, and funding opportunities for physical activity initiatives. HIA is a tool that can be disseminated to promote physical activity through evidence-based decisions. The reporting stage of an HIA involves disseminating information on the burden of disease as well as presenting recommendations to decrease and fairly distribute this burden.

Strategy 3: Integrate land-use, transportation, community design, and economic development planning with public health planning to increase active transportation and other physical activity. HIA can be applied to plans and development projects that result in collaborations between the public health and planning fields and inform planning and design efforts to increase physical activity opportunities such as active transportation and park development.

Lessons Learned

The collaborations that occurred within these three HIAs represent the partnerships commonly found in HIAs, which include representatives of local government departments, community organizations, university centers, public health experts, and local stakeholders (table 30.1). Through these partnerships, the HIA coordinators were better able to connect to decision makers, vulnerable populations, other previously unidentified stakeholders, and those in positions to bring about desired changes. In establishing and maintaining these relationships, HIA coordinators learned a number of lessons that could be useful for fostering cross-sectoral collaboration.

The key to developing all three of these collaborative efforts was identifying those who should participate in the collaboration and getting to know them. By asking who would be affected by the proposal, who had authority to make changes to the proposal, who was responsible for implementing the proposal, and who could provide the expertise needed to strengthen the proposal, the HIA coordinators identified potential members of the HIA team. Once these individuals were identified, the coordinators researched them further to determine what networks they commonly worked in, what their responsibilities and motivations were, and

their leadership style or overall personality. Having this knowledge helped the HIA coordinators determine whether to involve individuals in the collaboration and how to approach them in a way that would convince them to support the collaboration.

Another component of successful HIA collaboration is awareness of the political climate and context in which the HIA is being conducted. Finding a topic that all stakeholders can rally behind and identifying a political champion for the HIA or for public health in general can increase the success of the collaboration and the acceptance of the HIA's recommendations. In the Decatur Community Transportation Plan HIA, government officials and department leaders had already identified the need for incorporating an active living framework into their work and therefore were willing to support efforts to assess the potential health impacts of the plan. The discussion framework of public health also created an opportunity to shift the conversation from a competitive, resource-limited viewpoint of alternative transportation versus vehicle drivers to an opportunity-rich environment of transportation choice. Elected officials were given a chance to offer transportation choices instead of favoring one mode of travel at the expense of another.

Developing a common understanding of what an HIA is and how it can be used to improve the health impacts of a proposed policy or program also contributes to establishing a successful collaboration. For the Fort McPherson redevelopment HIA, providing an opportunity for all of the partners to meet and learn from each other proved to be a turning point. Follow-up meetings for smaller groups that focused on specific components of the HIA contributed to support for the process and the outcome.

To ensure continuation of the collaboration beyond the HIA's completion and acceptance of the recommendations by decision makers, it is crucial to prioritize the impacts considered within the HIA's scope and make sure that the team's objectives and recommendations are realistic. In particular, the comprehensive nature of the Atlanta BeltLine HIA required the team to limit its scope of work to the communities

Table 30.1   Partners, Stakeholders, and Decision Makers in Atlanta Case Studies

	Atlanta BeltLine	Decatur Community Transportation Plan	Fort McPherson Rapid HIA–Zoning in Interim Period
Lead organizations	Center for Quality Growth and Regional Development at Georgia Institute of Technology	Center for Quality Growth and Regional Development at Georgia Institute of Technology; Sycamore Consulting	Georgia Health Policy Center at Georgia State University
Main partners	Atlanta BeltLine, Atlanta Development Authority, BeltLine Partnership, MARTA, Park Pride, Path Foundation, Trust for Public Land, City of Atlanta (planning and community development, public works, watershed management, parks, recreation and cultural affairs)	City of Decatur (facilities maintenance, community and economic development, recreation and community service, police and fire, housing authority), DeKalb County Commissioners, Atlanta Regional Commission, Georgia Department of Transportation, Georgia Regional Transportation Authority, Georgia Division of Public Health, Agnes Scott College, City of Decatur Schools, neighborhood associations, nonprofit organizations (Georgia Conservancy, Decatur Preservation Alliance, PEDS), local businesses, churches	City of Atlanta Department of Planning and Community Development, McPherson Local Redevelopment Authority, and McPherson Action Community Coalition
HIA technical assistance	CDC (National Center for Environmental Health, Division of Unintentional Injury Prevention, Division of Nutrition, Physical Activity, and Obesity), Fulton County Department of Health and Wellness, Emory University	CDC, Georgia Tech Center for Quality Growth and Regional Development, DeKalb County Board of Health	CDC
Decision makers	City of Atlanta City Council, Fulton County Board of Commissioners, Atlanta Public School Board	Decatur City Commission	City of Atlanta Department of Planning and Community Development

within a half-mile (.8 kilometers) of the corridor and to highlight the most feasible and meaningful recommendations for decision makers.

Summary

Because overcoming barriers to increasing physical activity levels nationwide is such a complex and encompassing challenge, collaboration among multiple fields is necessary to create physically active, healthy, and vibrant communities for today's population as well as future generations. Health impact assessments are effective and should be considered when organizers are creating these types of collaborations, promoting physical activity, and achieving long-term public health goals such as those found within the National Physical Activity Plan.

Additional Reading and Resources

Georgia Health Policy Center, Fort McPherson rapid health impact assessment: Zoning for health benefit to surrounding communities during interim use. 2010. www.healthimpactproject.org/resources/document/FortMcPherson_at_ays_129.pdf.

References

Center for Quality Growth and Regional Development. 2007. Pathways to a healthy Decatur: A rapid health impact assessment of the City of Decatur Community Transportation Plan. www.decaturga.com/Modules/ShowDocument.aspx?documentid = 1211.

Center for Quality Growth and Regional Development. 2007. Atlanta BeltLine Health Impact Assessment. www.hiaguide.org/sites/default/files/beltline_hia_final_report.pdf.

County Health Rankings & Roadmaps. 2013. Health Factors: Built Environment. www.countyhealthrankings.org/our-approach/health-factors/built-environment

Healthy People 2020. 2012. *Social Determinants of Health.* http://healthypeople.gov/2020/topicsobjectives2020/overview.aspx?topicid = 39.

Hebert, K.A., A.M. Wendel, S.K. Kennedy, and A.L. Dannenberg. 2012. Health impact assessment: a comparison of 45 local, national, and international guidelines. Environmental Impact Assessment Review. 34:74-82.

National Association of County and City Health Officials. 2008. *Health Impact Assessment: Quick Guide.* http://activelivingresearch.org/files/NACCHO_HIA-QuickGuide_0.pdf

National Research Council. 2011. *Improving Health in the United States: The Role of Health Impact Assessment.* Washington, D.C.: The National Academies Press.

Ross, C. L. 2007. *Atlanta BeltLine Health Impact Assessment.* Atlanta: Center for Quality Growth and Regional Development, Georgia Institute of Technology.

Sycamore Consulting Inc., Kimley-Horn & Associates, Georgia Institute of Technology Center for Quality Growth and Regional Development. 2007. *Decatur Community Transportation Plan.* www.decaturga.com/index.aspx?page = 422

World Health Organization. 2013. *Social Determinants of Health.* www.who.int/social_determinants/en/.

CHAPTER 31

Move More Scholars Institute

Lori Rhew, MA, PAPHS
North Carolina Division of Public Health

Cathy Thomas, MAEd
North Carolina Division of Public Health

Kara Peach, MA
North Carolina Division of Public Health

Carolyn Dunn, PhD
*North Carolina Cooperative Extension,
North Carolina State University*

Jimmy Newkirk, Jr.
*National Society of Physical Activity
Practitioners in Public Health*

Dianne Ward, EdD
University of North Carolina at Chapel Hill

Amber Vaughn, MPH
University of North Carolina at Chapel Hill

NPAP Tactics and Strategies Used in This Program

Public Health Sector

STRATEGY 1: Develop and maintain an ethnically and culturally diverse public health workforce of both genders with competence and expertise in physical activity and health.

STRATEGY 2: Create, maintain, and leverage cross-sector partnerships and coalitions that implement effective strategies to promote physical activity.

The Move More Scholars Institute (MMSI) is a four-day training course for community-based physical activity professionals. It is the first state-level course modeled after the national Physical Activity and Public Health Practitioners (PAPH) course, offered annually by the Centers for Disease Control and Prevention (CDC) and the University of South Carolina. The MMSI was developed to create a statewide workforce skilled in addressing physical activity as a public health issue.

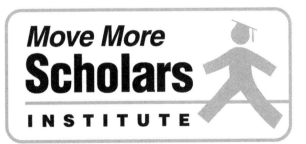

Reprinted, by permission, from the Physical Activity and Nutrition Branch, North Carolina Division of Public Health.

Program Description

Today's public health workforce requires the knowledge and skills needed to shape policies and environments that create access to and opportunities for physical activity. Public

Acknowledgments: We would like to acknowledge the Move More Scholars Institute Advisory Committee for their ongoing contributions to the course: Rich Bell, project officer, Active Living By Design; Phil Bors, project officer, Active Living By Design; Carolyn Crump, PhD, research associate professor, Department of Health Behavior and Health Education, Gillings School of Global Public Health, University of North Carolina at Chapel Hill; Carolyn Dunn, PhD, professor and nutrition specialist, North Carolina Cooperative Extension Service, North Carolina State University; Lisa Macon Harrison, director, Office of Healthy Carolinians and Health Education.

health professionals need to understand how administrative, organizational, and legislative policies affect physical activity; how the built environment influences physical activity; and how to build partnerships across sectors, including transportation, education, and community planning, to create policies and environments that support active living.

Physical Activity and Health: A Report of the Surgeon General, released in 1996, was a ground-breaking report that highlighted the association between physical activity and health (Franks et al. 2005). Since the release of this report, the evidence base for physical activity as a public health priority and the research base on how to increase physical activity have increased significantly. For example, in 2008 the first Physical Activity Guidelines for Americans were published, and in 2010 the first National Physical Activity Plan for the United States was released. In 2011, the National Prevention Strategy outlined the importance of prevention, recognized physical activity as a key health behavior, and noted the importance of interdisciplinary partnerships to address physical activity as a public health priority (National Prevention Council 2011). This increased emphasis on the importance of physical activity, coupled with increased evidence regarding strategies to increase physical activity and the need for an interdisciplinary approach, has created a unique set of competencies that public health practitioners need if they are to address physical activity as public health priority. In particular, practitioners need information about effective interventions and require skills for working with professionals from a variety of backgrounds to put successful strategies into practice.

Since 1996, the PAPH courses have been offered annually by the CDC and the University of South Carolina. The research course is designed to develop research competencies related to physical activity and public health, and the practitioner course is designed to increase the ability of practitioners to translate research to practice. In 2003, the Physical Activity and Health Branch at CDC established five benchmarks, outlining the areas of training and technical assistance that state health departments need to address to improve their

capacity to promote physical activity to the public (Martin and Vehige 2013). These benchmarks are (1) develop and sustain effective partnerships; (2) use public health data as a tool to develop and prioritize community-based interventions; (3) understand and implement a sound approach to planning and evaluation; (4) implement evidence-based strategies at the informational, behavioral, and social and environmental policy levels; (5) and develop an organizational structure that contributes to program growth and sustainability by encouraging and supporting professional development and fostering successful collaborations within and outside the health department (Martin and Vehige 2013). In 2005, the National Society of Physical Activity Practitioners in Public Health, in partnership with CDC, created core competencies, specific to physical activity and public health practice, that were based on these benchmarks (Dallman et al. 2009). Translating state-level benchmarks and competencies into community-based practice is an essential step for creating change that supports population levels of physical activity that will enhance health. This chapter describes how a state-level course, modeled after the national PAPH practitioners course, was created to train practitioners in the skills and competencies needed to address physical activity as a public health priority.

In 2006, the Physical Activity and Nutrition Branch of the North Carolina Division of Public Health, in partnership with the School of Public Health, University of North Carolina at Chapel Hill, developed a state version of the PAPH practitioner course, called the Move More Scholars Institute (MMSI). The MMSI is an intensive four-day training course for community-based physical activity professionals in North Carolina. It is the first state-specific course modeled on the PAPH course, integrating the core competencies established by the National Society of Physical Activity Practitioners in Public Health.

The development of the inaugural MMSI was guided by an expert advisory committee made up of representatives from the PAPH course, the North Carolina Division of Public Health, Active Living by Design, the University of North Carolina at Chapel Hill, and the University of Tennessee at Chattanooga. Committee members were chosen based on their expertise in policy and environmental change for physical activity and their knowledge of principles of adult learning. The committee's goal was to develop a course modeled after the PAPH course, with a curriculum specific to North Carolina that focused on policy and environmental initiatives.

MMSI was first conducted in the spring of 2006 and then again in 2008 and 2011. The course continues to be guided by an advisory committee that has grown to include representatives from North Carolina State University, the North Carolina Cooperative Extension, the University of North Carolina at Asheville, the Center for Health and Wellness, and the Office of Healthy Carolinians and Health Education. The advisory committee is instrumental in guiding the course to address national recommendations within the context of the needs of North Carolina.

The course is limited to 30 scholars to maximize opportunities for networking and interaction with faculty. A competitive application process, similar to that for the PAPH course, is used to select scholars. Applicants must submit three items: (1) a resume; (2) a letter explaining their role in their organization, experience partnering with other organizations to implement physical activity interventions, and what they plan to do as a result of attending the MMSI; and (3) a letter from their supervisor explaining why the applicant is a good candidate for the MMSI and how the agency will support the candidate in applying what he or she learns at the course. Applicants are selected to attend based on their experience, their ability to apply what they learn from the MMSI in their daily work, and their organization's support for their participation and application of the things they learn.

Scholars come from a variety of sectors, including health promotion coordinators from local health departments, family and consumer science agents from the North Carolina Cooperative Extension, local transportation planners, city and county planners, staff of parks and recreation departments, school staff, and staff of faith-based and nonprofit organizations. State-level professionals attend the course each time it is offered, including professionals from the North Carolina Division of Public Health, Parks

and Recreation; the Institute for Transportation, Research, and Education; and other agencies. A key goal of the MMSI is to help scholars connect with professionals across the state who work in a variety of settings. The combination of state and local participants provides an opportunity for increased learning about state and local perspectives.

Several factors contribute to the effectiveness of the MMSI. First, the course is based on adult learning principles. It includes both didactic and interactive sessions and provides time for interaction between faculty and scholars. Second, the course instructors are considered state-level, and frequently national-level, experts in physical activity and health. These instructors provide a state-of-the-art perspective on promoting physical activity through policy and environmental change. Third, faculty members focus the course material on the needs of North Carolina practitioners and provide examples specific to the state. The result is a statewide network of public health, transportation, parks and recreation, education, and other professionals who develop and engage in local and state efforts to increase physical activity.

Program Evaluation

The MMSI is assessed through daily evaluations, overall course evaluations, and a one-year follow-up evaluation. The results of these evaluations show that the MMSI is successful in increasing engagement, leadership, and partnerships that support physical activity. The daily and overall course evaluations indicate that the scholars appreciate the opportunity to interact with professionals with a variety of backgrounds. Scholars report that the connections established with other professionals are some of the most highly beneficial aspects of the course and that sharing and partnership development are key aspects of the course.

The one-year follow-up evaluations have been conducted for the 2006 and 2008 courses. Scholars reported that their level of work involvement in physical activity interventions has increased as a result of attending the MMSI, that their leadership role in physical activity promotion has expanded, and that they regularly apply what they learned at the MMSI to their work. In addition, they reported initiating professional contact with other scholars after the course, increasing their interactions with other professionals in their community as a result of attending the MMSI, and becoming more involved with statewide physical activity initiatives. Table 31.1 outlines these evaluation results.

Linkage to the National Physical Activity Plan

The MMSI addresses Strategy 1 of the Public Health Sector of the National Physical Activity Plan: *Develop and maintain an ethnically and culturally diverse public health workforce of* *both genders with competence and expertise in physical activity and health.*

Tactic: Support and expand training opportunities (e.g., Physical Activity and Public Health Course) based on core competencies for practitioners and paraprofessionals. Ensure interdisciplinary training such that physical activity and public health concepts are connected to other disciplines and also include leadership development and team-building. Augment the entry of physical activity professionals by engaging ethnic minority and disability organizations in public health, medicine, and related disciplines. The MMSI has trained more than 75 professionals from 11 disciplines to use a policy and environmental approach to increase population levels of physical activity in North Carolina. A key to the success of the course is to involve professionals from a variety of backgrounds

Table 31.1   Key Results from the Move More Scholars Institute Evaluation

OVERALL COURSE EVALUATION			
	2006 (*n* = 19)	**2008 (*n* = 26)**	**2011 (*n* = 19)**
Did the MMSI meet your expectations?	100% yes	100% yes	100% yes
Did the MMSI sessions fit well together?	100% yes	100% yes	100% yes

One-year follow-up evaluation

	2006 (*n* = 21)	**2008 (*n* = 17)**	**2011 not available**
How has your level of work involvement in physical activity interventions changed as a result of attending the MMSI?	57.1% increased	47.1% increased	
Have you become more involved with statewide initiatives as a result of attending the MMSI?	85.7% yes	64.7% yes	
Do you apply information from the MMSI to your work in physical activity promotion?	33.3% often 52.4% regularly	29.4% often 58.8% regularly	
Have you initiated any professional contact with any of the scholars since the MMSI?	85.7% yes	47.1% yes	
Has your leadership role in physical activity promotion increased since attending the MMSI?	76.2% yes	47.1% yes	
Have you increased your interaction with other professionals in your community as a result of attending the MMSI?	76.2% yes	64.7% yes	

and disciplines, which promotes informal and formal learning and networking among the scholars.

The MMSI also addresses Strategy 2 of the Public Health Sector: *Create, maintain, and leverage cross-sector partnerships and coalitions that implement effective strategies to promote physical activity.*

Tactic: Encourage public health professionals to both educate and learn from partners in order to strengthen the effectiveness of the partnership and the efforts of each member. A diverse advisory committee ensures that the course meets the needs of professionals from a variety of backgrounds. Advisory committee members have extensive technical expertise in adult learning and policy and environmental change and a strong understanding of the public health context in North Carolina.

Evidence Base Used During Program Development

The MMSI is built on the CDC benchmarks that outline the areas of training and technical assistance that state health departments need to address to improve their capacity to promote physical activity (Martin and Vehige 2013). It also incorporates the core competencies for physical activity and public health practice developed by the National Society of Physical Activity Practitioners in Public Health (Dallman et al. 2009). The result is a course based on national competencies that were established by experts in public health workforce and promotion of physical activity. Each time the course is offered, the curriculum is designed to align with current efforts in North Carolina. The goal is to increase engagement in statewide physical activity efforts.

Populations Best Served by the Program

The MMSI is targeted to community-based physical activity professionals in North Carolina. A community-based professional is anyone who partners with other organizations in his or her community to promote physical activity. The

course is marketed to attract professionals with a variety of professional backgrounds.

Lessons Learned

Key lessons learned through the process of creating and conducting the MMSI include these:

- Recruit a diverse advisory committee to guide curriculum development and participant recruitment.
- Limit the number of participants to maximize networking opportunities.
- Include peer-to-peer learning as a key aspect of the course.
- Include participants from different disciplines to enhance learning.
- Select quality speakers and those with expertise in state issues to ensure that information is immediately applicable.
- Provide time for interaction between scholars and faculty throughout the course.
- Adapt course content based on the needs of the participants.
- Select a high-quality venue that enhances the learning experience.

Tips for Working Across Sectors

A key to working across sectors for the MMSI was to ensure that the course content met the needs of public health professionals and then to gradually widen the range of professionals who attended the course. The inaugural MMSI focused on three specific groups of professionals who work in the area of community-based physical activity programming in North Carolina: (1) health promotion coordinators from local health departments, (2) coordinators of local physical activity and nutrition coalitions, and (3) family and consumer science agents from cooperative extensions. The course planners targeted these professionals because they play leadership roles in local communities' efforts to integrate physical activity interventions with policy-level and environmental-level change. These professionals were encouraged to share information about the course with any of their community partners who may have an interest in applying to attend. A majority of the inaugural scholars represented public health agencies or cooperative extensions.

The range of professionals who attend the MMSI has increased gradually each year. When the MMSI was offered in 2011, it had equal representation from public health, nonprofit, parks and recreation, and city and county planning agencies.

A key aspect to ensuring the relevance of the course across sectors was to avoid jargon and acronyms. In addition, the participant list and an example of a project on which each scholar is working are shared with the faculty prior to the course. This allows the faculty to better understand the background of the scholars and the work that they are doing.

Additional Reading and Resources

Schneider, L., D. Ward, C. Dunn, A. Vaughn, J. Newkirk, and C. Thomas. 2007. The Move More Scholars Institute: A state model of the physical activity and public health practitioners course. *Prev. Chronic Dis.* [serial online] www.cdc.gov/pcd/issues/2007/jul/06_0157.htm.

References

Dallman, A., E. Abercrombie, R. Drewette-Card, M. Mohan, M. Ray, and B. Ritacco. 2009. Elevating physical activity as a public health priority: Establishing core competencies for physical activity practitioners in public health. *J. Phys. Act. Health* 6:682-9.

Franks, A.L., R.C. Brownson, C. Bryant, K. McCormack Brown, S. Hooker, D.M. Pluto, et al. 2005. Prevention research centers: Contributions to updating the public health workforce through training. *Prev. Chronic Dis.* [serial online] /www.cdc.gov/pcd/issues/2005/apr/04_0139.htm.

Martin, S.L., and T. Vehige T. 2013. Establishing public health benchmarks for physical activity programs. *Prev. Chronic Dis.* [serial online] www.cdc.gov/pcd/issues/2006/jul/06_0006.htm.

National Prevention Council. 2011. *National Prevention Strategy.* Washington, DC: U.S. Department of Health and Human Services, Office of the Surgeon General.

CHAPTER 32

The National Society of Physical Activity Practitioners in Public Health

Elevating the Issue of Physical Activity; Equipping Professionals to Do So

Jimmy Newkirk, Jr.
National Society of Physical Activity Practitioners in Public Health

Amber Dallman, MPH, PAPHS
Minnesota Department of Health

Eydie Abercrombie, MPH, CHES, PAPHS
Public Health Institute

Jill Pfankuch, MS, MCHES, PAPHS
NSPAPPH Volunteer

NPAP Tactics and Strategies Used in This Program

Public Health Sector

STRATEGY 1: Develop the capacity of the public health workforce—addressed through conference offerings, webinars, networking, development and promotion of core competencies, and the PAPHS certification.

STRATEGY 2: Create, maintain, and leverage cross-sector partnerships—addressed by the practitioners themselves as well as the organization.

STRATEGY 3: Engage in advocacy and policy development—addressed by practitioners who work to educate decision makers, enabling them to more appropriately consider physical activity and health as they develop policy.

STRATEGY 4: Disseminate tools and resources—addressed by organizing more than 700 national, state, and local tools and resources in a web-based matrix that is searchable by setting, target audience, or state.

STRATEGY 5: Expand the monitoring (surveillance and evaluation) of PA and PA interventions—addressed by practitioners' evaluation and surveillance efforts with their state and local programs.

The National Society of Physical Activity Practitioners in Public Health (NSPAPPH) is working to elevate the issue of physical activity (PA) and help practitioners develop the skills and abilities to promote physical activity strategies. To achieve this goal, NSPAPPH builds the capacity of the public health workforce, leverages partnerships to promote physical activity, advocates, disseminates resources, and supports monitoring.

Acknowledgments: Since the writing of this chapter, the National Society of Physical Activity Practitioners in Public Health (NSPAPPH) has undergone a significant organizational shift. NSPAPPH has transitioned its entire operation, strategic plan, and capacity building efforts to a new organization, the National Physical Activity Society, to allow for improved service and impact. The content of this chapter remains accurate but is now assumed under the National Physical Activity Society. More information is available at: www.PhysicalActivitySociety.org.

Program Description

NSPAPPH began as an informal network of practitioners who recognized the need to share ideas, resources, and lessons learned across the profession to support and promote physical activity on a population level. It was created to meet the needs of practitioners (Kimber 2009).

NSPAPPH, now a developing nonprofit organization, focuses on elevating the issue of physical activity (PA) and equipping the practitioners who do so. These efforts lend themselves directly and indirectly to implementation of the National Physical Activity Plan (NPAP). Connections to the NPAP include building the capacity of the workforce, developing partnerships to promote PA, advocating, disseminating resources, and monitoring.

Core Competencies

NSPAPPH recognized that PA practitioners need to have both a specialized skill set to work with many diverse partners and a skill set common to public health. It also recognized that PA practitioners were coming to the field with diverse backgrounds and training. NSPAPPH worked with the Centers for Disease Control and Prevention (CDC) Division of Nutrition, Physical Activity and Obesity to develop a set of five core competency areas that are based on CDC's five benchmarks for physical activity and public health practice (Martin 2013). The core competency areas were later revised and a sixth area was added (Dallman 2009):

- Partnerships
- Data and scientific information
- Planning and evaluation
- Interventions
- Organizational structure
- Exercise science in the public health setting

These competency areas are subcategorized into 34 core competencies. Each of the core competencies is further subdivided, for a total of 129 knowledge, skills, and abilities (KSAs) (Dallman 2009).

The creation and promotion of these core competencies and KSAs add value to the practitioner, the employer, and the profession as a whole. Practitioners now have a reference point for their training, professional growth, and development. Employers now have a standard for hiring criteria, job descriptions, and work plans. And the profession as a whole, described as an "emerging subdiscipline" (Kohl et al. 2006), has a baseline for training and development of a workforce.

The field of physical activity is a critical component in public health. The original NSPAPPH core competencies defined the recommended essential competencies for public health staff assigned to physical activity efforts. The set has been revised and expanded with the American College of Sports Medicine (ACSM)–NSPAPPH Physical Activity in Public Health Specialist (PAPHS) certification, which calls them knowledge, skills, and abilities (KSAs); however, only the core competencies are here given space limitations. A competent physical activity practitioner should be in a position to review and advise the health department on all physical activity initiatives, to ensure that they are consistent, based on best available evidence, coordinated with each other, and likely to be effective. For a complete set of the core competencies with their associated KSAs, please visit http://physicalactivitysociety.org/wp-content/uploads/2010/08/approved_bod_cc_011410.pdf.

NSPAPPH Core Competencies: Essentials for Public Health Physical Activity Practitioners

Competency Area 1: Partnerships

Core Competency 1.1: Educate, collaborate, and engage with external partners from a variety of disciplines to promote physical activity at multiple settings and in a variety of populations.

Core Competency 1.2: Work with organizations and individuals to capitalize on complementary strengths, capabilities, resources, and opportunities for the promotion of PA.

Core Competency 1.3: Communicate appropriate public health physical activity messages to intended audiences through a variety of media channels.

Core Competency 1.4: Educate partners on the distinction between advocacy and lobbying and how they can take appropriate action to influence policy change.

Competency Area 2: Data and Scientific Information

Core Competency 2.1: Identify and use public health data as a tool to develop and prioritize community-based interventions, including policies, to promote physical activity.

Core Competency 2.2: Maintain professional knowledge of current trends, developments, guidelines, recommendations, and research in the field.

Core Competency 2.3: Review and recommend best and evidence-based practices and procedures for the development and implementation of PA promotion efforts.

Core Competency 2.4: Summarize data to illuminate public health issues in terms of disparity or access as well as other ethical, political, scientific, or economic determinations associated with physical activity.

Core Competency 2.5: Understand sources of data from professions outside of public health to address program needs (e.g., transportation data).

Core Competency 2.6: Use measurement and surveillance mechanisms to assess PA levels across populations.

Competency Area 3: Planning and Evaluating

Core Competency 3.1: Use theoretical frameworks and models to plan and evaluate physical activity interventions.

Core Competency 3.2: Serve as a technical advisor in the design, implementation, and evaluation of physical activity interventions to address chronic disease.

Core Competency 3.3: Address cultural, social, behavioral, and environmental factors that contribute to disease progression and health promoting behaviors as part of a physical activity program or intervention.

Core Competency 3.4: Identify internal and external issues, such as changes and trends in financing, regulation, legislation, and policies that may affect delivery of public health physical activity services.

Core Competency 3.5: Use social marketing principles to target and learn specifically about the population for physical activity intervention.

Core Competency 3.6: Oversee the development and implementation of a state physical activity plan, which includes goals, SMART objectives, and strategies.

Core Competency 3.7: Work with key staff to develop an evaluation plan for all physical activity related interventions.

Core Competency 3.8: Use both quantitative and qualitative analysis to determine process, impact, and outcome measures of physical activity programs.

Competency Area 4: Interventions

Core Competency 4.1: Recommend and translate effective intervention strategies to partners and other constituents.

Core Competency 4.2: Coordinate the efforts of local and community organizations (e.g. worksites, coalitions, agencies, schools, etc.) to create local policy and environmental changes that increase opportunities for physical activity.

Core Competency 4.3: Educate key stakeholders (participants, partners, implementers, and decision makers) to influence and effect policy and environmental change.

Core Competency 4.4: Understand and communicate the importance of using ecological approaches, and advise on evidence-based strategies to affect each of these levels.

Core Competency 4.5: Understand and communicate theories and mechanisms of policy development and appropriations, including how political and organizational agendas are set and pursued, to affect public health.

Core Competency 4.6: Collaborate with the media to communicate appropriate public health and physical activity messages to intended audiences.

Competency Area 5: Organizational Structure

Core Competency 5.1: Identify appropriate resources and continuing education for the implementation of a personal professional development plan, which includes training and ongoing technical assistance for promoting physical activity.

Core Competency 5.2: Establish partnerships with relevant partners at the federal, state, and local levels and other public and private sectors to promote physical activity as a critical health behavior.

Core Competency 5.3: Understand the budget management process related to policy and department budgetary processes (e.g., how funding allocations are made), budget appropriations, required budgetary reporting, and documentation.

Core Competency 5.4: Demonstrate and maintain knowledge in the roles of federal, state, and local government and specific legislative processes to address policy changes that affect physical activity.

Core Competency 5.5: Write and submit grant applications, reports, and manuscripts for professional and other publications and deliver presentations for programmatic and scientific meetings.

Competency Area 6: Exercise Science in Public Health Setting

Core Competency 6.1: Understand exercise physiology and related exercise science.

Core Competency 6.2: Understand health promotion and disease prevention.

Core Competency 6.3: Understand physical activity assessments.

Core Competency 6.4: Understand physical activity recommendations and programming.

Core Competency 6.5 Understand caloric balance and weight management related to physical activity.

Practitioners and Partnerships

In the relatively brief history of the PA practitioner in public health, most have been employed in health departments at the state or local level. These practitioners generally work with partners and organizations to increase physical activity opportunities in various settings. For example, practitioners may do the following:

- Work with land use and transportation planners to ensure that they see the impact of their efforts on the public's health. They often work to help create and promote Complete Streets policies, Safe Routes to School, land use or community design policies, and specific pedestrian and bicycle policies.

- Work with school administrators and educators to teach and reinforce lifelong physical activity skills of the whole child. Their collective efforts may increase the quantity or quality of physical education as well as PA opportunities before, during, and after the school day.

- Work with employers and economic leaders to ensure that a healthy community environment leads to increased marketability for business growth. They work to improve the health of employees, increasing productivity and reducing health care costs.

- Work with faith communities and other community-based organizations to serve as a resource and advocate within the community.

- Work with the media to convey that health is an individual choice that is heavily influenced by the policies and environments in which we live, and work to make the healthy choice the easy choice.

These examples provide a glimpse into the multifaceted work of practitioners. Similar activities are taking place across the United States with partners in parks and recreation, health care, and preschools.

The face of the practitioner continues to change, however. In increasing numbers, professionals and volunteers from these partnering industries are realizing that they too are PA practitioners and their work affects the physical activity behaviors and health of their target audience. As such, they are beginning to join the broad public health efforts to promote physical activity, not only for the sake of health but also because of its positive impact on their own work.

It is critical that practitioners document and evaluate their efforts. The nature of their work is unique, it has a long-term effect, it affects virtually 100 percent of the population, and yet it remains poorly funded. Practitioners usually conduct project-specific evaluation and support statewide surveillance efforts such as the Behavioral Risk Factor Surveillance System. In addition, NSPAPPH and its members have supported national evaluation efforts. For example, NSPAPPH assisted the Physical Activity Policy Research Network in the evaluation of the National Physical Activity Plan implementation.

Efforts to Support Practitioners

Practitioners have told NSPAPPH through needs assessments that networking and sharing among fellow practitioners are highly valued. Practitioners want to learn about and be connected with national efforts, to have readily identifiable resources, and to be supported as professionals. NSPAPPH has sought to provide for each of these practitioner needs.

In response, NSPAPPH adopted the following organizational priorities:

1. Increase membership and engagement.
2. Increase capacity building and certification.
3. Increase advocacy (education of decision makers).

Each of these priorities builds on and supports the others, as described next.

Increase Membership and Engagement

Increased membership and engagement serve two primary purposes. A larger body of practitioners creates an amplified, collective voice for PA strategies. It also creates a larger pool of practitioners with whom to network and share resources, challenges, and successes.

Build Capacity and Certification

Increased capacity building has taken several forms, including trainings, identification and promotion of resources, and the creation of a first-ever Physical Activity in Public Health Specialist certification.

The NSPAPPH annual conference has included a blend of national, state, and local speakers covering physical activity promotion strategies for persons of all ages and abilities, in all settings. For example, a speaker on national transportation issues may be followed by a local practitioner discussing local implementation and impact of national policies. Conference sessions, as well as webinar sessions, are selected to meet the specific requests and needs of the organization's members.

NSPAPPH has taken advantage of routine webinars, which allow great flexibility of topic and speaker. Current issues are presented in a timely manner, while ongoing issues can be examined from different perspectives and approaches. Single keynote speakers or panel combinations are constructed to ensure appropriate topic coverage. Webinar platforms are also carefully chosen to optimize interactive visual and voice presentations with audience participation.

Networking and learning from other members are essential to NSPAPPH as a society of practitioners. The organization has initiated an ongoing web-based PA resource matrix, which allows efficient sharing of resources among practitioners. More than 700 resources have been collected and made available to members on the organization's website: www.physical

activitysociety.org). These tools and resources have been created and used by practitioners nationwide as well as by national organizations. They are categorized into a matrix that is searchable by state, setting, or type of resource.

Capacity-building efforts, including the variety of training opportunities and resources, provide the foundation of an organizational newsletter called *NSPAPPH Matters*. This newsletter has assumed the functions of the previous CDC PA listserv and includes grant opportunities, job announcements, conference announcements, and newsworthy items.

NSPAPPH has taken capacity building to the next level with the creation of the Physical Activity in Public Health Specialist (PAPHS) certification. In collaboration with the ACSM, and building on the core competencies established with CDC (Dallman 2009), the PAPHS certification was launched as a new national standard for physical activity practitioners working for the health of the public (Newkirk 2010). The certification exam, available at more than 4,300 Pearson Vue testing centers, consists of 100 questions that evaluate domains of tasks and related knowledge, skills, and abilities to promote physical activity on a population level. The domains and the test percentages given for each area include partnerships (12 percent), data and scientific information (18 percent), planning and evaluating (23 percent), interventions (20 percent), organizational structure (10 percent), and exercise science in public health settings (17 percent). Partnerships, planning and evaluating, and organizational structure make up almost half of the exam. Additional information is available at www.paphscert.org.

The PAPHS certification adds value to individual professionals, to employers, and to the profession as a whole. Individuals benefit through achieving the certification, which demonstrates their knowledge, skills, and abilities and validates their qualifications. Employers benefit by using the PAPHS certification as a hiring or employment criterion, ensuring that candidates have a solid understanding of core competencies. Employers can also use the core competencies in job descriptions and work plans. The continuing education credits required for the PAPHS certification ensure professional growth and development. The PAPHS certification is comparable to the licensing and credentialing of other recognized professions, validating the significance of this young and emerging profession (Kohl 2006).

NSPAPPH's capacity-building efforts, although highly valuable, are not intended as an end unto themselves: They are designed to empower practitioners to effectively and efficiently influence physical activity behaviors. If NSPAPPH is to influence these behaviors, it must address policies, environments, and systems.

Increase Advocacy: Educating Decision Makers

Advocacy, which NSPAPH defines as educating decision makers (and is distinctly different than lobbying), is carried out by many practitioners and their organizations. NSPAPPH supports these efforts by building the capacity of practitioners to inform and educate on physical activity issues. Additionally, through membership and networking efforts, NSPAPPH is creating a collective, unified voice of PA practitioners, allowing them to join together on larger issues.

As the body of practitioners grows, and as individual and corporate capacity increases, the collective voice of PA practitioners will certainly have a great influence on physical activity behavior. NSPAPPH, as an organization, will continue to speak on behalf of practitioners and PA issues, but the unified voice of the members of the organization will be even more effective (Newkirk 2010).

Linkage to National Physical Activity Plan

NSPAPPH's efforts directly support the implementation of the National Physical Activity Plan. In particular, each of the Public Health Sector strategies is addressed:

Strategy 1: Develop the capacity of the public health workforce—addressed through conference offerings, webinars, networking, development and promotion of core competencies, and the PAPHS certification.

Strategy 2: Create, maintain, and leverage cross-sector partnerships—addressed by the practitioners themselves as well as the organization. NSPAPPH members work and collaborate with partners in all settings to promote and create opportunities for PA. As an organization, NSPAPPH is creating partnerships with cross-sector organizations.

Strategy 3: Engage in advocacy and policy development—addressed by practitioners who work to educate decision makers, enabling them to more appropriately consider physical activity and health as they develop policy. NSPAPPH will also continue to support education efforts from a national organizational level.

Strategy 4: Disseminate tools and resources—addressed by organizing more than 700 national, state, and local tools and resources in a web-based matrix that is searchable by setting, target audience, or state.

Strategy 5: Expand the monitoring (surveillance and evaluation) of PA and PA interventions—addressed by practitioners' evaluation and surveillance efforts with their state and local programs. Organizationally, the strategy is supported by partnering with Physical Activity Policy Research Network and other researchers to expand PA monitoring.

In addition to making direct contributions to the public health strategies, NSPAPPH indirectly supports many other NPAP strategies by building the capacity of members to promote PA in other sectors, such as transportation and schools.

Evidence Base Used During Program Development

In developing the core competencies, practitioners conducted a literature review and referenced related competencies and certification (Dallman 2009). The benchmark areas were organized under CDC's five benchmarks for physical activity and public health practice (Martin et al. 2013). For training opportunities, such as webinars or conference presentations, the evidence base is specific to the topic and, therefore, varies greatly from presentation to presentation.

Lessons Learned

The development of core competencies was beneficial to establishing a baseline of knowledge, skills, and abilities for PA practitioners. These will likely continue to evolve given the changing definition and profile of practitioners. As such, our capacity-building efforts, advocacy, and support for practitioners will continue to develop.

Monthly webinars and annual conferences sponsored by NSPAPPH are linked to our knowledge, skills, and abilities to ensure that individuals seeking PAPHS continuing education credits meet ACSM requirements and are awarded credits for attending training sessions at no additional cost. NSPAPPH's professional development committee continually evaluates training sessions to confirm that we are addressing the core competency areas and meeting the continuing education needs of our members. Needs assessments have identified additional training topics requested by our members, and continuing education credits are offered when training is scheduled. NSPAPPH partners with other organizations to offer continuing education credits for PAPHS-certified individuals for other approved trainings.

One notable challenge for practitioners in general, and an area of continued learning, is determining how to assess the impact of and tell the story of the PA practitioner. Much of the PA practitioners' policy, environment, and systems change work is completed through partnerships, making it difficult to directly attribute their specific impact. Additionally, assessing the impact of policy, environment, or systems changes on physical activity behavior is problematic because of the inherently lengthy process and the potential impact of numerous other factors. The difficulty in directly demonstrating impact and long-term outcomes creates challenges not only in evaluation but also in terms of justifying the value of the effort to funders. Through networking, and the sharing of ideas, successes, and struggles, we will work through this challenge that is inherent to the profession.

To build the profession, NSPAPPH's initial efforts concentrated on PA practitioners within public health. Now these efforts are expanding to include other disciplines, even those that do not consider PA to be their primary focus. For example, transportation planners may not have health as their primary goal; however, they may see PA as a strategy to achieve transportation efficiency goals. By working together, both parties may achieve their desired outcomes.

NSPAPPH has worked to meet the professional development and capacity-building needs of its members by soliciting feedback and input through a needs assessment process. As the field of PA interventions continues to grow and as new evidence-based and promising practices emerge, it is crucial that professional development opportunities meet the needs of the practitioners. As NSPAPPH membership further evolves and becomes increasingly professionally diverse, ongoing input and feedback from practitioners are critical. To maintain and increase the perceived value of the organization, NSPAPPH will continue to use a member needs assessment to create a professional development and training framework.

Populations Best Served by the Program

The networking, advocacy, and capacity-building activities of NSPAPPH are suited to anyone who promotes physical activity. Although oriented toward those addressing policy, systems, or environmental changes, the organizational offerings also include individual and interpersonal approaches. In the 2011 Physical Activity Policy Research Network survey, more than 34 percent of respondents indicated that they were not employed primarily as a physical activity practitioner (www.unc. edu/~kevenson/_NSPAPPH_SurveySummary. pdf). NSPAPPH welcomes anyone who wishes to promote physical activity, whether employed or volunteer, and whether at the local, state, national, or international level.

Tips for Working Across Sectors

Practitioners routinely work across sectors to find the win-win solution, identifying strategies

that partners have in common, even though there may be different purposes for the intervention. Practitioners recognize how promoting physical activity fits into a variety of settings. With NSPAPPH's support, PA practitioners work with partners to advance policy, systems, or environmental changes that support and encourage regular physical activity in a variety of settings.

As an example, in Minnesota a PA practitioner worked with transportation, education, and nonprofit partners to support legislators in establishing the Safe Routes to School program in the 2012 legislative session. The PA practitioner, as a technical expert and resource, provided partners with information about what was happening across the state related to health improvement efforts in schools. This vital contributory role led to the passage of the legislation.

While working with partners outside of public health it is important to recognize that language matters. For example, the words *intervention* and *surveillance* can be perceived differently outside of public health. When practitioners discuss the most common forms of physical activity—walking and bicycling—they may be interpreted differently by partners. For example, to transportation partners, walking and bicycling could mean nonmotorized transportation; to parks and recreation partners, walking and bicycling could mean leisure-time exercise opportunities. Either way, PA practitioners must be skilled in adapting to promote physical activity among diverse partner and stakeholder groups.

Program Evaluation

NSPAPPH is continually assessing how business is done and is adapting to the evolving field of physical activity promotion among diverse populations and settings. Members are surveyed biannually to determine their technical assistance and training needs to promote physical activity. This survey assists planners in selecting training webinars and topics for the annual conference.

PA practitioners who have completed the certification provide another snapshot of existing capacity. The certification exam allows NSPAPPH to get a better picture of what competency areas are strongest among practitioners and where more training is needed. The number of candidates who have sat for the certification is another indicator of how NSPAPPH is growing the field of physical activity promotion. In the first three years since the certification was established, and with virtually no marketing, more than 237 practitioners have become PAPHS certified.

To assist our members in capacity building, NSPAPPH and its partners provide resources to self-assess PA in public health competency levels. These resources include the NSPAPPH monthly webinars; continuing education online courses (www.acsm.org); the core competencies–KSA document; a 15-question free practice exam (www.acsmlearning.org); the PAPHS certification exam; the PAPHS certification informational (www.PhysicalActivitySociety.org); and the more than 700 resources provided to members on the NSPAPPH website.

The ACSM–NSPAPPH PAPHS Certification Exam Preparation Course was recently released. This course, which was developed in conjunction with the ACSM and NSPAPPH, is a perfect resource for PA practitioners and other health professionals looking to better understand the role of physical activity in public health as well as those seeking continuing education credits. The online course includes the *Foundations of Physical Activity and Public Health* (Kohl and Murray 2012) textbook. To learn more, visit www.physicalactivitysociety.org.

NSPAPPH is elevating the issue of physical activity by uniting a new profession, educating decision makers, and building the capacity of practitioners to influence all levels of decisions that affect physical activity. NSPAPPH will continue its efforts to support its members—PA practitioners—who are themselves leaders for the implementation of the National Physical Activity Plan in their communities and states and across the nation.

Additional Reading and Resources

The complete set of core competencies, titled *Core Competencies and Knowledge Skills and Abilities: Essentials for Public Health Physical Activity Practitioners,* can be found at http://physicalactivitysociety.org/wp-content/uploads/2010/08/approved_bod_cc_011410.pdf.

References

Kimber, C., E. Abercrombie, J.N. Epping, L. Mordecai, J. Newkirk, Jr., and M. Ray. 2009. Elevating physical activity as a public health priority: Creation of the National Society of Physical Activity Practitioners in Public Health. *Journal of Physical Activity and Health* 6:677-81.

Dallman, A., E. Abercrombie, R. Drewette-Card, M. Mohan, M. Ray, and B. Ritacco. 2009. Elevating physical activity as a public health priority: Establishing core competencies for physical activity practitioners in public health. *Journal of Physical Activity and Health* 6:682-9.

Kohl, H.W., III, I-M. Lee, I.M. Vuori, F.C. Wheeler, A. Bauman, and J.F. Sallis. 2006. Physical activity and public health: The emergence of a sub discipline. *Journal of Physical Activity and Health* 3:344-64.

Kohl, H.W., III, and T. Murray. 2012. *Foundations of Physical Activity and Public Health,* Champaign, IL: Human Kinetics.

Martin, S.L., and T. Vehige. 2013. Establishing public health benchmarks for physical activity programs. *Prev. Chronic Dis.* [serial online] www.cdc.gov/pcd/issues/2006/jul/06_0006.htm.

Newkirk, J. 2010. The NSPAPPH: Answering the call. *Journal of Physical Activity and Health* 7(Suppl. 1):S7-8.

CHAPTER 33

Successful Cross-Sector Partnerships to Implement Physical Activity

Live Well Omaha Coalition

Kerri R. Peterson, MS
Live Well Omaha

Mary Balluff, MS, RD, LMNT
Douglas County Health Department

Brian Coyle, MPH, PAPHS
*Nebraska Department of Health
and Human Services*

NPAP Tactics and Strategies Used in This Program

Public Health Sector

STRATEGY 2: Create, maintain, and leverage cross-sector partnerships and coalitions that implement effective strategies to promote physical activity. Partnerships should include representatives from public health; health care; education; parks, recreation, fitness and sports; transportation, urban design, and community planning; business and industry; volunteer and non-profit organizations; faith communities; mass media; and organizations serving historically underserved and understudied populations.

STRATEGY 3: Engage in advocacy and policy development to elevate the priority of physical activity in public health practice, policy, and research.

Live Well Omaha (LWO) is a long-term collaborative effort of individuals and organizations, both public and private, representing all levels of government, schools, health care, public health, faith-based organizations, community organizations, and businesses. These strategic partners share a vision to improve the overall health of area residents and position Omaha as a thriving community for the future. LWO serves as a catalyst for discussions about community health issues and guides partners to collaborate, facilitate infrastructure changes, and address policy opportunities to create and sustain a healthier community. The mission of LWO is to improve the community's health,

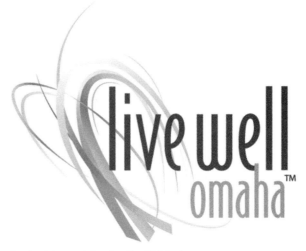

Reprinted, by permission, from Live Well Omaha.

through a forum of organizations, positively affecting health outcomes for all individuals and families.

Program Description

Beginning in 1995, the Douglas County (Nebraska) Health Department collaborated with Alegent Health, a large hospital and health system, to create a local healthy community movement. That same year, 18 organizations came together to form LWO. This group included both public and private partners that were interested in addressing community health needs. Priorities for LWO were based on a community health assessment that identified health needs. The assessment was a coordinated effort between local public health agencies and the LWO board of directors and staff. These initial organizations included the local health department, hospital and health systems, insurance companies, and other public and private corporations such as Blue Cross and Blue Shield of Nebraska, Union Pacific, and Valmont Industries. This innovative partnership fostered new collaborations and leveraged funding to support health initiatives specific to increasing physical activity and healthy eating to prevent obesity.

In the early 2000s, as initiatives and partnerships grew, LWO became a separate entity from the Douglas County Health Department. However, a strong, collaborative relationship remained between the two organizations.

In 2002, LWO used vital statistics, a community health assessment, and Behavior Risk Factor Surveillance System data to describe the current health status of the community. This was the first LWO biannual Community Report Card, which served as a wakeup call for the community. The report card indicated an increase in the number of community members who were either overweight or obese (59 percent were overweight or obese compared with the Healthy People 2010 goal of less than 15 percent). Twenty-seven percent had high blood pressure, compared with the Healthy People 2010 target of 16 percent or less. Only 43.7 percent of adults reported 20 minutes or more of vigorous physical activity three or more times a week (Live Well Omaha Community Report Card 2002). Seeing evidence that indicated an imminent obesity epidemic in Omaha, LWO focused its efforts on increasing the community's capacity to mobilize resources to address obesity prevention, with an emphasis on physical activity, by facilitating communication among key stakeholders such as health care agencies, nonprofit organizations, and major employers.

Omaha's built environment provided both challenges to and opportunities for active living. Omaha had experienced rapid westward growth in recent decades. Unfortunately, the city was unable to build and expand certain infrastructure (e.g., public transportation, sidewalks, trails, bike lanes) at the same pace. Many neighborhoods, both new and old, lacked the necessary infrastructure for sidewalks. Bike trails had only recently been constructed. Although there were more than 60 miles (96.5 kilometers) of recreational trails in Omaha, they were not well connected. Other factors that limited active living behaviors included traffic conditions, aggressive drivers, poor street design, lack of bike lanes, hilly terrain, and harsh winters. Because of these factors, few residents engaged in active living, specifically bicycling. Most bicycle trips in Omaha were recreational only. Transportation-related trips were rare because of the lack of east-west trail connectivity.

Early funding was secured through the Omaha Community Foundation, Blue Cross and Blue Shield of Nebraska, and Nebraska Department of Health and Human Services and featured joint efforts between local public health and LWO. The first of many major milestones for the LWO was a funding opportunity called Active Living by Design, which was created by the Robert Wood Johnson Foundation. This grant funding focused on increasing physical activity options through community design. By providing support for changes in community design, specifically related to land use, transportation, parks, trails, and greenways, the Active Living by Design initiative was intended to make it easier for people to be active as part of their daily routines. Active Living by

Design's community action model provided five active living strategies, known as the 5Ps, targeting community change through preparation, promotions, programs, policy influences, and physical projects. The 5P model provided a comprehensive approach to increasing physical activity through short-, intermediate-, and long-term community changes. In November 2003, LWO was 1 of 44 communities in the United States to receive $300,000 for a five-year funding period. The new initiative, under the LWO umbrella, was branded LWO: Activate Omaha and focused primarily on promotional efforts. The inclusive 5P model facilitated the integration of policy approaches, physical projects, and a vast number of programmatic efforts specific to active living. The program, promotion, and partnership-building efforts that were part of LWO: Activate Omaha helped to build credibility for the active living movement and generated support for infrastructure and policy change.

The mission of LWO: Activate Omaha was to create awareness, advocacy, and excitement about activity and to highlight the importance of designing the community for active lifestyles. LWO: Activate Omaha is a community-wide initiative designed to encourage community members to incorporate activity into daily living and to support changes in urban design, land use, and transportation policies to cultivate and support active living. A 2004 health report card released by LWO found no change in obesity or physical activity levels (Live Well Omaha Community Report Card 2004). Initial programmatic efforts were aimed at increasing citizen awareness of the benefits of physical activity and the range of activities that could increase physical activity. Several campaign messages were used: Physical activity can be fun, physical activity can be done any time and in many places, and physical activity works best as a part of everyday living. As the campaign messages continued to show success, efforts changed and LWO: Activate Omaha became the resource for physical activity opportunities and initiatives in the community. Perhaps LWO: Activate Omaha's most successful effort was the commuter challenge, which encouraged businesses to support teams of bicyclists to ride to

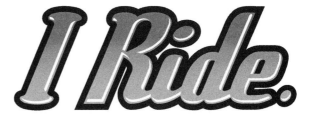

Funding for these items was made possible (in part) by the cooperative agreement award 1U58DP002394-01 from the Centers for Disease Control and Prevention. The materials do not necessarily reflect the official policies of the Department of Health and Human Services.

work and log their miles. The project featured maps noting routes across the city and provided awards to company teams with the most miles. LWO: Activate Omaha provided the technical support, route identification, incentives, and program maintenance.

As the number of activities and grant opportunities increased, LWO: Activate Omaha created a number of subcommittees, including media, Safe Routes to School, policy, and fund-raising (see figure 33.1). This allowed volunteer members to use their expertise, skills, and resources to create a more effective and efficient partnership. In the third year of the Active Living by Design grant, local organizations expressed an interest in forming a bicycle-friendly community design coalition under the umbrella of LWO: Activate Omaha. LWO: Activate Omaha used programs and promotions to build community demand and establish rapport with community members in order to influence policy change. The partnership worked with partners to promote active living policies by providing resources and information to community members about how to become well-informed citizens and advocates for change, often through existing programs. LWO: Activate Omaha continues to implement small- and large-scale environmental changes through the following policies and programs, among others:

Bicycle-Pedestrian Advisory Committee

This technical advisory group (composed of city planners, local health department personnel, cycling advocates, and others) advises the mayor on issues such as improving conditions for bicycling, walking, and other forms of alternative transportation.

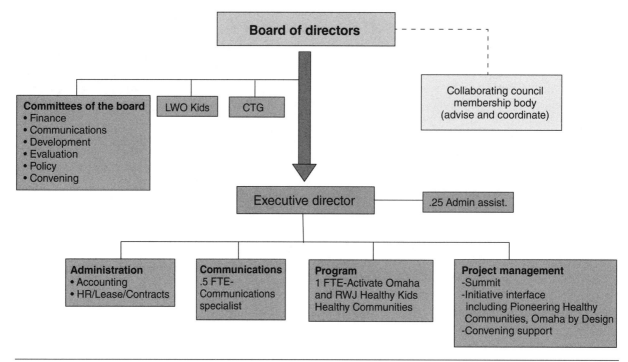

Figure 33.1 Live Well Omaha organizational chart.

Funding for these items was made possible (in part) by the cooperative agreement award 1U58DP002394-01 from the Centers of Disease Control and Prevention. The materials do not necessarily reflect the official policies of the Department of Health and Human Services.

Land Use and Street Design Policy

- The city council unanimously passed a package of revisions and additions to the city's zoning and subdivision code structure for streetscapes, signage, landscaping, building design, pedestrian networks, public spaces, and connections between city neighborhoods, commercial centers, and civic districts.

- The partnership supported this effort by providing information and encouraging residents to write letters and attend meetings.

Bicycle and Pedestrian Loop

The partnership received funding to develop a 20-mile (32-kilometer) bicycle and pedestrian loop in Omaha as a pilot project to increase physical activity. The partnership hoped that the success of the pilot project would encourage the funder to invest additional resources in expanding the loop and would serve as the groundwork for a citywide transportation master plan. Subsequently, in 2012, the city planning board approved a transportation plan.

Bike Amenities

- LWO: Activate Omaha increased community demand for bicycle lanes and other bicycle infrastructure such as bike racks and parking amenities.

- The partnership identified streets that needed to be redesigned and requested that bike lane signage and striping be incorporated. The partnership targeted streets that could easily accommodate bike lanes.

- More than 20 miles (32 kilometers) of on-street enhancements were in design phases as a result of funding provided by a number of private foundations. Federal transportation enhancement funds were also secured through the city planning office for "road diets" (i.e., a reduction in traffic lanes), bicycle lanes, and other amenities.

- The city planning and public works departments agreed to allocate an additional 10 feet (3 meters) of right-of-way on all road-widening projects.
- In collaboration with local bicycle shops, LWO: Activate Omaha offered inexpensive bicycle racks to businesses throughout the city.
- Bike racks were added to all buses and trains that were part of the metro area transit system.

LWO Kids

As the momentum began to build around combating obesity, another key partnership occurred. Alegent Health made a significant investment in the community in 2006 when it committed more than one million dollars in funding and staff resources to create a community coalition dedicated to fighting childhood obesity in Omaha and surrounding communities. The initiative was moved under the LWO umbrella. This ensured strategic alignment across LWO: Activate Omaha and LWO: Kids and prevented duplication.

Following are examples of successful projects that have been led by LWO Kids:

- Physician training to measure patients' body mass index at every office visit.
- Implementation of a social marketing campaign called 54321Go! This program, which was modeled after a Chicago program, focuses on the number of healthy behaviors kids should engage in each day.
- A school-based physical activity during recess initiative funded by the Robert Wood Johnson Foundation.

As LWO grew in partnership and experience, so did the opportunities to affect community health efforts through new collaborative efforts and funding opportunities over the years. Omaha became 1 of 45 communities that participated in the Pioneering Healthier Communities efforts in 2007. This was a national initiative from the YMCA Activate America program. In 2008, the Robert Wood Johnson Foundation awarded a Healthy Kids Healthy Communities grant to the Douglas County Health Department and LWO Kids. In 2009, the Douglas County Health Department with the LWO collaboration was awarded funding from the Communities Putting Prevention to Work (CPPW), a grant opportunity from the Centers for Disease Control and Prevention that is part of the American Recovery and Reinvestment Act. This $5.7 million grant was possible because of the leveraged community partnerships and capacity created by the LWO collaboration.

The CPPW funding addressed multiple health issues, including healthy eating and active living. This allowed LWO and the Douglas County Health Department to move existing efforts forward as well as to create new activities. The funding broadened the scope of after-school programs and provided training for Safe Routes to School and bike pedestrian safety initiatives. As a new venture it added a revision to the transportation element of the city's master plan. These funding opportunities and the alignment of community efforts have built and facilitated a strong foundation for the recently released Community Transformation Implementation Grants provided by the Centers for Disease Control and Prevention. As of September 27, 2011, Douglas County Health Department was 1 of 61 funded organizations to receive this grant funding. The funding focuses on tobacco-free living, active living, healthy eating, and provision of high-quality clinical and preventive services.

LWO uniquely exemplifies an aligned effort across community coalitions working to eliminate childhood obesity, encourage active living, and promote healthy eating. The infusion of CPPW funding into the Omaha community, along with the leveraging of community-based funding, has allowed for the collaboration to make a significant step in solving some of the health issues affecting the city. To be strategic and efficient, the LWO coalition serves as the umbrella organization to guide and unite four existing collaborative initiatives to create community-wide, sustainable change.

Linkages to the National Physical Activity Plan

LWO's successes in addressing Strategy 2 for the Public Health Sector can be directly linked to the cross-sectoral partnerships that have been created, maintained, and leveraged. In collaboration with the Douglas County Health Department, LWO has built an exceptional community model that began with the engagement of nonprofit organizations and a large health care–based organization. Buying into the vision of LWO and providing funding allowed the coalition to come together in a unified effort to address poor nutrition, physical inactivity, obesity, and other identified health issues. Through continuous leveraging of resources and partners, LWO has developed a large network that can address physical activity strategies within the areas of public health, health care, education, parks, recreation, transportation, urban design, community planning, worksites, nonprofit organizations, faith communities, and underserved populations. These strategic partners also help to carry out other strategies found in the National Physical Activity Plan, specifically the Business and Industry; Education; Mass Media; Transportation, Land Use, and Community Design; and Volunteer and Nonprofit Sectors.

Building on these cross-sectoral partnerships has allowed LWO to address two additional strategies in the National Physical Activity Plan, Public Health Sector. Drawing on Strategy 3 of this sector, the partnership has helped LWO create a policy and advocacy agenda to improve the health of the citizens of Douglas County. An example of this work was the recently approved citywide transportation master plan, which includes a Complete Streets policy approach that highlights the need for an integrated transportation system that is available for all citizens. This policy work was accomplished through collaboration of various key partners from public health, community planning, public works, local coalitions, local government agencies, and the public. Regarding Strategy 3 of the Public Health Sector, Activate Omaha has extensive experience in developing, disseminating, and promoting tools to improve individual- and community-based physical activity habits. Many of the tools and resources help to promote bike and pedestrian efforts, such as the commuter challenge, Safe Routes to School programming, and policy and advocacy efforts.

Evidence Base Used During Program Development

The combined effects of society, family, and individual factors intensify the causes of obesity (Davison and Birch 2001; DeMattia and Denney 2008). Research suggests that environmental change is critical at all levels of the ecological model to support individual change (Budd and Hayman 2008; Ferreira et al. 2001; Sallis and Glanz 2006). Throughout this collaborative process, the primary goal was to create a community that supported physical activity. The collaborative used three models to produce such an environment: an ecological model, a health policy model, and the Robert Wood Johnson's Active Living by Design 5P model. The ecological model served as the cornerstone and clearly defined the scope of work needed to create meaningful results. The ecological model requires planners to identify elements in the community that affect a behavior, from personal elements such as homes and work to public elements such as faith-based organizations and legislative bodies.

The second model used in the planning process was the health policy model. According to Richmond and Kotelchuck (1991, 1993), in order to effectively implement system change across a community, planners must develop a knowledge base, gain political will to support change, and create a social strategy to accomplish change. An adequate knowledge base is needed to facilitate decision making. Political will provides a mechanism by which communities' needs are heard and resources allocated. The way in which knowledge is applied and the political will is built is the social strategy. These social strategies may help to reset behaviors and contribute to sustained change.

The third model that helped to integrate the LWO: Activate Omaha was the 5P model, The

5P model, created by Active Living by Design, a national program of the Robert Wood Johnson Foundation, featured preparation, partnership, promotion, policy, and physical environment focuses. The model establishes innovative approaches to increase physical activity through community design, public policies, and communications strategies (Bussel, et al. 2009). The model suggests that a community that engages in a range of activities, from partnerships to programming and policy change, creates lasting sustainable change.

Populations Best Served by the Program

LWO serves the entire Omaha metropolitan area and focuses on Douglas County. The U.S. Census Bureau's 2010 population estimate for the City of Omaha is 408,958; the estimate for Douglas County is 510,199. The population of Douglas County is diverse (72 percent white, 12 percent Black, 11 percent Hispanic, and 5 percent other racial and ethnic groups) and faces a number of challenges, including poverty, health disparities, and health risks related to poor nutrition, physical inactivity, and other chronic disease risk factors.

Omaha's health ranking is extremely low— 142 out of 182 metropolitan cities, according to 2009 data from the Behavioral Risk Factor Surveillance System. Five indicators contribute to this classification: current smokers, binge drinkers, physical activity levels, consumption of fruits and vegetables, and overweight and obesity (Centers for Disease Control and Prevention 2009). Douglas County exceeds the 2009 national rates for diabetes-related deaths and overweight youth. The county's rankings (University of Wisconsin Population Health Institute 2011) indicate that only 77 percent of Douglas County residents have access to healthy foods such as fruits and vegetables, compared with 92 percent nationally. In a 2008 random survey of 894 Douglas County youth ages 12 to 19 years, more than 50 percent reported that they rarely ate fresh fruits and vegetables and less than 10 percent reported eating five servings of fruits and vegetables each day (Wang et al. 2009). In

addition, 77 percent of students reported that they never biked or walked to school, attributable in great part to a lack of infrastructure connecting schools to trails, bike paths, green spaces, and parks.

Lessons Learned

LWO used several strategies that contributed to its early successes. The strongest keys to success thus far have been (1) building on a history of partnerships, (2) creating awareness by setting an agenda for change, (3) following a planning model in developing programs, and (4) implementing some activities on a rolling basis.

Building on a History of Partnerships

Central to LWO's success has been the history of the Douglas County Health Department and LWO partnerships with other organizations in the community and the ability to leverage existing activities in the community. Before the introduction of CPPW funding, the network of 19 partners and members of Omaha's business community had engaged in several early collaborations to address obesity and physical activity in the community. Many of these early activities laid the groundwork for LWO's CPPW current objectives and activities, allowing it to build on the existing efforts and interests of the community and to hit the ground running at the time of the award. A key to success has been the joint effort by the two organizations to leverage funding opportunities by aligning the leadership processes and plans with the strengths of each organization.

Creating Awareness Through Media and Setting an Agenda for Change

Another key to success noted by LWO CPPW staff is the use of media to engage members of the community. The media campaign's early messages to the community regarding Omaha's poor health ranking caught people's attention

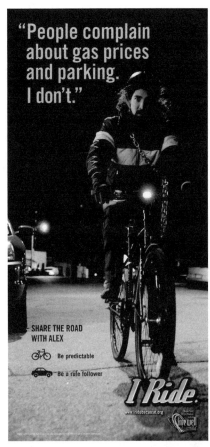

"People complain about gas prices and parking. I don't."

SHARE THE ROAD WITH ALEX

Be predictable

Be a rule follower

I Ride.

www.iridebecause.org

Live well omaha

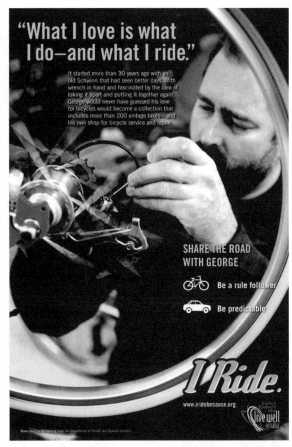

"What I love is what I do—and what I ride."

It started more than 30 years ago with an old Schwinn that had seen better days. With wrench in hand and fascinated by the idea of taking it apart and putting it together again, George would never have guessed his love for bicycles would become a collection that includes more than 200 vintage bikes – and his own shop for bicycle service and repair.

SHARE THE ROAD WITH GEORGE

Be a rule follower

Be predictable

I Ride.

www.iridebecause.org

Live well omaha

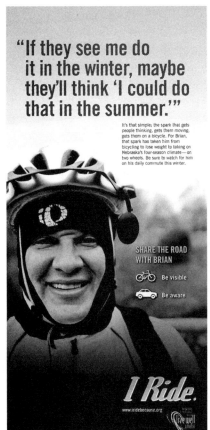

"If they see me do it in the winter, maybe they'll think 'I could do that in the summer.'"

It's that simple: the spark that gets people thinking, gets them moving, gets them on a bicycle. For Brian, that spark has taken him from bicycling to lose weight to taking on Nebraska's four-season climate—on two wheels. Be sure to watch for him on his daily commute this winter.

SHARE THE ROAD WITH BRIAN

Be visible

Be aware

I Ride.

www.iridebecause.org

Live well omaha

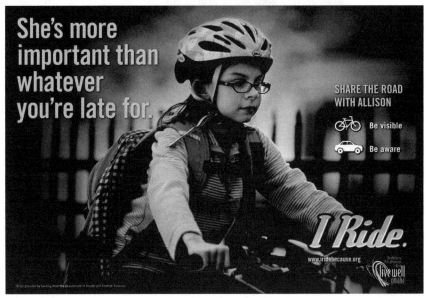

She's more important than whatever you're late for.

SHARE THE ROAD WITH ALLISON

Be visible

Be aware

I Ride.

www.iridebecause.org

Live well omaha

Funding for these items was made possible (in part) by the cooperative agreement award 1U58DP002394-01 from the Centers for Disease Control and Prevention. The materials do not necessarily reflect the official policies of the Department of Health and Human Services.

292

and spurred greater interest and involvement. As explained by one LWO CPPW staff member, the overall goal of the media activities is not just to inform people about health issues but also to create a movement for improving health in the community. Central to this strategy has been branding LWO CPPW across the set of project activities so that people in the community associate the individual or smaller environment, policy, or systems change activities with a much larger effort to improve the community and its health.

Following a Planning Model in Developing Programs

LWO CPPW staff found that their experience using the Robert Wood Johnson Foundation 5P model for change was helpful. LWO was introduced to this model through its participation in the Robert Wood Johnson Foundation Active Living by Design community grant program and has used its basic approach with subsequent projects. Using the model prompted staff to think about policy as a part of change and to draw on a holistic framework for evaluating and addressing health issues in the community. By using this model in designing programs, LWO CPPW staff are better able to strike a balance between working directly on policy change and creating public education, interest, and involvement, which they believe is required for changes in policy to be enacted.

Implementing Activities on a Rolling Basis

Several LWO CPPW strategies have been implemented on a rolling basis; some organizations and communities participated in or completed program efforts in the first year and others became engaged in the second year. Although the intent of this design was mostly to make these activities more manageable, this phased-in approach has allowed LWO staff to gain experience and refine their efforts and has provided opportunities for staff to present success stories to potential future partners and the city as a whole.

Tips for Working Across Sectors

In working across sectors, program leaders must define key concepts, strategies, and outcomes. These definitions require a common vision, resulting in a common language. Finding a common language is key as new partners join an initiative: The language a public health officer uses may be different than that used by a planner.

- Align project duties with an organization's agendas and strengths. In order to make projects simple, they should contain clearly delineated duties for every partner, depending on each partner's expertise. This allows partners to work in tandem with others doing the same functions, and their combined work contributes to the common good. When partners use similar strategies aimed at a common goal, their combined efforts create a more robust product. An example is the installation of bicycle lanes. These lanes could be viewed by public health officers as a means to increase physical activity, whereas public works planners may consider bicycle lanes as a means of promoting public safety and reducing car traffic. Further, planners and developers may view bicycle lanes as an engaging design element.

- Create meaningful dialogue that acknowledges the importance of the project in each partner's overall scope of work. This requires mutual respect and an open dialogue that honors all partners' points of view and contributions. Respectful dialogues allow partners to discuss the value of their achievements with each other and with the greater community. Remember that what might seem trivial to one group can be important to another.

- Persevere in your efforts to communicate. Success requires continuous and positive engagement.

References

Budd, G.M., and L.L. Hayman. 2008. Addressing the childhood obesity crisis. *MCN. Am. J. Matern. Child Nurs.*33(2):111-8.

Bussel, Leviton, and Orleans. 2009. Active living by design: Perspectives from the Robert Wood Johnson Foundation. American Journal of Preventive Medicine. (37):6S2.

Centers for Disease Control and Prevention. 2009. *Behavioral Risk Factor Surveillance System Survey Data*. Atlanta, GA: U.S. Department of Health and Human Services, Centers for Disease Control and Prevention.

Davison, K.K., and L.L. Birch. 2001. Childhood overweight: A contextual model and recommendations for future research. *Obes. Rev.* 2(3):159-71.

DeMattia, L. and S.L. Denney. 2008. Childhood obesity prevention: Successful community-based efforts. *Ann. Am. Acad. Pol. Soc. Sci.* 615:83-99.

Ferreira, I., K. van der Horst, W. Wendel-Vos, S. Kremers, F.J. van Lenthe, and J. Brug. 2001. Environmental correlates of physical activity in youth: a review and update. *Obes. Rev.* 8(2):129-54.

Live Well Omaha Community Report Card. 2002. Omaha, NE: Douglas County Health Department.

Live Well Omaha Community Report Card. 2004. Omaha, NE: Douglas County Health Department.

Richmond, J.B., and M. Kotelchuck. 1991. Co-ordination and development of strategies and policy for public health promotion in the United States. In: *Oxford Textbook of Public Health*. W.W. Holland, R. Detels, and G. Knox, Eds. Oxford, UK: Oxford Medical Publications.

Richmond, J.B., and M. Kotelchuck. 1993. Political influences: Rethinking national health policy. In: *Handbook of Health Professions Education*. C. Mcquire, R. Foley, A. Gorr, and R. Richards, Eds. San Francisco: Jossey-Bass.

Sallis, J.F., and K. Glanz. 2006. The role of built environments in physical activity, eating, and obesity in childhood. *Future Child.* 16(1):89-108.

University of Wisconsin Population Health Institute. 2011. *County Health Rankings & Roadmaps*. Madison, WI: Robert Wood Johnson Foundation.

Wang, H.M. et al. 2009. Youth physical activity and dietary behavior in Douglas County survey findings. www.livewellomahakids.org.

CHAPTER 34

Tracking and Measuring Physical Activity Policy

Amy A. Eyler, PhD, CHES
Washington University in St. Louis

Kelly R. Evenson, PhD
University of North Carolina

Ross C. Brownson, PhD
Washington University in St. Louis

NPAP Tactics and Strategies Used in This Program

Overarching Strategies

STRATEGY 3: Disseminate best practice physical activity models, programs, and policies to the widest extent practicable to ensure Americans can access strategies that will enable them to meet federal physical activity guidelines.

STRATEGY 4: Establish a center for physical activity policy development and research across all sectors of the National Physical Activity Plan.

For decades, health professionals have recommended regular physical activity as a way to improve health and prevent disease. Despite the proven health benefits of regular physical activity, about half of adults in the United States do not participate in physical activity at recommended levels, and about 25 percent do not participate in any leisure-time physical activity (Centers for Disease Control and Prevention 2008). Because participation rates have changed very little over time, public health, medical, and other concerned organizations are promoting new and broader strategies to help people become more active. These new strategies focus less on individual or small group changes, since these approaches are not very efficient and the changes often don't last (Brownson et al. 2006). Current strategies include changing policies and the environment, which has the potential to affect physical activity at the population (rather than individual) level (Centers for Disease Control and Prevention 2011). The objectives of this chapter are (1) to define physical activity policy, (2) to describe and provide examples of aspects of physical activity policy surveillance within the National Physical Activity Plan, and (3) to provide examples of mechanisms for physical activity policy surveillance.

Program Description

Physical activity policies are legislative actions, organized guidance, or rules that may affect the environment or behaviors related to physical activity (Schmid et al. 2006). These policies can be in the form of formal written codes (e.g., state legislation requiring physical education) or standards that guide choices (e.g., a bicycle or pedestrian master plan for a community).

Physical activity (PA) policies involve many disciplines. Public health, education, recreation, urban planning, transportation, and advocacy groups are some of the key stakeholders. Examples of PA policies include those within schools, such as required physical education, recess policies, and active transport policies, and those within worksites, such as policies that reward PA or flexible schedules that allow employees to exercise. Municipalities may develop and maintain quality public spaces, such as parks and trails, and implement policies that encourage their use. Transportation policies, when they consider all users of transportation resources, including bicyclists and pedestrians, can promote physical activity in a community.

Research on and surveillance of these policies can help determine best practices for improving population levels of PA. This is consistent with the aim of the National Physical Activity Plan (NPAP) to "create a national culture that supports physically active lifestyles" (National Physical Activity Plan Coordinating Committee 2010).

Linkage to National Physical Activity Plan

PA policy and surveillance are integral to the NPAP. Two of the overarching strategies of the NPAP encompass the need for best practices in PA policies and policy information dissemination.

Strategy 3: Disseminate best practice physical activity models, programs, and policies to the widest extent practicable to ensure Americans can access strategies that will enable them to meet federal physical activity guidelines.

Strategy 4: Establish a center for physical activity policy development and research across all sectors of the National Physical Activity Plan.

Additionally, each of the eight sectors within the NPAP includes at least one priority strategy that relates to policy research, development, advocacy, or action. To best accomplish these

strategies, participants must learn more about existing (or missing) policies.

PA Policy Surveillance

Public health surveillance is a cornerstone of public health (Lee and Thacker 2011). The United States has surveillance or tracking systems that provide excellent data for estimating the person, place, and time dimensions of physical activity. Although these are helpful, it is also important to identify and track policies that have the potential to influence population PA. Information provided by policy surveillance systems can be an enormous asset when planners are developing new policies or when trying to solicit support for policies. For example, a school district representative can examine data on rates of physical activity for a community and its schools to justify the development of a joint-use policy. Databases for existing and successful joint-use agreements can provide important guidance and language in policy development.

Physical activity policy surveillance involves three steps: identifying policies, identifying policy content, and exploring implementation.

Identifying Policies

The first step in determining the most effective PA policies is to identify what policies exist. Identification is challenging because of the broad and complex scope of policies that can influence PA. Obtaining information on the policies can be difficult, because each level of government (state, county, municipal) and each sector may have its own tracking and data system. For example, a state may have a database that provides information on physical education, including a list of physical education policies enacted or in place within a certain time frame at the state level. At the local level, however, few comprehensive databases or tracking tools exist for compiling or examining policies. Surveillance of local policies often requires the use of secondary data sources, such as school district policy documents or municipal websites. Following is a brief case study of policy identification.

Case Study: Complete Streets Policy Surveillance

For many PA policy topics, no single, easy method exists for gathering information. However, by using several methods and data sources and some creative thinking, interested individuals or organizations can collect information on PA policies. A good example is collecting Complete Streets policy information. A Complete Streets policy supports the premise that transportation planners and engineers should design and operate the entire roadway with all users in mind—including bicyclists, pedestrians of all ages and abilities, and public transportation vehicles and riders (National Complete Streets Coalition 2010). By way of these policies, people will have more options for active travel and therefore may increase their physical activity. An inventory of such policies can show geographical trends, identify gaps and opportunities for dissemination, and provide important information for active transportation advocates.

Surveillance of Complete Streets policies can be complex, because such policies can be enacted at state, regional, and local levels. In 2010, the National Complete Streets Coalition found that more than 100 jurisdictions—state, local, and regional—had adopted Complete Streets policies (National Complete Streets Coalition 2010). This organization defines model policies and attempts to identify emerging and existing policies for surveillance purposes. Despite national efforts, achieving a comprehensive list of these policies can be difficult. State legislative databases can provide information on existing statutes (state laws), legislation that has been introduced, or resolutions. For a local perspective, assessments of metropolitan planning organizations within states may provide information on the presence of Complete Streets policies. Another potential way to inventory Complete Streets policies is to glean information from advocacy groups within states that focus on the built environment or transportation improvements. These agencies often track local

and regional policies as a measure of advocacy progress.

Identifying Policy Content

The second step in PA policy surveillance is identifying policy content. Content included in a policy can determine effectiveness. Assessing the content for the inclusion or lack of an evidence base is important for evaluation and improvement. A policy that mandates proven strategies will more likely have expected outcomes than will a policy not based on evidence. Additionally, content analysis on policies can show trends and patterns over time. For example, content analysis can show trends in how evidence is disseminated into both policy and practice. Last, examining content of PA policies can help in the development of model legislation. An assessment of many policies on a certain topic usually will reveal a range of quality in terms of policy content. The best policies may be used to develop model policy language.

Case Study: Evidence-Based Content in State Physical Education Policies

Public health and education professionals increasingly agree that policy-based approaches targeting the school environment, such as physical education (PE), may have the greatest impact on child and adolescent physical inactivity and childhood obesity (Masse et al. 2007). PE is a policy area for which specific evidence-based components exist, and aspects of PE are known to increase the quality and quantity of PA in children and adolescents. National recommendations include (1) a minimum requirement for PE minutes, (2) an increase in moderate to vigorous activity in PE class, (3) a recommendation for PE teacher qualifications, and (4) access to a sufficient environment and equipment for PE (Centers for Disease Control and Prevention 2011; National Association for Sport and Physical Education 2004). To assess to what extent these four evidence-based components are included in state PE legislation, Eyler and colleagues (2010) used online state legislation databases to collect a list of all state bills (introduced and enacted). More than 800 bills were identified during the time period 2000-2007. Each bill was read and coded for the four evidence-based components, and the levels of content across the bills were analyzed. Researchers concluded that many state-level PE policies were not evidence based. Only 272 contained at least one of the four evidence-based components. Enactment rates of bills with and without evidence-based components varied. Forty-three of the 272 bills with at least one evidence-based element were enacted (16 percent), compared with 23 percent for the rest of the bills in the sample (Eyler et al. 2010).

Exploring Implementation

The third step in PA policy surveillance is exploring implementation. Once a policy is enacted, it is important to assess how and to what extent it is being put into action. This step involves gaining information on the implementation process. Implementation analysis could include the following:

- Information on barriers and enablers of implementation
- Necessary stakeholders
- Successful methods of media advocacy
- Best practices for implementation

Analysis of this type of process information involves collecting data in a variety of ways. Key informant or stakeholder interviews, focus groups, or event observations can be used to assess what it takes for a PA policy to be implemented.

Case Study: Analysis of Policy Implementation for Development of Community Trails

Strategy 2 in the Transportation, Land Use, and Community Design Sector of the NPAP calls for the development of trails. A trail is defined as a travel way established either by construction or use that is passable by a variety of modes, such as walking, bicycling, in-line skating, and wheelchairs (Federal Highway Administration 2005). Community trails provide healthy and safe recreation, transportation, and physical activity opportunities for people of all ages. They also connect people with social destinations or points of interest and ensure sustained opportunity for physical activity (Rails to Trails Conservancy 2013). Developing a community trail often involves policies across scales and sectors. Some policies within communities can facilitate trail development (e.g., an established bicycle and pedestrian plan), whereas others can hinder it (e.g., restrictive zoning policies).

The Physical Activity Policy Research Network conducted a case study on the policy process of trail development by examining six trails in several states (Eyler et al. 2008). The goals of this case study were to identify the policy influences on trail development, explore the roles of key players in trail development, and compare and contrast findings from the different trails. Drawing from 46 key informant interviews, researchers found that policies at all governmental levels were apparent in trail development. Both federal and state funding policies and design standards were reported by representatives in all trail projects studied. Local policies that addressed funding and land acquisition were also important. Leadership, advocacy, community group involvement, and residential input were all factors in the success of the trail projects (Eyler et al. 2008).

Case Study: Evaluation of the National Physical Activity Plan

National plans that address health problems are meant to demonstrate the extent of the problem and recommend multilevel strategies to improve the specific health condition within the population. These strategies are often divided by sector and include many aspects of policy and environmental change. Additionally, such plans can increase visibility of the issue at the political level and allow stakeholders to follow common objectives and strategies for improvement (Daugbjerg et al. 2009). The U.S. National Physical Activity Plan is one such example. This plan followed the release of the 2008 Physical Activity Guidelines for Americans (U.S. Department of Health and Human Services 2008). Although the guidelines provided evidence-based recommendations on the types and amounts of PA that are needed to yield health benefits, the national plan detailed changes that were needed to put those recommendations into place (Pate 2009).

With the development of physical activity plans in the United States and around the world, several groups have called for the need to evaluate these national plans (Bornstein et al. 2009). To accomplish this goal for the U.S. national plan, several initial activities have occurred. The evaluation team created an evaluation strategy guided by the theoretical underpinnings of the Diffusion of Innovations Theory (Rogers 2004) and the RE-AIM model (reach, effectiveness, adoption, implementation, maintenance) (Glasgow et al. 2006). The evaluation team identified three major, measurable activities for the initial, short-term evaluation of the National Physical Activity Plan: (1) sector reports, (2) survey of the members of the National Society of Physical Activity Practitioners in Public Health, and (3) case studies.

Lessons Learned

The most important, yet the least explored, aspect of PA policy surveillance is determining the outcomes of the policy. Outcomes can be defined in many ways. Behavioral outcomes (e.g., increased PA in school children) as a result of specific policies (e.g., PE policies) are of interest to researchers, advocates, and policy makers. These behavioral outcomes can reach beyond PA and potentially influence health conditions, such as diabetes or obesity. However, without the use of complicated study methods, it is extremely difficult to say with certainty that the policy brought about the outcome. Economic outcomes are another potential measure of PA policy effectiveness, but they too are difficult to measure precisely, given the complex nature of these policies.

Other outcomes could include environmental or culture change as a result of PA policy. These types of outcomes may be indirectly related to physical activity. For instance, if policies promote the increase of active transportation, this could reduce the number of automobiles on the road and thus increase physical activity but could also lower air particulates. A cultural change as a result of more opportunities for active transportation may include better acceptance of walking or cycling for short errands. As in the case of both behavioral and economic outcomes, environmental and cultural changes are difficult to measure and to quantify in terms of their relationship to the policy.

Evidence Base Used During Program Development

As exemplified in the case study examples, many resources and sources of information exist for identifying PA policies. These resources vary in scope of information, comprehensiveness, and relative ease of use.

• Databases: For information on policies at the state or federal level, subscription-based databases can provide an easy way to search federal and state legislation by topic and state. Additionally, each state has its own legislative search website available for free access, although these vary in the amount of information available and search capabilities.

• National organizations: National organizations that promote or support PA can be a source for policy surveillance. For example, the National Conference of State Legislatures provides comprehensive information on many physical activity policy topics. Advocacy associations such as the American Alliance for Health, Physical Education, Recreation and Dance provide information on school-specific policies (e.g., PE, recess). Disease-specific organizations, such as the American Heart Association, are involved in PA policy advocacy and have included policy information on their websites and in reports.

• National surveillance: Survey systems such as CDC's School Health Policy and Programs Study and its Behavioral Risk Factor Surveillance System include some information about PA behavior and policy. Other surveillance systems, such as the National Household Travel Survey and the American Time Use Survey, can provide comparative PA data.

• Research networks: The Physical Activity Policy Research Network is a CDC-funded network of academic professionals and their community affiliates who study effective elements and outcomes of policies that have the potential to improve population physical activity rates. Although this network is not a comprehensive database for PA policy, the products from the network's research studies can provide information on evidence-based policies and other background information that can inform policy advocacy or practice.

Active Living Research is an organization funded by the Robert Wood Johnson Foundation to provide a platform for quality active living research and dissemination, particularly focusing on policy and environmental change. The organization has an extensive resource list on its website that includes academic articles, policy briefs, and other PA policy-related information.

• Miscellaneous resources: Many topic-specific resources for PA policy surveillance exist. Advocacy agencies that promote increases in the use of Complete Streets policies, Safe Routes to School, and joint use, for example, all have policy resources on their websites. These websites vary in scope but can provide a good baseline of policy information devoted to the topic of interest.

Summary

Policies are an important part of a comprehensive strategy to improve population PA. These policies are complex and span many sectors and levels of government. Assessing the policies, their content, and implementation through surveillance is essential for gathering evidence for effective policies, informing policy development, and advocating for policy support.

Surveillance and assessment of PA policies can help inform future efforts to implement the NPAP and contribute to the growing body of literature on best practices and evidence-based policy strategies to increase populations PA. Despite its importance, there are several gaps in current surveillance efforts:

• Policy measurement and surveillance are not at the capacity needed to address the increasing recommendations for policy interventions by authoritative bodies, including NPAP.

• Some high-quality sources of national and state PA policy information exist, but local policies are often difficult to assess because of a lack of a unified data source.

• Assessing the evidence base in policy content is important to this developing field.

• There is a need for better assessment of policy implementation in order to inform evaluation of outcomes.

References

Bornstein, D.B., R.R. Pate, and M. Pratt. 2009. A review of the national physical activity plans of six countries. *J. Phys. Act. Health* 6(Suppl. 2):S245-64.

Brownson, R.C., D. Haire-Joshu, and D.A. Luke. 2006. Shaping the context of health: A review of environmental and policy approaches in the prevention of chronic diseases. *Annu. Rev. Public Health* 27:341-70.

Centers for Disease Control and Prevention. 2008. *Behavioral Risk Factor Surveillance System: National Center for Chronic Disease Prevention and Health Promotion.* Atlanta: Centers for Disease Control and Prevention.

Centers for Disease Control and Prevention. 2011. Guide to community preventive services. Promoting physical activity: Environmental and policy approaches. www.thecommunityguide.org/pa/environmental-policy/index.html.

Daugbjerg, S.B., S. Kahlmeier, F. Racioppi, et al. 2009. Promotion of physical activity in the European region: Content analysis of 27 national policy documents. *J. Phys. Act. Health* 6(6):805-17.

Eyler, A., R. Brownson, S. Aytur, et al. 2010. Examination of trends and evidence-based elements in state physical education legislation: A content analysis. *J. Sch. Health* 80(7):326-32.

Eyler, A., R. Brownson, K. Evenson, et al. 2008. Policy influences on community trail development. *J. Health Polit. Policy Law.* 33(3):407-27.

Federal Highway Administration. 2005. *Safe, Accountable, Flexible, Efficient Transportation Equite Act: A Legacy for Users.* Washington, DC: U.S. Department of Transportation.

Glasgow, R., L. Klesges, D. Dzewaltowski, P. Estabrooks, T.M. Vogt. 2006. Evaluating the impact of health promotion programs: Using the RE-AIM framework to form summary measures for decision making involving complex issues. *Health Educ. Res.* 21:688-94.

Lee, L.M., and S.B. Thacker. 2011. The cornerstone of public health practice: Public health surveillance, 1961-2011. *MMWR. Morbid. Mortal. Wkly. Rep.* 7(60):15-21.

Masse, L., J. Chriqui, J. Igoe, et al. 2007. Development of a Physical Education-Related State Policy Classification System (PERSPCS). *Am. J. Prev. Med.* 33(4 Suppl.):S264-76.

National Association for Sport and Physical Education. 2004. *Moving Into the Future: National Standards for Physical Education.* Reston, VA: McGraw-Hill.

National Complete Streets Coalition. 2010. Complete the streets. http://www.completestreets.org.

National Physical Activity Plan Coordinating Committee. 2010. National Physical Activity Plan. www.physicalactivityplan org.

Pate, R. 2009. A national physical activity plan for the United States. *J. Phys. Act. Health* 6(Suppl. 2):S157-8.

Rails to Trails Conservancy. 2013. Plan, design, build: Accessibility. www.railstotrails.org/ourwork/trail-building/toolbox/informationsummaries/accessibility.html.

Rogers, E.M. 2004. A prospective and retrospective look at the diffusion model. *J. Health Commun.* 9(Suppl. 1):13-19.

Schmid, T., M. Pratt, and L. Witmer. 2006. A framework for physical activity policy research. *J. Phys. Act. Health* 3(Suppl. 1):S20-9.

U.S. Department of Health and Human Services. 2008. *Physical Activity Guidelines for Americans.* Washington, DC: U.S. Department of Health and Human Services.

Transportation, Land Use, and Community Design

Mark Fenton, MS

Tufts University, Friedman School of Nutrition Science and Policy

This section takes a somewhat surprising approach to sharing two critical lessons with readers. The chapters are written primarily by professionals in fields other than the traditional physical activity promotion fields. These authors demonstrate the broad range of disciplines and backgrounds that must come together to implement true policy and environmental approaches to increasing population levels of physical activity. One author, Ray Sharp, is a public health community planner in Houghton, Michigan. Kerri R. Peters and Julie T. Harris are part of Live Well Omaha, a nonprofit public-private partnership focused on sustainable community health. Ian Thomas works with PedNet, a pedestrian and bicycle advocacy nonprofit in Columbia, Missouri. Leslie A. Meehan and Michael Skipper are planners with Nashville's Metropolitan Planning Organization. Jennifer J. Selby is a transportation engineer who shares work she did with the Urbana, Illinois, Department of Transportation. Only Sharp is in a traditional public health role, and even his chapter emphasizes the need to partner with the city manager, public works department, planning officials, economic developers, and school officials.

You might expect a chapter on transportation, land use, and community design to espouse the virtues of well-known pedestrian-friendly cities such as Boston, New York, and Chicago or high-profile models of bicycle-oriented design such as Portland, Oregon; Boulder, Colorado; and Davis, California. Although worthy of accolades and study, Boston, New York, and Chicago have the advantage of having developed decades or even centuries before widespread automobile use, and Portland, Boulder, and Davis have the advantage of a 10- to 20-year focus on bicycle-oriented policies and infrastructure. Instead, this section visits wintry Houghton, in Michigan's Upper Peninsula, where post-mining economic decline and long, snowy winters would seem to fly in the face of investment in infrastructure to support physical activity. The section also visits Omaha and Nashville, models of so many middle-American cities that once enjoyed a hearty core but in the latter 20th century were economically eviscerated by automobile-oriented sprawl spilling out into the surrounding farmlands and forests. The most walkable, bike-friendly parts of these cities were undermined as the middle class migrated out into an indistinguishable and unwalkable landscape of housing tracts, strip malls, and big box stores. Columbia and Urbana are college towns that illustrate how transportation challenges, from school-induced traffic jams to inefficient roadways, can be resolved in ways that systematically increase opportunities for regular walking, bicycling, and transit use among all residents, from elementary school students to adults.

Two lessons described in the chapters in this section are especially notable. The first is that establishing partnerships outside traditional health roles is critical to building a community that supports increases in routine physical activity across the population. The second lesson is that communities must pursue environmental and policy approaches to increasing physical activity. These lessons frame the approaches that all communities must use to build healthier lifestyles for all residents.

CHAPTER 35

Institutionalizing Safe Routes to School in Columbia, Missouri

Ian Thomas, PhD
PedNet Coalition

Mark Fenton, MS
Tufts University

NPAP Tactics and Strategies Used in This Program

Transportation, Land Use, and Community Design Sector

STRATEGY 1: Increase accountability of project planning and selection to ensure infrastructure supporting active transportation and other forms of physical activity. Tactic: Support annual reporting by all schools of their transportation mode split.

STRATEGY 2: Prioritize resources and provide incentives to increase active transportation and other physical activity through community design, infrastructure projects, systems, policies, and initiatives. Tactic: Support and increase incentives for the adoption and expansion of "safe routes" initiatives such as Safe Routes to School, Bike to Work, and other active transportation programs.

STRATEGY 3: Integrate land-use, transportation, community design, and economic development planning with public health planning to increase active transportation and other physical activity. Tactic: Support the development of standards and identification of "best practices" for the dissemination and adoption of "safe routes" initiatives such as Safe Routes to School, Bike-to-Work, and other active transportation programs.

STRATEGY 4: Increase connectivity and accessibility to essential community destinations to increase active transportation and other physical activity. Tactic: Expand Safe Routes initiatives at national, state, county. and local levels to enable safe walking and biking routes to a variety of destinations, especially to schools.

In 2006, West Boulevard Elementary School in Columbia, Missouri, conducted a moderately successful "walking school bus" program with support from PedNet Coalition, a pedestrian and bicycle advocacy organization and its partners. However, only a fraction of the students eligible to walk and bike to school did so. This was in part because of traffic congestion around the school, which many parents believed created unsafe conditions for pedestrians and cyclists. Ironically, many of those parents then opted to drive their children to school, thus worsening the very traffic they found concerning.

The goal of the Safe Routes to School (SRTS) program was to use a comprehensive approach to increase the number of children walking and cycling to school. The program attempted to increase physical activity for as many students as possible, even those who typically took the school bus or were driven by car. The effort began with a community workshop and walkabout that identified the possibility of having bus drivers and parents drop students off at a park adjacent to the school. Students could then walk to school on a one third of a mile (half a kilometer) pathway connected to the school grounds. Several major steps were taken to develop the program:

- Several "test days" were held to allow parents and bus drivers to try dropping students off at the park.
- All key stakeholders were involved, including school administrators and faculty; planning, public works, and parks and recreation staff; public safety and health professionals; parents and students; and members of the school board.
- A two-day design and planning charrette was conducted during which walking and bicycling advocates shared current Safe Routes to School best practices, students provided feedback, and adult stakeholders developed recommendations based on the 5E model: evaluation and planning, engineering, education, encouragement, and enforcement.
- A more sustained test of the remote drop-off area at the park was conducted for bus riders.

Key results of this process included a renewed effort around all components of the 5E model, including the development of an additional crosswalk near the park and a more direct pathway through the park to the school entrance. The school then adopted the remote drop-off as formal school policy for designated days and seasons, giving all bus riders a short daily walk to school, while strongly encouraging parents to drop off at this area as well. Together with other traffic and pedestrian safety measures over two years, these steps helped promote walking and bicycling to school for nearby students (attributable in part to an easing of the traffic in front of the school) and increased physical activity for students riding the bus.

Program Description

In the past 30 to 40 years, a dramatic change has occurred in how children travel to school. A study by Ham and colleagues (2008) showed that more than 40 percent of children walked and biked to school in 1969, whereas only about 15 percent traveled by car. By 2001 those numbers had practically reversed, with fewer than 15 percent walking and cycling and nearly 50 percent arriving by car. But now a handful of studies and an increasing body of practical experience suggest that a structured Safe Routes to School approach can turn the tide on this trend, by increasing the percentage of students walking, cycling, and taking the bus.

In 1997, the Partnership for a Walkable America, a coalition of government, private, and nonprofit transportation, safety, and health organizations, launched an annual Walk to School Day. The National Center for Safe Routes to School at the University of North Carolina (www.saferoutesinfo.org) promotes an annual Walk to School Day (usually the first Wednesday in October) and Bike to School Day (in early May), provides technical assistance and extensive information on safe routes best practices, and maintains a national registry of participating schools. Along with the National Safe Routes Partnership (a coalition of organizations supporting Safe Routes to School efforts across the United States; www.saferoutespartnership.org), these groups recommend not only launching one-day events but also creating comprehensive programs that address all five components of the 5E model in an ongoing effort to get more children walking and cycling regularly:

- Evaluation and planning: Best when done as the first of the 5Es, this includes measuring travel modes; conducting parent, student, and school staff surveys; and examining traffic, speed, and crash data, development patterns and plans, and similar information collected by local officials.
- Education: This entails teaching students and adults safe behavior, proper procedures (e.g., for arrival and dismissal), and the personal and community benefits of routine walking and cycling.
- Encouragement: People are encouraged to participate through programs and events to reward walking and cycling (such as punch cards, prize drawings, and healthy breakfasts), as well as adult-led walking and bicycling groups and safety measures, which can help

allay parental concerns, especially for students considered too young to walk or bike alone.

• Enforcement: Components of a program can be enforced by reducing speed with improved markings and information (e.g., speed feedback signs), enhanced fines, and increased presence of officers, crossing guards, and volunteers.

• Engineering: The physical infrastructure can be improved in ways such as using signs and crosswalk paint, constructing sidewalks and multiuse pathways, installing bicycle lanes and covered bike parking, and using traffic calming measures (e.g., roundabouts and median islands).

The PedNet Coalition of Columbia, Missouri, is a nonprofit pedestrian and bicycle advocacy group that began its Safe Routes to School efforts by organizing one-day walk-to-school events in 2003. The coalition participated in International Walk to School Day, which allowed local organizers to promote the benefits of routine walking and cycling to school, includ-

ing better student health, improved academic performance and behavior, positive environmental impacts, and reduced traffic congestion and associated safety risks at school arrival and dismissal times. The event also allowed PedNet to evaluate current conditions and learn what was needed to increase walking and bicycling, using the following steps:

• Conducting show-of-hands tallies on pupil travel modes preceding and on Walk to School Day ("Raise your hand if you walked to school today. Rode your bike. Took the school bus. Came by car.")

• Asking parents and students to complete walkability or "bikeability" checklists, reviewing the conditions on their walk or bike trip to school, and identifying challenges and opportunities.

• Conducting surveys of parents and students regarding their attitudes about walking and cycling to school and what would

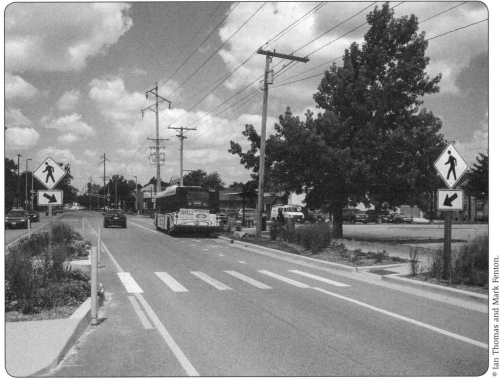

© Ian Thomas and Mark Fenton.

Parents and children should assess available walking and cycling routes, including the presence of quality crosswalks.

be needed for them to walk or bike more routinely.

Concerns regarding their children's safety is often cited as the reason many parents don't allow their children to walk or bike to school. In response, PedNet launched its daily "walking school bus" program in spring 2005. The premise of a walking school bus is to designate a route to the school that is walked by an adult leader on a schedule, picking up student walkers along the way. Communities have taken various approaches to finding walking school bus leaders, such as parent volunteers on a rotating schedule, retirees, hired leaders (similar to crossing guards), and college students fulfilling community service obligations.

Most of the participating children lived within one mile (1.6 kilometers) of the school, but that was only a fraction of those eligible to walk. An ongoing challenge has been to increase participation of those within a mile of school and to include children living farther away. At many schools the pick-up and drop-off traffic is substantial and chaotic enough to intimidate potential pedestrians. Also, the ideal program would provide physical activity opportunities for all students, not just those within walking and bicycling distance.

With the federal government's authorization of the U.S. SRTS program and a growing partnership between PedNet, the Columbia Public School district, West Boulevard Elementary School, and the City of Columbia, an opportunity arose in 2006 to apply for a "noninfrastructure" SRTS grant. The grant would be used to explore the idea of developing a remote bus and car drop-off program that could potentially allow 100 percent of children to engage in at least some physical activity during the daily trip to school. A park immediately next to the school offered an ideal location for the drop-off area, as the students could then walk through the park directly to the school, never crossing a roadway. PedNet and its school and community partners saw this as an opportunity to execute a case study at one elementary school, using a comprehensive planning process that could then be replicated at schools throughout the city.

The model Safe Routes to School program at West Boulevard Elementary School moved through several phases, including one-day walk-to-school events, the launch of walking school buses, community workshops to build consensus on ways to increase routine walking and cycling to school, and implementation of those tactics in a phased approach.

The first phase was the initial launch of Walk to School Day events at elementary schools around the city, which began in 2003 at just four schools. PedNet, the city's nonprofit pedestrian and bicycle advocacy organization, took the leading role in launching these events. This phase grew over time to include two Walk to School Days a year (October and May) with 2,000 to 3,000 students participating.

The positive reaction to the one-day events led to a walking school bus program, launched in 2005. PedNet's walking buses began with just 30 children walking to school along four supervised routes over a six-week period. Since then, the program has grown to include more than 400 registered children at 14 different schools, walking on 60 routes under the supervision of 120 trained volunteers, many of them college students earning credits or community service hours. Businesses have sponsored T-shirts to help create program identity. Frequent walker cards, on which a punch or mark is made for every day a child walks or bikes, allows kids to earn incremental incentives to stay with the program and to enter drawings for bigger prizes such as a bike or skateboard. "Walk stop" (as opposed to bus stop) signs mark locations in neighborhoods where students can meet their walking school bus; these signs also increase program visibility in the community. The program has even used banner ads on public buses, an inexpensive way to advertise the program, to recruit both volunteers (used on university bus routes) and student participants (used on neighborhood bus routes).

One of the target schools for this effort, West Boulevard Elementary, implemented a walking school bus program, but only a fraction of the eligible students participated. One concern of parents was traffic congestion at the school during arrival and dismissal, making it unsafe

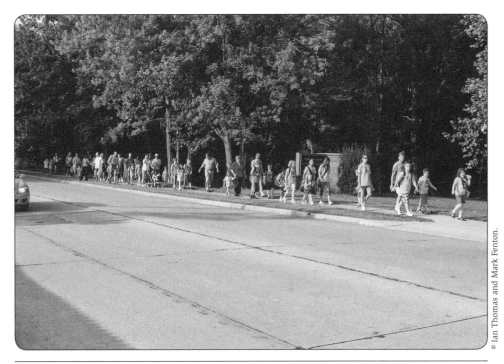

A walking school bus on the way to West Boulevard Elementary School.

for pedestrians. In 2004 PedNet hosted a Healthy Community Design workshop in a location near West Boulevard Elementary. During a walk audit of the area, walking advocates and community members recognized that Again Street Park abuts the school grounds and that a very nice trail through the park could allow students to walk to school after being dropped off at the far side of the park. This led the community to submit a grant application to the state's department of transportation SRTS program for funds to execute a more comprehensive SRTS planning effort around the school in 2007-2008. This planning process included a brief trial of the remote drop-off idea and a highly collaborative design workshop (called a *charrette*).

For the practice "remote drop-off," school buses dropped children off at the far side of the park and allowed them to walk to the school with adult guides. This allowed everyone to gauge student reaction and to assess what needed to be done if the remote drop-off was to be used regularly.

The community charrette was then held to plan the program in detail. The goal was to use a highly open, transparent, inclusive process with as many stakeholders as possible participating, along with the media. Participants included the school principal and superintendent, school board members, teachers, parents, students, health care and public health professionals, the mayor, city council members, law enforcement officials, traffic engineers, city planners, and PedNet advocates. The following elements were included to ensure success of the charrette; these are strongly recommended for similar planning efforts:

- Engage an energetic, upbeat, and technically knowledgeable facilitator. The facilitator's job is first to teach the fundamentals of Safe Routes to School and then to stimulate constructive dialogue among participants, making it inspiring and engaging for everyone. (Providing food can promote a collegial environment.)

- Open with an educational component for all participants. In this case, an opening PowerPoint presentation highlighted proven SRTS tools and principles but used local photos to illustrate how the proven methods could be applied to local challenges and opportunities. This was done before the facilitator asked for feedback, so all participants started with a similar base of knowledge.

- Engage the full group in developing and sharing ideas in the form of smaller round-table working groups. As the working groups report to the full group, the facilitator should respond positively to every idea and constructively to every challenge; the existing body of SRTS experience (see the Additional Readings and Resources at the end of the chapter) provides many excellent solutions to common challenges and concerns.

- Conclude with full-group sharing to find areas of consensus and pull together specific action ideas for moving forward.

- Engage students. In this case the students who had tried the drop-off at the far side of the park took part in a focus group in which they drew pictures and told stories about their experiences. Their enthusiasm for the walk through the park was critical in convincing adults to move forward and make it a more regular opportunity.

- Have the professional team (in this case the facilitator, planning and engineering staff, and PedNet advocates) spend an intensive session analyzing and organizing the community input and create a comprehensive presentation of recommendations. This presentation need not be elaborate (e.g., fancy graphics aren't necessary) but it should display direct quotations and evidence of community input, such as sketches participants created of alternative vehicle routings or maps of walking routes.

- Invite everyone to review and respond to the summary and recommendations. Produce a final report with specific, detailed action items and next steps, and send it to all of the key stakeholders within a few weeks.

- Tie policy and environmental changes to programmatic and outreach activities in the plan. In this plan, for example, having buses drop students off at a staging post

on the far side of the park and increasing promotion of the walking school bus were combined with more funding for sidewalks around schools, new traffic-calming cross-walk devices, and model design guidelines for Complete Streets around schools.

Following the workshop, a number of stakeholders, including school administrators, the PedNet team, and city staff in planning, public works, and parks and recreation, followed up on implementing many of the recommendations. The premise of the plan was to use a phased approach to shift vehicle traffic away from the front of the school to ease dangerous and uninviting traffic conditions, improve walking and bicycling infrastructure, and renew efforts to promote those travel modes over time. The plan recommended priority actions for each component of the 5E model.

Evaluation and Planning

Begin measuring and reporting travel mode split at the school twice per year, through a show-of-hands survey. Continue to reach out to parents and learn why some choose not to let their children walk and bike, and identify what would make them more comfortable. Most important, share the findings of this evaluation with parents, administrators, and the school board so that they can more effectively implement policies supporting walking and cycling.

Enforcement

Begin by inviting adults who drive students to voluntarily drop off at the far side of the park, and have two school buses (of the four that serve the school) drop off alternately at the park each day (two buses one day, the other two the next). Over time, evolve from voluntary use of the remote drop-off to restriction of automobile drop-off in front of the school (e.g., limit it to children with physical needs or those carrying heavy or cumbersome items). One policy approach to shifting pick-up to the remote location is to institute a five-minute safety delay on cars picking up at the school, holding cars until all pedestrians, bicyclists, and buses have cleared the school zone. This dramatically reduces potential vehicle-pedestrian conflicts, and it creates an incentive for kids to urge their parents to use the remote pick-up location, because most students would prefer to be dismissed with the pedestrians rather than wait for the automobile pick-up line.

Engineering

Pursue funding to construct a trail through the park from the drop-off area to the school, to improve pathway connections to the surrounding neighborhood, to paint bicycle lanes, to repaint crosswalks and increase their visibility, and to study other possible traffic calming measures.

Education

Offer SRTS education initiatives designed to reach teachers, students, and parents. Provide teachers with information on the link between student physical activity and academic performance and with curricular materials on the health and environmental benefits of walking and cycling. Provide students with increased bicycle and pedestrian safety instruction (e.g., in physical education classes and during assemblies). Reach out to parents directly, and teach students the arrival and dismissal procedures.

Encouragement

As traffic adjacent to the school eases, promote walking school buses with renewed vigor. Use frequent walker cards, which are punched or marked every day a child walks to school. Once filled, a card can be turned in for a small prize (a pencil or zipper pull) and entered into a drawing for a large prize (e.g., a donated bike, iPod) at the end of the year.

A comprehensive approach to encouraging walking and cycling is ongoing. Successes include construction of the direct walking path through the park and creation of an enhanced crosswalk approaching the park. These environmental changes provide a lasting benefit to the community, beyond the Safe Routes to School program.

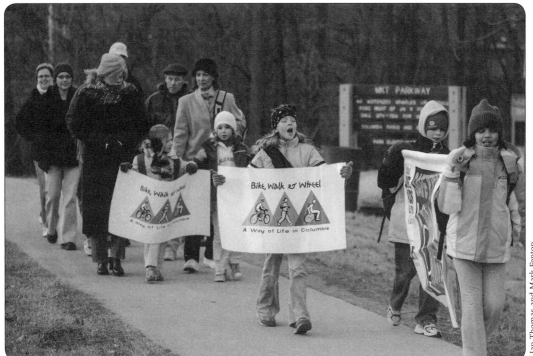

A large walking school bus in Columbia avoids the traffic congestion surrounding the school.

© Ian Thomas and Mark Fenton.

Linkage to the National Physical Activity Plan

The Safe Routes to School approach is mentioned explicitly in four of the strategies identified in the National Physical Activity Plan's Transportation, Land Use, and Community Design Sector. The work in Columbia aligns with all of those recommendations:

Strategy 1: Increase accountability of project planning and selection to ensure infrastructure supporting active transportation and other forms of physical activity. Tactic: Support annual reporting by all schools of their transportation mode split. The SRTS design charrette recommended creating physical infrastructure to support walking and cycling, including a new trail through the park adjacent to the school and creation of a bus pull-out area on the quiet street along the park, farthest from the school, for minimum traffic impact. Other recommendations included routinely measuring and reporting travel mode split at the school as well as painting bicycle lanes and constructing missing sidewalks, crosswalk markings, and neighborhood links to the trail in the park.

Strategy 2: Prioritize resources and provide incentives to increase active transportation and other physical activity through community design, infrastructure projects, systems, policies, and initiatives. Tactic: Support and increase incentives for the adoption and expansion of "safe routes" initiatives such as Safe Routes to School, Bike to Work, and other active transportation programs. This campaign moved well beyond a one-day event by creating procedural changes that provide much greater incentive for routine walking to school for all students. For example, on days the remote drop-off area is used, students arriving by bus have no choice but to get a 10- to 15-minute walk through the park to school.

*Strategy 3: Integrate land-use, transportation, community design, and economic development planning with public health planning to increase active transportation and other physical activity. Tactic: Support the development of standards and identification of "best practices" for the dissemination and adoption of "safe routes" initia-*tives such as *Safe Routes to School, Bike-to-Work, and other active transportation programs.* The design charrette and interventions at West Boulevard Elementary have been used as a model at other elementary schools in Columbia; customized SRTS plans and initiatives have been developed for each of these schools.

Strategy 4: Increase connectivity and accessibility to essential community destinations to increase active transportation and other physical activity. Tactic: Expand Safe Routes initiatives at national, state, county. and local levels to enable safe walking and biking routes to a variety of destinations, especially to schools. This project helped connect residents not only with the neighborhood elementary school but also with the adjoining park. The increased activity in the park and the development of the walking trail made the park more inviting and accessible to many nearby residents.

Evidence Base Used During Program Development

An increasing number of publications and position statements recommend the use of Safe Routes to School to increase physical activity among youth. Comprehensive programs provide other benefits as well, such as reducing traffic congestion and improving air quality at schools, improving behavior and academic performance among students, and potentially lowering transportation costs when fewer students require bus service. The reference list at the end of this chapter includes review papers (Active Living Research 2007; Centers for Disease Control and Prevention 2010; Davison and Lawson 2006; Fenton 2012), position statements (Environmental Protection Agency 2003, 2012; Institute of Medicine 2009), and original research (Centers for Disease Control and Prevention 2005; Heelan et al. 2009; Staunton et al. 2003) that detail the case for SRTS initiatives.

Although the review papers make clear that the built and policy environments have a substantial impact on children's levels of physical activity, the Institute of Medicine and Environmental Protection Agency make the case that conscious policy decisions must be made in support of routine walking and bicycling to school, including choices about where schools are located and the construction of the surrounding infrastructure for walking and bicycling. Summaries by the Centers for Disease Control and Prevention and Active Living Research confirm that more active and physically fit children perform better academically and see fewer disciplinary problems.

Some studies suggest that SRTS efforts can have a significant impact on a school's travel mode split. Heelan and colleagues (2009) showed that over a two-year period, schools with a walking school bus program had 27 percent more frequent walking to school by students compared with a control school, and that frequent walkers engaged in 25 percent more physical activity on average while gaining 58 percent less body fat. Staunton and colleagues (2003) conducted research on the decade-long Marin County comprehensive SRTS program that showed a 64 percent increase in walking, a 114 percent increase in bicycling, a 91 percent increase in carpooling, and a striking 39 percent reduction in the number of vehicles driving one child to school.

Populations Best Served by the Program

A unique aspect of this SRTS effort was that it benefited children beyond those who lived within walking and bicycling distance of the school. The addition of the remote drop-off area means that even children who ride the bus or are driven to school have an opportunity for physical activity via their walk to the school through the park. In general, the reach of the SRTS efforts in Columbia varied by grade level:

- Walk to School Day events and walking school bus program: grades K through 5
- Bicycle skills courses and the bike brigade (a dedicated group that rides bikes to school every day for an entire year, right through winter!): grades 6 through 8
- Education on public policy advocacy, encouraging students to become active advocates for more and safer pedestrian

and bicycle accommodation: grades 9 through 12

Lessons Learned

A number of key lessons were learned from the work on this Safe Routes to School Program. The first two lessons are the most important. Creating a truly interdisciplinary team and focusing on policy and infrastructure changes are absolutely necessary conditions for long-term success in shifting more students to routine walking and cycling.

- Create a fully diverse partnership for a healthy community and welcome everyone. Not just the obvious partners—school officials, parent organizations, public health officials, and planning and public works staff—but also other stakeholders such as law enforcement agencies, parks and recreation staff, neighborhood groups, local business owners, historical society members, and others.

- Focus on policy and infrastructure change. Encouragement programs can get the ball rolling, but the ultimate goals must be to create physical infrastructure (e.g., sidewalks, trails, bike parking), set policies (e.g., defining districts and walking zones), and establish practices that promote walking and cycling as the default travel choice for as many students as possible.

- Commit significant effort to media and community outreach and focus on positive outcomes. Show everyone how SRTS benefits them: healthier, better-performing students; less traffic congestion in neighborhoods near schools; less money spent on student busing.

- Identify heroes. Let everyone know about the great leadership or commitment of the principal, superintendent of schools, director of the public works department, mayor, or wealthy philanthropist. This helps spread the credit for success, lets key players know they are appreciated for their efforts, and rewards their courage.

- Make children into advocates. Equipping students to conduct community surveys, take photos, provide feedback in focus groups, and even provide testimony before key decision makers (board of education, city council, planning commission) can be a powerful tool in helping adults to truly understand the stakes and take meaningful action.

• Identify confident kids who are comfortable being a bit "different," and help them become role models. Kids who are willing to begin bicycling, walking, or skateboarding to school before it's the norm can be the critical "early adopters" who demonstrate to others that it's more fun, they are more independent, and it's cooler than riding in the car.

Tips for Working Across Sectors

A successful SRTS program will not be completed by one sector or group in a community. It is important to maintain a politically balanced team throughout the effort. In Columbia, some of the early adopters were more politically liberal, but with careful framing, attractions for conservative partners were identified, including the local community focus, provision of greater transportation choices, and the fiscal benefits of the program.

It requires a conscious effort to bring a variety of organizations and agencies together to work toward a common goal, including continual education on the benefits of SRTS and identification of the common goals they share. Engaging other entities in the community provides easy, almost turnkey ways for them to support SRTS.

• The school district can include walking school bus leaders and other volunteers in its routine background check process.

• A college or university nutrition, health promotion, sports, recreation, or exercise science program can give students academic credit for serving as volunteer walk group leaders.

• A local bike shop can send a mechanic to bike classes to fix problems, teach skills, and generate relationships with next-generation cyclists.

• A local Rotary Club or other service organization can lead a coat, hat, mitten, and boot drive to ensure that all children

are equipped with adequate clothing for walking or bicycling through the winter. (Lack of proper clothing can keep parents in lower-income households from allowing their children to walk in the colder weather.)

• Local businesses can sponsor frequent walker prizes, as simple as notebooks and pencils, colored shoelaces, and zipper pulls for backpacks.

Additional Readings and Resources

The following describes two invaluable, practical resources. Both provide an archive of webinars on relevant topics, ranging from launching your program to dealing with liability and safety concerns.

National Center for Safe Routes to School: www.saferoutesinfo.org

This center has a lot of useful information on organizing a Safe Routes to School program and specific materials such as sample press releases and program announcements, parent and student survey materials and tally sheets (for doing show-of-hands surveys in the classroom and observation counts outside the school), and curricular materials. It also maintains a national registry of participating schools, so you can find a school doing this work in your region or state.

National Safe Routes to School Partnership: www.saferoutespartnership.org

This national coalition supports SRTS programs at the state and local level, providing regional coordinators and technical assistance to community efforts across the United States as well as national advocacy for continued federal funding and program support. Your state or region likely has an SRTS partnership that can provide technical assistance as you launch your program.

References

Active Living Research. 2007. Physical education, physical activity, and academic performance. www.activelivingresearch.org/files/Active_Ed.pdf.

Centers for Disease Control and Prevention. 2005. Barriers to children walking to or from school—United States, 2004. *MMWR. Morbid. Mortal. Wkly. Rep.* 54:949-52.

Centers for Disease Control and Prevention. 2010. The association between school-based physical activity, including physical education, and academic performance. www.cdc.gov/healthyyouth/health_and_academics/.

Davison, K.K., and C.T. Lawson. 2006. Do attributes in the physical environment influence children's physical activity? A review of the literature. *Int. J. Behav. Nutr. Phys. Act.* 3:19.

Environmental Protection Agency. 2012. School siting guidelines. www.epa.gov/schools/siting.

Environmental Protection Agency. 2003. Travel and environmental implications of school siting. EPA report 231-R-03-004. www.epa.gov/smartgrowth/school_travel.htm.

Fenton, M. 2012. Community design and policies for free-range children: Creating environments that support routine physical activity. *Child. Obes.* 8(1):44-55.

Ham, S.A., S. Martin, and H.W. Kohl, III. 2008. Changes in the percentage of students who walk or bike to school—United States, 1969 and 2001. *J. Phys. Act. Health* 5:205-15.

Heelan, K.A., B.M. Abbey, et al. 2009. Evaluation of a walking school bus for promoting physical activity in youth. *J. Phys. Act. Health* 6(5):560-7.

Institute of Medicine. 2009. Local government actions to prevent childhood obesity. www.iom.edu/Reports/2009/Local-Government-Actions-to-Prevent-Childhood-Obesity.aspx.

Staunton, C.E., D. Hubsmith, and W. Kallins. 2003. Promoting safe walking and biking to school: the Marin County success story. *Am. J. Public Health* 93(9):1431-4.

CHAPTER 36

Local Public Health Leadership for Active Community Design

An Approach for Year-Round Physical Activity in Houghton, Michigan

Ray Sharp, BA

Western Upper Peninsula Health Department

NPAP Tactics and Strategies Used in This Program

Transportation, Land Use, and Community Design Sector

STRATEGY 1: Increase accountability of project planning and selection to ensure infrastructure supporting active transportation and other forms of physical activity.

STRATEGY 3: Integrate land-use, transportation, community design and economic development planning with public health planning to increase active transportation and other physical activity.

STRATEGY 4: Increase connectivity and accessibility to essential community destinations to increase active transportation and other physical activity.

Almost everyone who influences public policy decisions represents a particular interest group—taxpayers, property owners, developers, preservationists, environmentalists, walkers, cyclists, ATV riders, parents, retirees, business owners, and public sector workers. Public health professionals, in contrast, work for and on behalf of all residents. The only agenda of health department staff is to help people live longer, healthier lives by advocating for decisions and policies that improve everyone's health and quality of life. When public health professionals make recommendations to city councils, planning commissions, and city staff based on best practice and scientific evidence, it helps policy makers make tough decisions and do the right thing for their communities. And when it comes to preventing heart disease, stroke, diabetes, and other chronic diseases, the right thing is to work for local policy and environmental changes that support an active lifestyle.

Although many important public health policies are decided by state and federal lawmakers and agencies, the creation of a community that encourages physical activity depends heavily on local professionals and policy makers who are not in the health department. In many cases the best approach is to work with a city, township, neighborhood, or school district, where many policies that directly affect people's daily lives are crafted. Often a local public health professional can be a "big fish in a small pond," someone others in the pond know and respect. To illustrate how such an approach can work, this chapter discusses how health department staff, key city staff in nonhealth disciplines, and elected and appointed officials can lead the way for positive change at the local level.

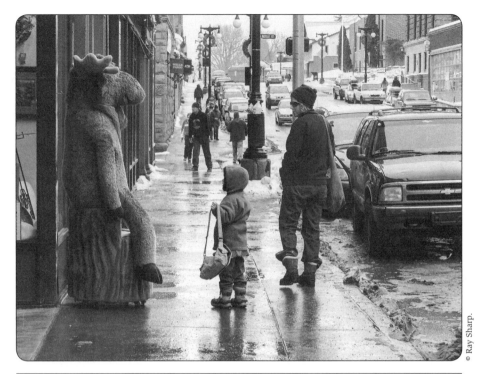

© Ray Sharp.

Houghton's historic downtown district is pedestrian friendly, with a mix of small shops, restaurants, offices, and upstairs apartments that attract residents and visitors of all ages.

Programmatic Approach— Focus on Local Policy

Admittedly it seems like an unlikely proposition—to create a pedestrian- and bike-friendly community in the rugged and remote Western Upper Peninsula region of Michigan. Houghton, a small city of 8,000 residents located near Lake Superior, 200 miles (322 kilometers) north of Green Bay, Wisconsin, faces many challenges to active community design, including long winters that deliver an average of 250 inches (6 meters) of snow, extremely hilly terrain, and a stagnant economy.

The Western Upper Peninsula Health Department (WUPHD) is the local public health agency, serving the 70,000 residents of five rural counties bounded by Wisconsin on the south and Lake Superior on the north. The health department provides public health services aimed at preventing disease in the general population. With obesity on track to become the leading preventable cause of chronic disease and premature death, the public health com-

munity, including WUPHD staff, is committed to providing leadership in policy, systems, and environmental strategies to increase physical activity. Houghton's efforts of the last few years exemplify these efforts and are closely linked to strategies from the National Physical Activity Plan. But this effort did not begin in a vacuum, and at its heart it was focused on making every city professional and even elected officials understand and consider the health impacts of their routine decisions.

Healthy Community Planning: Help Build a Vision

Houghton's commitment to active community design has evolved over 40 years, since the closing of the copper mines in 1968 left the region searching for new focus and vitality. The consequences of land use decisions made in the 1970s and 1980s to maintain public access to Houghton's waterfront, a long-time emphasis on nonmotorized trail development to attract and retain a young and active work force, and coordinated policy and environment initiatives

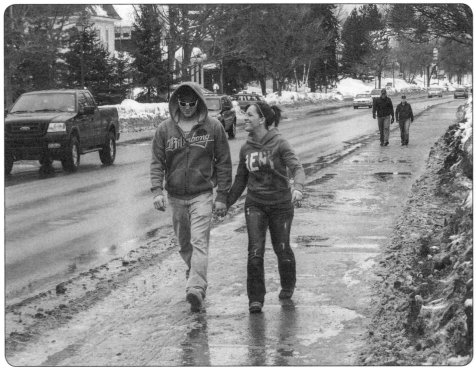

© Ray Sharp.

Houghton receives 200 to 300 inches (5-7 meters) of snow per year. Snow removal on principal pedestrian routes, like this wide sidewalk connecting Michigan Tech University to the downtown area, is done by the city workers with small trucks and mini-plows.

established since 2002 have helped Houghton burnish its reputation as one of the most livable small towns in the Upper Midwest. Houghton has avoided the fate of many declining Rust Belt towns by envisioning a healthy and vibrant future that includes year-round access to physical activity and working to make it a reality.

Houghton City Manager Scott MacInnes has worked for the City of Houghton since graduating from Michigan Tech University with a degree in engineering in the mid-1970s, so he has seen first-hand the process of gradually reinventing the city. When MacInnes was a student at Michigan Tech, students were warned to stay away from the city's waterfront along Portage Lake (a navigable waterway connected to Lake Superior) because the submerged piers and dilapidated warehouses, remnants of the copper mining boom, were hazardous. As happened in many American cities that began along the water but turned their backs on the shoreline as they grew outward, with rings of suburbs designed around the automobile and

made possible by cheap and plentiful gasoline, Houghton's waterfront became a neglected shambles. The adjacent downtown business district declined as well, with shopping malls and big box stores springing up at the city's periphery, where real estate was more affordable. As locally owned businesses lost customers to national chains and residents gradually stopped walking their main street, many cities, especially in the northern Midwest, lost their identity and reason to exist.

The Houghton city council and its planning commission, however, envisioned a different future. They sent delegations to visit other lakeshore cities, such as Traverse City, Michigan, to learn from their successes (and regrets). After several of these fact-finding missions, the council and planners reached a decision—to preserve the shoreline for public access instead of selling out to private development—so that all citizens would benefit. In the ensuing decades, the city gradually acquired most of the shoreline property in the two-mile (3.2-kilometer) stretch from west of the business district, past the downtown area, all the way to the Michigan Tech campus on the east. The industrial ruins were removed and replaced with parks, marinas, a new public library, and a paved bicycle and pedestrian trail that is used by hundreds of walkers, bikers, skaters, and stroller-pushers daily. In a survey of residents conducted by the city as part of its master planning process, the waterfront trail ranked as the most-used city facility, with an average of 36 days of use per respondent. Some residents use it almost daily for commuting, recreation, or exercise.

When asked whether city leaders knew the trail would become some so popular, MacInnes said the original intent was to cover just a short section of decommissioned railroad tracks with asphalt for safety and aesthetic reasons. However, so many residents started using the path that there was an outcry for the city to finish the job, and it eventually paved the railroad grade, little by little, all the way to the town line on both ends, a distance of five miles (8 kilometers). Houghton's experience was not unusual

in this regard. Studies show that when a new sidewalk or bike path is constructed—even in the absence of any health promotion campaign—significantly more residents will report getting 30 minutes of exercise per day, a true case of "build it and they will come."

Public Health Can Support Economic Health

In the 1990s, MacInnes and local architect Pat Coleman, founder of the international Winter Cities Institute, engaged city planners in designing streetscapes that better served residents year-round, even in long, harsh, and very snowy winters. In 1997, Houghton hosted the Winter Cities Institute annual conference, attended by urban planners from as far away as Russia, Scandinavia, and Japan, who came to talk about how cities and residents can endure, and thrive, in far-northern climates. Practical measures implemented by Houghton include smaller, more cost-effective vehicles for clearing snow from pedestrian routes; textured paving

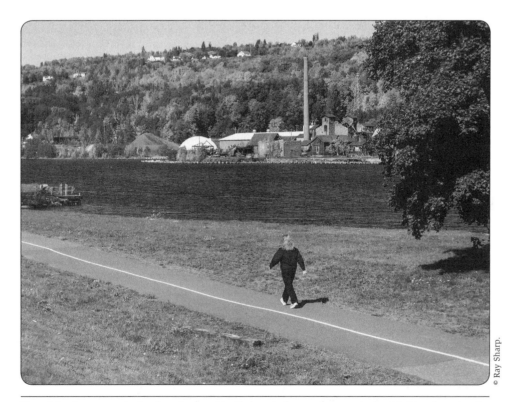

© Ray Sharp.

Houghton's nonmotorized waterfront trail, located on a former industrial land and rail corridor, extends nearly five miles (8 kilometers), connecting the city center to parks and residential districts.

to provide pedestrian safety in slippery conditions; and covered stairs and walkways in public areas, such as connecting routes from parking structures to shopping areas. Awnings over doorways of stores and restaurants are another simple feature that makes a destination more inviting to pedestrians and helps keep sidewalks clear of snow. Details like these often go unnoticed when they work well, but they go a long way toward making walking more convenient and comfortable in winter.

Another factor that makes winter cities more livable is the presence of facilities such as public ice rinks and ski and snowshoe trails where residents can remain physically active in winter. Houghton has many indoor and outdoor skating venues, from small neighborhood parks to large arenas, owing to its legacy as "the birthplace of professional hockey." Cross-country skiing is increasingly popular and offers the advantage that it can be enjoyed at any age, alone or with friends. The university developed a world-class ski and snowshoe trail system over the

last 10 years, which has hosted regional and national championship events but is also used by hundreds of residents who will never ski a competitive race in their lives. The system features more than 20 miles (32 kilometers) of groomed Nordic ski trails; approximately 5 miles (8 kilometers) of trails are lit for night skiing. The same terrain is used for mountain biking in summer. Houghton now has more miles of off-road trails than paved streets, providing ample recreational opportunity and attracting people seeking a fun and healthy place to live.

As residents become more physically active, they naturally turn to their local government officials with ideas for further improving active transportation infrastructure. At the urging of the West Houghton Neighborhood Association in 2002, Houghton's planning commission developed a walkability plan. The city inventoried sidewalks and assessed traffic accidents involving pedestrians and then took public comments at neighborhood forums. Planning staff developed a plan for pedestrian facilities,

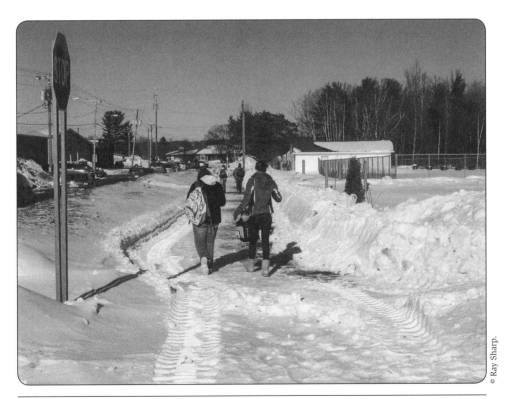

© Ray Sharp.

The city plows the sidewalks when it snows. Snow removal is a constant battle from Halloween to Easter.

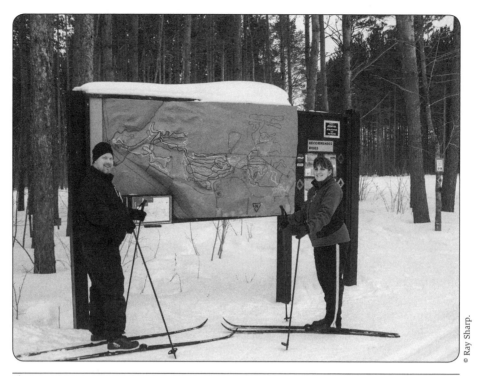

© Ray Sharp.

Houghton has more miles of bicycle, walking, ski, and snowshoe trails than city streets.

including a pedestrian tunnel under a principal roadway so residents could reach waterfront parks and trails. That project was funded by the state highway department and has alleviated a dangerous crossing of a five-lane highway.

In 2007, bike commuters contacted the city to express interest in creating a bicycle plan. That fall, the Houghton Bike Task Force was formed as an ad hoc group to study the issue and report to the city council. The task force created a short online survey to ask residents about their summer and winter bike commuting routes. An astounding 384 people completed the survey, more than 5 percent of the city's population. The group created maps showing summer and winter use patterns and compiled and evaluated comments about safety concerns. A city bike plan, with routes and projects identified, was submitted to the city council and approved.

Program Evaluation

Despite the economic, topographic, and weather challenges, Houghton has developed bike and pedestrian plans, expanded its network of bike lanes and side paths, conducted Safe Routes to School assessment and planning, was named a Bicycle Friendly Community by the League of American Bicyclists, passed an innovative bike-parking ordinance, and enacted a Complete Streets ordinance that requires accommodating the needs of pedestrians, cyclists, and transit users of all ages and abilities in roadway design. Today in Houghton, residents and visitors will find new bike lanes, connector trails, bike racks, and midblock pedestrian crossings; more miles of off-road recreation trails than paved city streets; and a local public health department that is a partner in all these initiatives, contributing staff time, training, grant funding, and a rationale for building a healthier community. The effort that led to these changes did not focus solely on a specific infrastructure improvement. Rather, the goal has been to incorporate consideration of health outcomes in all city infrastructure and policy actions.

The power of the change in processes outlined here is well illustrated by this case study of Safe Routes to School planning and implementation. Staff from the Western Upper Peninsula Health Department in Michigan attended a small meeting with the Houghton-Portage

Township School Wellness Team, in the city of Houghton. The meeting was a group planning session, called a *charrette* in the parlance of urban design. The school wellness team brought together members of the school's Safe Routes to School team and the City of Houghton's bike and pedestrian committee to hash out routes and identify priorities for construction projects to make school travel safer for walkers and bikers. Both the Safe Routes to School planning initiative and Houghton's commitment to Complete Streets (Houghton passed a Complete Streets ordinance in 2010, described later in the chapter) came about with a push from the Western Upper Peninsula Health Department. Health department staff had convened planning groups at the city and school district, provided training and technical assistance, and helped the city win small grants from state and federal sources to improve infrastructure with new bike racks and signage and striping for bike lanes.

Also attending the charrette were the Houghton city manager, the police chief, the director of public works, the school superintendent and middle school principal, a school board member, and teachers, parents, students, and community members with an interest in student health and safety. The students and their parents were the most important stakeholders in the process. The students described where they normally walk and bike to and from school, and the parents shared their concerns about dangerous roads and intersections. The city manager showed a map of the city streets and presented optional routes leading from the school to three nearby neighborhoods. By the end of the meeting, the participants had agreed on four streets that should be designated as principal routes to school, and which needed sidewalks, and three intersections that needed better crosswalks plus center islands to act as traffic-calming devices and give students a midstreet refuge while crossing.

These recommendations were reported to the rest of the city's bicycle and pedestrian committee, discussed at neighborhood forums, and incorporated into the nonmotorized transportation plan that was to be adopted as part of the city's new master plan. The city manager pledged to start the search for sidewalk funding and believed he could complete the three enhanced intersections in the near future.

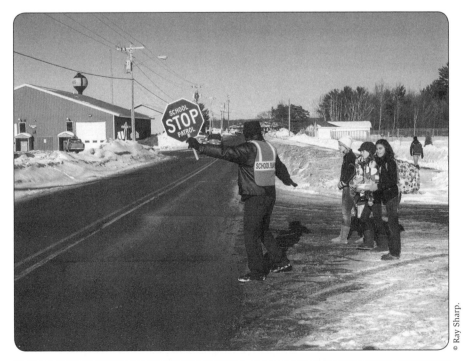

© Ray Sharp.

The Houghton-Portage Township School District is a partner with city and public health officials in Safe Routes to School planning.

Although that one meeting resulted in a number of positive changes, the meeting was in large part the culmination of months of work by the health department. This work helped community committees form, grow, build trust, and work together toward the common goal of a healthier community where all residents have access to safer routes for active transportation.

Linkage to National Physical Activity Plan

The Western Upper Peninsula Health Department is working to embrace all of the principles of the Transportation, Land Use, and Community Design Sector of the National Physical Activity Plan. However, it has found particular traction in working on the following three strategies from that sector, given the engagement of allies in planning, economic development, public safety, and engineering.

Strategy 1: Increase accountability of project planning and selection to ensure infrastructure supporting active transportation and other forms of physical activity. The health department is taking a leading role in encouraging the integration of physical activity infrastructure into community design, land use planning, and transportation network development, especially through work on Complete Streets and efforts to extend the community's trail network.

Strategy 3: Integrate land-use, transportation, community design and economic development planning with public health planning to increase active transportation and other physical activity. As part of its mission to reduce the prevalence of chronic diseases such as heart disease, cancer, and diabetes and to improve well-being and quality of life, WUPHD works with local government officials, transportation agencies, planning commissions, police departments, schools, bike and pedestrian advocates, neighborhood associations, environmental groups, state and federal health and transportation agencies, private foundations, and faculty and students from Michigan Tech University to make it safer and more convenient for people to walk and bike as part of their daily lives. With leadership from

the health department, Houghton is taking steps toward a faraway but attainable goal—reversing the epidemic of childhood and adult obesity and inadequate physical activity.

Strategy 4: Increase connectivity and accessibility to essential community destinations to increase active transportation and other physical activity. The health department and its partners have established short-term objectives, including increasing the number of children and adults walking or biking to school, work, and errands; reducing traffic congestion and automobile emissions; and improving pedestrian and cyclist safety. Anticipated long-term community benefits include healthier residents, a healthier environment, sustainable economic development, and improved quality of life. Houghton's Complete Streets law and other policies will guide transportation and land use planning, resource allocation, engineering design, and the creation of a network of active transportation routes connecting neighborhoods, schools, parks, work sites, shopping, and other destinations.

Tips for Working Across Sectors

Houghton's story has been driven by many players, not just public health professionals; visionary leaders who have targeted economic redevelopment have been central to the city's success. In fact, public health professionals traditionally had not played a role in city planning. But faced with compelling and incontrovertible evidence that our vehicle-centric cities and suburbs are slowly killing Americans through inactivity-related chronic disease, many public health professionals are beginning to see the connections between clean sidewalks and clean arteries, healthy networks of bicycle pathways, and healthy children.

In 2010, WUPHD pursued and was awarded grants from several public and private sources to work with community partners to reduce chronic disease through local policy initiatives. The health department was given a seat on the community's Bicycle Task Force, which was exploring trends in active living design and studying what the nation's leading bike-friendly communities, such as Portland, Oregon; Boulder, Colorado; and Madison, Wisconsin, have done to make their communities safer and more convenient for cycling. One of the first policy successes was a bike-parking ordinance, adapted from an innovative policy from Madison and presented to the planning commission. The ordinance, passed by the city council after a public hearing in April 2010 and amended to the parking section of the city zoning code, calls for the provision of adequate parking facilities for bikes, with specifications based on the size of business or apartment building.

The next order of business was to assess the city's status with regard to cycling infrastructure and programs. A bike-friendly community survey developed by the League of American Bicyclists was used to perform a gap analysis. The instrument is a detailed 84-section survey that is completed online after gathering information about the community's status in five domains, called the 5 Es—evaluation and planning, engineering, education, encouragement, and enforcement. The Bicycle Task Force gath-

ered data about miles of bike lanes and trails, classes, community events, and police programs and then asked city leaders to pass a Bicycle Friendly City Resolution, allowing submission of an application in July 2010. In September 2010, Houghton was designated a bronze-level Bicycle Friendly Community.

Part of the local health department's grant funding came from the state health department's cardiovascular disease section and was designated to promote collaboration with the city to pass a Complete Streets policy. A Complete Streets training session was organized in September 2010 for 30 local government officials and citizen advocates, with help from state health and transportation experts. In October and November, the health department worked with the planning commission and Bicycle Task Force on Complete Streets ordinance language. The city manager determined where to insert Complete Streets language into the city's existing codes for street and subdivision design. By December, the city council took up the proposal, and after two meetings and public hearings to review the costs and benefits of the law, Houghton adopted it on December 22,

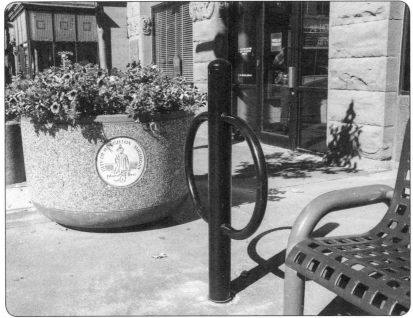

Downtown Houghton sidewalk furnishings include benches, bike racks and planters.

2010, becoming the sixth Michigan city, and the first in the Upper Peninsula region, to enact a Complete Streets ordinance.

Lessons Learned

Health educators often hesitate to wade into the unfamiliar waters of public policy. Two elements of the Houghton effort, along with seven tips for success, suggest a way forward, even for health departments that have never participated in healthy community design.

Jump Into Current Efforts, and Build on Existing Momentum

Admittedly, in Houghton the public health department was lucky to join the Complete Streets effort well into what was truly a 30-year process. Houghton's vision of public access along the waterfront, creation of a waterfront trail, attention to the details of winter cities design, and citizen involvement in bike and pedestrian planning all contributed to readiness to pass a Complete Streets ordinance. But Houghton certainly was not unique in this regard. Many school districts around the nation participate in Safe Routes to Schools planning, using the same 5 Es approach as the Bicycle Friendly Communities program. Most cities update their master plans every five years and hold forums to get citizen input on streets, sidewalks, and parks. Existing groups such as cycling clubs, parent-teacher organizations, and neighborhood committees are natural allies in active communities planning. Cities, townships, and counties have planning commissions that routinely consider changes to building codes, zoning, and land use plans. And increasingly, in Michigan and many other states, highway funding allocations favor projects that include enhancements for pedestrians, cyclists, and transit users. State and local highway departments are in the midst of a generational change, defined not by age but by interest in new Complete Streets approaches to transportation planning. When public health professionals attend a meeting to talk about active communities

planning, they may be pleasantly surprised to find that policy makers are ready to listen to information on the health benefits of sidewalks and bike lanes.

Speak the Language That Key Stakeholders Hold Dear

Don't restrict the discussion to arguments about health and safety. It is rare to meet an elected official who doesn't favor the concept of a healthier community for all residents, especially when health includes social, environmental, and economic health. But the inevitable first question will be "How much is this going to cost us?" Health professionals should be prepared to pivot from health and safety to discussions of tourism, economic development, job creation and employee retention, and increased property values, all benefits of bicycle- and pedestrian-friendly community designs. When speaking before a city council or town hall meeting, health professionals should provide one-page color handouts on the health and economic benefits of Complete Streets, bike lanes, and non-motorized trails, with enough copies for policy makers, members of the media, and the public. Health advocates should provide arguments, in clear and succinct language, in a form that others can share with friends and coworkers. (Many of the resources at the end of this chapter provide such facts and talking points.) When city council members, police officers, school principals, business owners, and friends and neighbors are all talking about the benefits of active community design, it will be clear that the public health department has played a leadership role in shaping the conversation about a healthier future.

Use Seven Tips for Success

Some of these final lessons may seem obvious, but can ease the transition of public health into a leading role in creating a healthy community.

1. Public health is not a narrow interest group. It represents everyone who is concerned with health, safety, and quality of life.

2. All policy is local. Work with schools, neighborhood groups, park districts, cities, and townships in your jurisdiction; wherever you can be a big fish in a small pond.

3. Begin with a vision based on the public's sense of what its community should become, a vision that is large enough to inspire yet is practical and achievable.

4. Build it and they will come. New parks, trails, sidewalks, and bike routes will be used if they are well designed and lead to places people want to go.

5. Discuss community health in the broadest terms—physical, social and emotional, economic, and environmental—to broaden support for healthy communities policies and projects.

6. Measure the effectiveness of your work (through evaluation) and celebrate successes to strengthen the coalition and public support.

7. Policy and built-environment changes are stickier than health promotion programs. Exercise classes come and go with the seasons, but a multi-use trail lasts a lifetime.

Additional Reading and Resources

Maintained at the University of California at San Diego, this is an outstanding resource library and bibliography of the latest research and practical information on factors leading to active community environments; it is an ideal first stop if you're looking for the best evidence supporting policy efforts: www.activelivingresearch.org

The National Complete Streets Coalition has a wealth of information on Complete Streets, including fact sheets, model ordinances, news, and advocacy: www.completestreets.org

This describes the League of American Bicyclists' Bicycle Friendly Communities program, with criteria, applications, and lists of honorees: www.bikeleague.org/programs/bicyclefriendlyamerica

The Rails-to-Trails Conservancy is a national body in the United States; many states have chapters or similar organizations: www.railstotrails.org

The Michigan Trails & Greenways Alliance is a state-level nonprofit agency dedicated to rails-to-trails projects: www.michigantrails.org

The Michigan Complete Streets Coalition is one of an increasing number of statewide coalitions; this website includes local and state news, such as reports on the Michigan Complete Streets Advisory Council, and a compendium of local ordinances, resolutions, and policies: www.micompletestreets.org

This Michigan-based website is one of the best sources for plans, policies, fact sheets, and links to other helpful resources: www.mihealthtools.org/mihc/CompleteStreetsResources.asp

The Houghton city website has bike and pedestrian plans and ordinances, as well as information on trails, parks, community gardens, and other healthy communities facilities and plans: www.cityofhoughton.com

Beyond the Blue Building: Partnerships for a Healthier Western Upper Peninsula Region is the Western Upper Peninsula Health Department's blog about initiatives and partnerships promoting healthy living: http://healthywup.wordpress.com.

This site provides information on how the Western Upper Peninsula Health Department and its community partners are working to prevent childhood obesity through multiple strategies with support from the Robert Wood Johnson Foundation's Healthy Kids, Healthy Communities grant program: www.healthykidshealthycommunities.org/communities/houghton-county-mi

The National Center for Safe Routes to School is loaded with information on creating 5E plans for schools and answers to common questions: www.saferoutesinfo.org

The Winter Cities Institute links northern cities worldwide in the pursuit of sustainable designs for active living: www.wintercities.com

CHAPTER 37

A Road Diet for Increased Physical Activity
Redesigning for Safer Walking, Bicycling, and Transit Use

Jennifer J. Selby, PE
Foth Infrastructure and Environment

NPAP Tactics and Strategies Used in This Program

Transportation, Land Use, and Community Design Sector

STRATEGY 1: Increase accountability of project planning and selection to ensure infrastructure supporting active transportation and other forms of physical activity.

STRATEGY 2: Prioritize resources and provide incentives to increase active transportation and other physical activity through community design, infrastructure projects, systems, policies, and initiatives.

STRATEGY 4: Increase connectivity and accessibility to essential community destinations to increase active transportation and other physical activity.

In 2005, the new mayor and city council of Urbana, Illinois, set a goal to "get Urbana bicycling." As the first step in reaching that goal, they created a Bicycle and Pedestrian Advisory Commission. The commission's first major task was to oversee the development of a citywide bicycle master plan.

The Urbana Bicycle Master Plan, approved in April 2008, set forth three goals for the city:

1. Increase the percentage of persons using bicycles for transportation in Urbana by 50 percent in the next five years.

2. Achieve a Bicycle Friendly Community award through the League of American Bicyclists.

3. Substantially expand the bicycle network.

The end product of the bicycle master plan was a defined network of recommended bikeways—such as bike lanes, bike routes, and shared-use paths—that, when implemented, would connect all of the neighborhoods in the city. One of the many benefits would be an increase in the number of people able to use bicycling for routine trips and thus get more physical activity as a part of their daily tasks.

One of the first priorities was the conversion of Philo Road, along a stretch from Colorado Avenue to Florida Avenue, from a four-lane cross section to a three-lane cross section with bike lanes. Often referred to as a "road diet," this was the first master plan project that the city implemented. Although the Philo Road project would help the city reach the goals set forth in the bicycle master plan, city leaders also hoped that the road diet would allow the city to improve mobility and access for all roadway users.

Program Description

From the 1960s through the 1980s, Philo Road between Colorado Avenue and Florida Avenue served as a regional retail center. The corridor contained a shopping center with a grocery

329

store and a drug store as anchors as well as a large discount retail store and a second grocery store in the vicinity.

Until the late 1970s, Philo Road was a two-lane road. Because of the many businesses and resulting increased traffic, the city widened part of the road from two lanes to four in the late 1970s. Following additional retail construction in the 1980s, the entire road from Colorado Avenue to Florida Avenue was widened to four lanes.

In 1991, Philo Road lost its designation as Illinois Route 130 to High Cross Road, a north-south corridor to the east. High Cross Road became a major artery serving regional traffic, and Philo Road became a minor artery serving neighborhood traffic. Additional changes to the retail market in Urbana and Champaign in the 1990s led retail traffic to move away from Philo Road. By 2003, two of the three grocery stores and the large discount retail store were gone.

Soon, Philo Road became a blighted commercial area with several large vacant buildings, vast underused parking lots, and many unused parcels. Litter and loitering became problems, and the community, city council, and mayor became concerned about the area. The city

undertook several initiatives during 2003 and 2004 to combat the demise of this area. All of these efforts were commendable, but the area remained blighted. Although residents were patronizing businesses in the area because of loyalty and convenience, the public consensus was that the existing buildings needed to be updated, with better signage and lighting, and that the overall appearance, landscaping, and security of the area needed to be improved.

Linkage to National Physical Activity Plan

Developers believed that the area had the image of an aging, inactive, and open area and that the marketability was fair to poor. They thought that road improvements—such as wider, multilane roads with boulevards—would improve the appearance of and access to the area and could help with revitalization. Fortunately, the city took a more enlightened view and developed a strategic approach that aligns with several strategies in the Transportation, Land Use, and Community Design Sector of the National Physical Activity Plan.

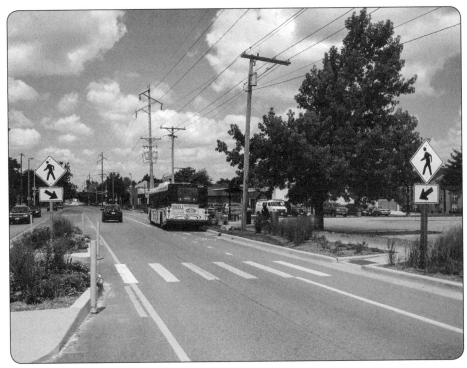

© Jennifer J. Selby.

Photo of Philo Road bus stop.

Strategy 1: Increase accountability of project planning and selection to ensure infrastructure supporting active transportation and other forms of physical activity. City leaders did not believe that widening the road to improve access for vehicles was the solution. In January 2005, city council adopted the Philo Road Business District Revitalization Action Plan. The plan proposed redevelopment policies and programs to be implemented through specific action elements. One of the action elements recommended planning and constructing infrastructure improvements, including rebuilding Philo Road south of Colorado Avenue and reducing the number of lanes to three, improving pedestrian crossings, and extending bike trails. This approach specifically considered not just the motor vehicle functionality but also the bicycle and pedestrian functionality of the roadway. The city council noted that the road's average daily traffic was only about 11,000 vehicles per day. Transportation planners acknowledged that three lanes, properly designed, are quite sufficient for this traffic volume.

Strategy 2: Prioritize resources and provide incentives to increase active transportation and other physical activity through community design, infrastructure projects, systems, policies, and initiatives. In the summer of 2006, the section of Philo Road south of Colorado Avenue was improved to provide better access between southeast Urbana—which had the fastest growing neighborhoods in the city—and the commercial district between Colorado Avenue and Florida Avenue. Following completion of these improvements, the city developed a beautification plan for Philo Road, which included converting the four lanes on Philo Road between Florida Avenue and Colorado Avenue to three lanes, with possible inclusion of bike lanes. These improvements would promote a more pedestrian- and bike-friendly and safer environment.

In presenting the beautification plan, city staff noted that the current budget included no funding for such improvements. Two months later, the city council and mayor revised the annual budget ordinance, reducing the capital improvement fund by $125,000 in order to set aside the funds to construct infrastructure improvements on Philo Road.

Strategy 4: Increase connectivity and accessibility to essential community destinations to increase active transportation and other physical activity. In early 2008, the Urbana Bicycle Master Plan identified Philo Road between Colorado Avenue and Florida Avenue as a priority project for implementation. Members of

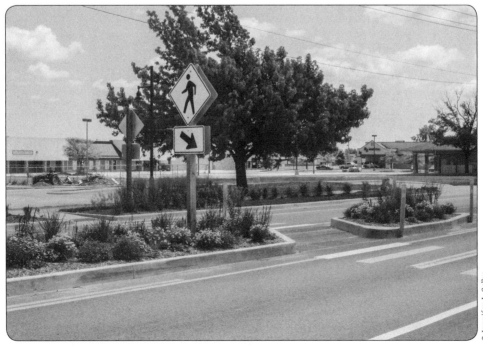

© Jennifer J. Selby.

Photo of Philo Road median.

the public were requesting installation of bike lanes in this segment, primarily because of the destinations it served, both commercial and residential. The commercial corridor contained a large grocery store, a drug store chain, restaurants, banks, and office space surrounded by single-family and multifamily homes, including several senior assisted living facilities. Further, this segment of the road would provide a key link (or connectivity) in the bicycle network by connecting with a shared-use path to the south and planned future bike lanes to the north.

In summer 2008, Philo Road between Colorado Avenue and Florida Avenue was resurfaced and restriped from four lanes of vehicle traffic (two lanes in each direction) to one lane of vehicle traffic in each direction, a continuous two-way left turn lane in the center, and one bike lane in each direction. The bike lanes connected to an existing shared-use path on the east side of Philo Road south of Colorado Avenue and, in the future, would connect to bike lanes planned for north of Florida Avenue (constructed in 2010).

Other types of transportation, particularly bus transportation, also benefitted from the improvements. The city constructed bus stop pads that complied with the Americans with

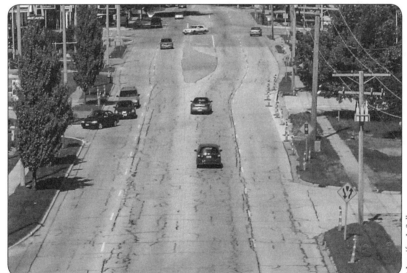

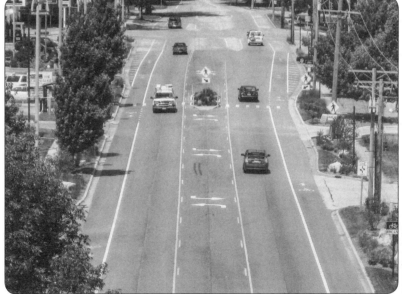

Philo Road before and after the addition of bicycle lanes.

Disabilities Act (ADA) to better accommodate waiting, boarding, and accessibility. The new bus stops included shelters, benches, trash cans, recycling cans, and real-time signs to indicate when the bus would arrive. The new bus stop locations were shifted slightly and offset so that the midblock crosswalks were behind the bus stop. This placement prevented buses from obstructing pedestrians' view of oncoming traffic when they were crossing the street, and it allowed bus drivers to pull away from the stop without danger that pedestrians were attempting to cross in front of them.

The city constructed a raised landscaped median in the two-way left turn lane at the midblock bus stop crossing. The median broke what used to be a complex four-lane crossing into two simpler one-lane crossings. This shorter crossing distance reduced pedestrian exposure time, making the crossing safer, especially important given that many of the transit riders in this corridor are seniors. An added safety element of the raised median involved constructing an angled crossing in the median. Because the crossing is angled, pedestrians who are crossing through the median are facing the traffic that is approaching them.

Separate from the street improvement project, a major landscaping project was undertaken that included planting perennials, ornamental grasses, and trees; regrading and sodding turf areas; installing ornamental boulders; installing ornamental benches and trash cans; and installing pedestrian lighting on the east side of the street. Finally, the city added an art component to the project. Concrete pads were constructed at two locations along the corridor and two sculptures that enhanced the prairie theme of Philo Road were installed.

In October 2008, the city held a press conference and ribbon cutting announcing completion of the first bike lanes implemented from the Urbana Bicycle Master Plan. The ceremony was attended by business owners and residents of the Philo Road area and city staff.

Program Evaluation

The city achieved several of its goals with the project. The changes improved mobility and access for all roadway users. The renovated

road is much safer for pedestrians, because the reduced number of travel lanes and the raised median shorten the crossing distance and reduce exposure time. Reducing the travel lanes from four to two often reduces speeds, because the first car sets the pace. Speed is an important factor for pedestrian safety, because as vehicle speeds decrease, the chance of a pedestrian surviving a crash significantly increases.

The addition of bike lanes improved mobility for bicyclists. The bike lanes dedicate a space for bicycles, making it easier for bicyclists and motorists to share the road. The bike lanes also benefit pedestrians by creating a buffer between pedestrians on the sidewalk and motorists on the street.

The addition of a raised median and marked midblock crosswalk at the bus stops improved mobility and access for transit riders. The continental-style crosswalk markings and crosswalk warning signage brought attention to the fact that pedestrians cross at this location and motorists should be aware.

The changes to Philo Road resulted in significant revitalization of the area, one of the primary goals of the project. During the road work, a new shopping center was completed and a national drug store chain moved onto the street. Subsequently, a new bank, three cell phone stores, a fast food restaurant, and other businesses were constructed or remodeled. The existing shopping center underwent façade improvements, the vacant drug store space was remodeled into a specialty shop, and a new restaurant opened.

As for the goals set forth in the Urbana Bicycle Master Plan, the city was named a Bronze-level Bicycle Friendly Community in May 2010. Approximately four more miles (6.4 kilometers) of bike lanes and two miles (3.2 kilometers) of shared lane markings were installed to expand the bicycle network. The shared lane markings were installed on Philo Road south of Colorado Avenue in 2009 to help bicyclists and motorists share the road, even though an off-street side path is also present in that stretch. The bike lanes north of Florida Avenue to Washington Street were constructed in 2010, completing the Philo Road corridor recommended in the bicycle master plan.

Evidence Base Used During Program Development

An increasing number of design guidelines and manuals identify road diets as one of the many tools that can improve the built environment for walking, bicycling, and transit while improving motor vehicle safety and efficiency. Public health and physical activity advocates can use the following materials as references while making the case for considering a road diet, whereas engineers and planners can refer to them for more detailed design guidance.

Populations Best Served by the Program

Philo Road is now a complete street, which benefits all roadway users. Pedestrians cross shorter distances and are protected by slower speeds, fewer lanes, and median and bike lane buffers. Bicyclists and transit riders particularly have benefited from the improvements. Bicyclists benefit from dedicated on-street space with the addition of bike lanes, and transit riders benefit from shorter crossing distances, angled crossings, better crosswalks, and ADA-compliant bus stop shelters. Perhaps the biggest benefactors of the improvements are the senior adults who live in adjacent neighborhoods and who can now walk, cycle, and use the buses more safely.

Lessons Learned

Start with roads that are well suited to a diet. City governments, road planners, and pedestrian, bicycle, and health advocates should look for roads that meet some of the following criteria:

- Currently a four- or five-lane profile, with two travel lanes in each direction
- A concern regarding rear-end and side-swipe collisions
- Average daily traffic fewer than 20,000 vehicles a day
- Transit corridors with bus service

- Popular or essential bike or pedestrian routes
- Commercial reinvestment areas
- Main or historic streets, often in or near central business districts

Implement bike lanes whenever the opportunity presents itself. Much of the negative feedback from the public about the bike lanes was that they "didn't go anywhere." The section of Philo Road between Colorado Avenue and Florida Avenue was only .4 miles (643 meters) in an almost 2-mile (3.2-kilometer) corridor. The bike lanes north of Florida Avenue were not constructed until 2010. However, waiting until 2010 to stripe the bike lanes on Philo, when it was being resurfaced in 2008, would not have been the right decision. A bicycle network cannot be constructed overnight— it must be constructed in pieces, as it was here.

Get residents invested in the project. The road diet and bike lane ideas were presented at several public meetings called *charrettes,* design gatherings in which many approaches may be considered, that were held at a neighborhood church. Local business owners, neighborhood association representatives, and residents attended the charrettes. Everything from the road diet to the landscaping to the lighting was discussed, and these gatherings were crucial in both revealing the community's priorities and building public support for the project. Physical activity advocates can play a critical role in convening such meetings and ensuring a constructive environment. Perhaps most important, health advocates can ensure that the long term community-wide physical activity benefits of such a project can be kept in clear focus throughout the process.

Tips for Working Across Sectors

Although physical activity advocates may easily embrace the notion of a road diet, the concept may be counterintuitive to those unfamiliar with the idea. Many people assume that a three-lane road cannot carry as much traffic as a four-lane road and that adding pedestrian and bicycle facilities will make problems even worse. Therefore, physical activity supporters must be ready with an evidence-based case for this type of improvement, and the argument must be based on factors that are important to key collaborators, such as elected officials, transportation planners, engineers, local business owners, and residents.

Additional Reading and Resources

FHWA proven safety countermeasures. "Road diet" (roadway reconfiguration) http://safety.fhwa.dot.gov/provencountermeasures/fhwa_sa_12_013.pdf

FHWA summary report: Evaluation of lane reduction "road diet" measures and their effects on crashes and injuries. www.fhwa.dot.gov/publications/research/safety/humanfac/04082/04082.pdf

National Complete Streets Coalition: completestreets.org/complete-streets-fundamentals/factsheets/health/ and www.completestreets.org/webdocs/factsheets/cs-health.pdf

Road diet handbook: Setting trends for livable streets, Jennifer Rosales. www.ite.org/emodules/scriptcontent/Orders/ProductDetail.cfm?pc = LP-670

Road diets: Fixing the big roads, Dan Burden and Peter Lagerway. www.walkable.org/assets/downloads/roaddiets.pdf

Road diets: Designing streets for pedestrians and bicyclists, Michael Ronkin. www.smartgrowthonlineaudio.org/np2007/310c.pdf

Incorporating Physical Activity and Health Outcomes in Regional Transportation Planning

Leslie A. Meehan, AICP
Nashville Area MPO

Michael Skipper, AICP
Nashville Area MPO

NPAP Tactics and Strategies Used in This Program

Transportation, Land Use, and Community Design Sector

STRATEGY 1: Increase accountability of project planning and selection to ensure infrastructure supporting active transportation and other forms of physical activity.

STRATEGY 2: Prioritize resources and provide incentives to increase active transportation and other

physical activity through community design, infrastructure projects, systems, policies, and initiatives.

STRATEGY 3: Integrate land-use, transportation, community design, and economic development planning with public health planning to increase active transportation and other physical activity.

STRATEGY 4: Increase connectivity and accessibility to essential community destinations to increase active transportation and other physical activity.

P hysical activity plays an important role in combating preventable diseases and improving overall health. In general, states in the southeastern United States have the lowest rates of physical activity and experience the highest rates of preventable diseases. In 2010, Tennessee ranked first among the states in adult inactivity, second in the rate of overweight adults (more than 68 percent), third in the rate of obese adults (over 30 percent), fourth in extreme obesity, and fifth in the percentage of children ages 10 to 17 who are overweight or obese (Centers for Disease Control and Prevention 2010).

The opportunity to include physical activity as part of travel requires that the places people want to go are connected by safe, convenient, and reliable transportation facilities such as sidewalks, bike lanes, greenways, and public transit. The rise of automobile travel and the movement toward building automobile-oriented

communities caused many Americans to rely on the car as the dominant mode of transportation and created an environment in which transportation funding is almost exclusively focused on improving the flow of vehicular traffic (U.S. Department of Transportation 2009).

However, public policy makers are increasingly acknowledging the strong connection between the built environment and the health of citizens. Specifically, researchers and urban planners are recognizing the relationship between transportation and land use and observed levels of physical activity. The types of transportation infrastructure built in a community, and the modes of travel supported, may enhance or inhibit physical activity as part of the local travel experience. Opportunities exist to change transportation policy at the federal, state, and local levels to be more inclusive of health-related objectives and to provide greater opportunities for citizens to be physically active as part of local travel.

Providing Opportunities for Physical Activity as Part of Transportation

Providing increased opportunities for physical activity as part of transportation trips begins with building infrastructure that supports active transportation. Active transportation is a term used to describe modes of transportation that require physical activity as part of the mode (Walkable and Livable Communities Institute 2011). Active transportation typically refers to walking, bicycling, and taking transit, since transit trips routinely involve a walk or bicycle trip to a transit stop or station.

People who take active transportation trips may obtain significant amounts of physical activity. Studies show that nearly one third of transit riders get their daily recommended physical activity by walking to and from a transit bus stop or station. Other factors, such as a reduction in traffic crashes, are significant public health benefits of transit (Lachapelle and Frank 2009; Litman 2010). Several studies have found that users of public transit reduce their body mass indices and are less likely to become obese (MacDonald et al. 2010; Morabia et al. 2010). Similar studies show that physical activity obtained from bicycling can increase overall health and add to life expectancy (Besser and Dannenberg 2005; de Hartog et al. 2010; Pucher et al. 2010).

According to the 2009 National Household Travel Survey, 41 percent of all trips taken in the United States are three miles (4.8 kilometers) or less and nearly 19 percent are one mile (1.6 kilometers) or less (Litman, 2011). The average person can walk one mile in approximately 20 minutes and can bicycle the same distance in less than 10 minutes. However, nearly 60 percent of trips of one mile or less are taken by car (Federal Highway Administration 2009). One of the primary reasons for taking short trips by car is the absence of safe and convenient transportation facilities for bicycle and pedestrian modes of travel.

On average, states spend only 1.2 percent of federal transportation dollars on walking and bicycling facilities (Alliance for Biking and Walking 2010). To encourage more spending on infrastructure for these modes, an increasing number of transportation plans and reports are recommending the construction of facilities, such as sidewalks, bike lanes, and greenways, that provide opportunities for transportation, recreation, and physical activity. However, transportation policies and funding mechanisms generally do not align with these recommendations.

Linkage to National Physical Activity Plan

The National Physical Activity Plan calls for communities, agencies, and organizations to prioritize physical activity in planning, programming, and initiatives. The Transportation, Land Use, and Community Design Sector addresses the fact that transportation systems, land use patterns, and the ways communities are designed affect physical activity as part of daily routines, such as getting to work or school or doing errands within a community. The plan includes four strategies designed to help transportation and land use increase physical activity levels. These strategies relate to incorporating physical activity outcomes into transportation policy, planning, and funding and creating connectivity between travel modes and destinations in transportation systems.

The Nashville Area Metropolitan Planning Organization (MPO) has emerged as a national leader in supporting the strategies prioritized in the National Physical Activity Plan by emphasizing increased physical activity as the center of the MPO's policies and funding mechanisms.

Strategy 1: Increase accountability of project planning and selection to ensure infrastructure supporting active transportation and other forms of physical activity. The Nashville Area MPO addresses this strategy by adopting project scoring criteria for roadway projects in which more than half of the points are awarded for improving opportunities for physical activity, increasing safety for all modes, and providing a variety of transportation options. The restructuring of the project scoring criteria has placed an emphasis on health and safety as priority outcomes of a transportation network.

Strategy 2: Prioritize resources and provide incentives to increase active transportation and other physical activity through community design, infrastructure projects, systems, policies, and initiatives. In addition to adopting the scoring criteria mentioned previously, which are used to allocate several billion dollars in federal transportation funds, the MPO created a reserved portion of funding to be spent on active transportation. This funding comes from the MPO's surface transportation program allocation and reserves 15 percent off the top for projects that provide active transportation infrastructure or education. These projects are conducted in addition to active transportation infrastructure provided as part of roadway projects.

Strategy 3: Integrate land-use, transportation, community design, and economic development planning with public health planning to increase active transportation and other physical activity. The MPO is addressing this strategy by including a land-use allocation model as part of its transportation analysis tools and by coding areas that have high rates of minority, elderly, and impoverished households as populations that are more likely to have high rates of health disparities and chronic diseases as well as lower physical activity levels. Additionally, the MPO analyzed food environments by mapping existing grocery and convenience stores in the region in proximity to high concentrations of at-risk populations while analyzing the surrounding active transportation infrastructure. The Nashville Area MPO is placing a strong emphasis on the health outcomes of transportation planning, highlighting the ways that transportation systems provide access to important destinations, such as food stores, and provide opportunities for physical activity.

Strategy 4: Increase connectivity and accessibility to essential community destinations to increase active transportation and other physical activity. The MPO addresses this strategy through its Regional Bicycle and Pedestrian Study, which created a proposed network consisting of more than 1,000 miles (1,600 kilometers) each of bikeways and sidewalks; planners placed priority on segments of bikeways and sidewalks that provided connections to existing facilities and connected important community destinations such as schools, community centers, parks, stores, jobs, and transit.

Nashville Area MPO

The Nashville Area MPO is one of 385 federally designated regional transportation planning organizations, called metropolitan planning organizations, in the United States. MPOs were established by Congress in the 1960s to coordinate transportation planning on a regional level. Regions are defined by urbanized areas with populations greater than 50,000 residents.

The primary purpose of MPOs is to help local governments prioritize improvements to the transportation system to efficiently move people and goods throughout a region. MPOs also help governments allocate funding from federal, state, and local sources to transportation projects. The process of prioritizing and programming transportation projects is outlined in the federation transportation bill and is conducted in the development of a long-range plan for each region that estimates funding revenues and assigns funding to transportation projects for spans of 20 or more years. The plan, often referred to as a long-range or regional transportation plan, must be updated every four to five years. The process is guided by a technical coordinating committee, typically consisting of municipal planners and engineers in the MPO region, as well as an executive board made up of elected officials of the jurisdictions located within the MPO boundary and with populations of at least 5,000 people (U.S. Department of Transportation 1992).

The Nashville Area MPO consists of 22 city and county governments in addition to local and regional transit authorities and the Tennessee Department of Transportation. The region is home to approximately 1.3 million people and this population is expected to increase by 1.3 million people in the next 25 years (Nashville Area MPO 2010). The policies and programs of the MPO affect all those who live and work in the MPO region. The MPO is involved in funding hundreds of transportation projects, including interstates, roadways, transit systems, sidewalks, bikeways, and greenways, as well as intelligent transportation infrastructure such as traffic signals and electronic message boards.

Documenting the Need to Increase Opportunities for Active Transportation

To increase opportunities for active transportation, the case first has to be made that residents in the area are interested in having access to such facilities. To provide this evidence, the Nashville Area MPO conducted the region's first bicycle and pedestrian study from 2008 to 2009, which created a strategic vision for a network of walking and bicycling facilities throughout the greater Nashville area. This strategic vision feeds into the MPO's 2035 Regional Transportation Plan and provides the foundation on which future funding priorities of the MPO are established for bicycle and pedestrian accommodations.

The study was guided by public input in the form of public meetings, stakeholder meet-ings, surveys, and a bicycle and pedestrian advisory committee consisting of community members and representatives from local governments (figure 38.1). Working with local governments, businesses, nonprofit organizations, and the general public, the Nashville Area MPO designed the study to gain a better understanding of bicycle and pedestrian needs within the region. The study looked at the many advantages of bicycle and pedestrian facilities, such as the ability to make transportation trips by nonmotorized modes, the benefits for congestion and air quality, and the benefits for physical activity levels. The study served several functions:

- Provided a comprehensive inventory of existing and proposed on- and off-road bicycle and pedestrian facilities in greater Nashville

- Increased the region's understanding of how nonmotorized transportation adds to the capacity of the transportation system by improving connectivity between residential areas, employment centers, schools, retail centers, recreational centers, and other attractions (with an emphasis on short-distance trips)

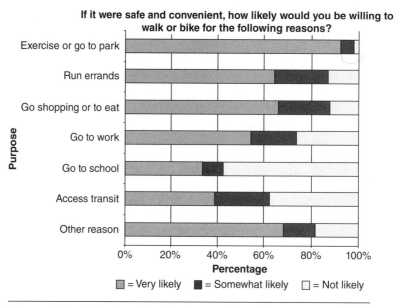

Figure 38.1 Bicycle and pedestrian study: public input.
Reprinted, by permission, from Nashville Area Metropolitan Planning Organization.

- Served as a framework for identifying and selecting bicycle and pedestrian projects for the 2035 Regional Transportation Plan
- Provided guidance for engineering, education, enforcement, encouragement, and evaluation activities to help improve the safety of nonmotorized travel modes

The Regional Bicycle and Pedestrian Study provided the MPO an opportunity to make transportation policy recommendations to improve physical activity levels and overall population health.

Addressing Health and Health Disparities

MPO staff were particularly interested in prioritizing bicycle and pedestrian facilities in areas

with populations that engaged in low levels of physical activity and experienced high rates of health disparities and chronic diseases. Staff members focused on sections of the MPO region with high concentrations of minority, senior adult, and impoverished populations, because these populations tend to experience high rates of preventable chronic diseases. For this reason, MPO staff used census data to help prioritize regional improvements for active transportation facilities to improve population health (Surface Transportation Policy Project 2011; U.S. Department of Health and Human Services 2001). Areas with above-average prevalence of these populations were identified and mapped, so that areas with high concentrations of all three groups could be identified. These were labeled as high health impact areas and received priority consideration for active transportation facilities to improve population health (figure 38.2).

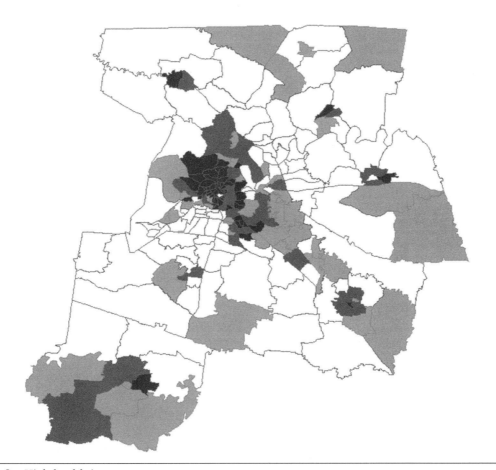

Figure 38.2 High health impact areas.
Reprinted, by permission, from Nashville Area Metropolitan Planning Organization.

Prioritizing Bicycle and Pedestrian Facility Needs

The high health impact areas were one of six factors upon which the regional prioritization of bicycle and pedestrian facilities was based. Staff used five additional factors to analyze more than 3,300 miles (5,310 kilometers) of roadway throughout the MPO region to determine which areas should receive priority for bicycle and pedestrian facilities. Staff determined (1) whether a roadway was congested and could benefit from nonmotorized travel options; (2) whether a new bicycle or pedestrian facility would connect to a network of existing facilities; (3) whether a proposed sidewalk or bikeway had been identified in a local government plan as a priority for a community; (4) whether a high number of bicyclists and pedestrians were expected to make trips in an area (based on the outputs of a latent demand Bicycle and Pedestrian Travel Demand Model); and (5) how well a current roadway was safely serving bicycle and pedestrian trips (figure 38.3).

The project evaluation method and process were developed based on citizen input and the objectives and strategies of the Regional Bicycle and Pedestrian Study. The prioritization method continues to provide a consistent yet flexible means for selecting bicycle and pedestrian facility improvement projects for funding. The process provides the MPO with an objective and quantifiable way of assessing walking and biking project needs that are consistent with the MPO's regional goals and objectives. Feedback from the public about the need for bicycle and pedestrian facilities in the region, and the quantitative tools developed by the study to help prioritize where facilities should be located, were then incorporated into the MPO's 2035 Regional Transportation Plan.

The MPO's strategic vision for walking and bicycling emphasizes roadways that serve as major commuting corridors and commercial corridors and connect communities, activity centers, transit, and major destinations throughout the region. These roadways serve as the backbone for other roadways and streets in the region that, combined with local sidewalks and streets, link neighborhoods, businesses, and other community facilities to one another.

Adopting Policy to Support Active Transportation

During the development of the 2035 Regional Transportation Plan in 2009 to 2010, planning staff provided the public and interested stakeholders with a variety of opportunities to share ideas for improving walking and bicycling in their communities. During the course of that community outreach, several themes regarding obstacles, challenges, and solutions surfaced consistently. Residents mentioned the need for more sidewalks and bicycle lanes and the need to make sure that these facilities connect with other facilities and destinations and do not end abruptly. There was also a strong desire to create a culture among roadway users and law enforcement that is supportive of walking, bicycling, and transit in Nashville. Residents want walking and bicycling to be accepted modes of travel by the community and want to feel encouraged and supported to take these modes. This could include feeling more respected on the roadway and feeling as though law enforcement officers will enforce laws that protect the rights of bicyclists and pedestrians. Combining the public input with peer reviews, best practice research, and the results of the Regional Bicycle and Pedestrian Study, the MPO established regional objectives for advancing active transportation choices and providing a platform for the development of walkable and bikeable communities that support increased physical activity.

In December 2010, the Nashville Area MPO adopted the 2035 Regional Transportation Plan, formally responding to the need for increasing opportunities for bicycle and walking trips by making infrastructure recommendations and prioritizing policy and funding for these modes. Supporting active transportation and walkable communities was one of three policy initiatives in the plan, along with creating a bold

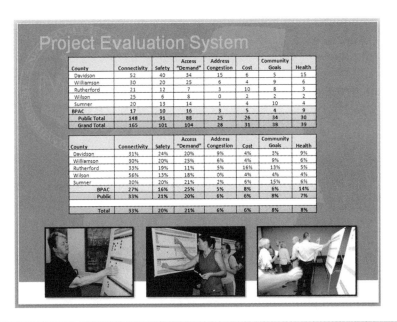

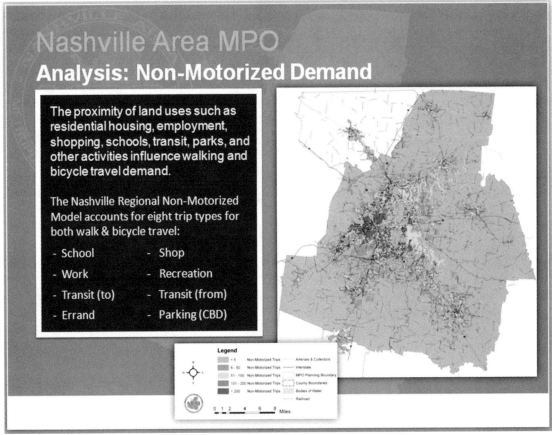

Figure 38.3 Creating a scoring system to evaluate bicycle and pedestrian projects.
Reprinted, by permission, from Nashville Area Metropolitan Planning Organization.

new vision for mass transit and preserving and enhancing existing roadways first versus building new infrastructure. The policies, project scoring criteria, and funding levels included in the plan marked a significant shift to increase the support for active transportation projects.

Scoring Transportation Projects: Including Physical Activity

To ensure that transportation projects include infrastructure for bicyclists and pedestrians, the MPO adopted a systematic process by which candidate roadway projects are evaluated, scored, and ranked by how well they serve the needs of bicyclists and pedestrians. This prioritization process is based on the six evaluation factors developed as part of the Regional Bicycle and Pedestrian Study and is used to assist the MPO as it considers funding bicycle and pedestrian investments throughout the region.

As part of the 2035 Regional Transportation Plan, the MPO developed new scoring criteria on which to rank roadway improvement project proposals seeking funding from the MPO's largest highway funding source—the Federal Highway Administration Surface Transportation Program (STP) funds. Sixty of the 100 points on which roadway transportation projects were scored were based on positive outcomes for air quality, provision of active transportation facilities, improvement of personal and environmental health, injury reduction for all modes, and equity of transportation facilities in underserved areas. More than 400 roadway projects, such as new roads and roadway widenings, were submitted for the plan and were scored according to the new criteria. MPO staff saw a significant shift in the type of transportation projects submitted for the estimated $6 billion dollars in available funding, with 75 percent of the submitted roadway projects including an active transportation element such as a bikeway, sidewalk, or greenway. In the final regional transportation plan, 70 percent of the adopted roadway projects have active trans-

portation infrastructure, up significantly from the estimated 2 percent of projects in the 2030 plan (figure 38.4)

Dedicated Funding for Active Transportation

In addition to adopting a new set of scoring criteria for the plan, the MPO reserved 15 percent of the STP funds for additional active transportation projects. Projects eligible for the reserved funds include active transportation infrastructure projects, such as sidewalks and bikeways, that were not included as part of a submitted roadway project, and noninfrastructure projects such as bicycle and pedestrian safety classes. The reserved STP funds for active transportation are intended to support the objectives of the Regional Bicycle and Pedestrian Study—provide facilities, build support, create policies and programs, and increase awareness for bicycle and pedestrian travel. Example expenditures could include adding sidewalks or bikeways to an infrastructure project that does not have a budget for these facilities; funding stand-alone, multiuse facilities such as greenways; supporting education programs such as Safe Routes to School; providing classes on bicycle and pedestrian safety; and purchasing gear to be provided in bicycle and pedestrian safety classes, such as helmets and reflective safety items.

The MPO reserved 10 percent of STP funds to be combined with grants from the Federal Transit Administration to be used for transit-related improvements. Including this funding with that of the criteria-ranked projects and the 15 percent active transportation funding, the MPO is programming a significant portion of federal funding for active transportation infrastructure and education.

Lessons Learned

One of the most important lessons learned by staff in the development of the 2035 Regional Transportation Plan was how to frame the issues. Staff began the conversation by invit-

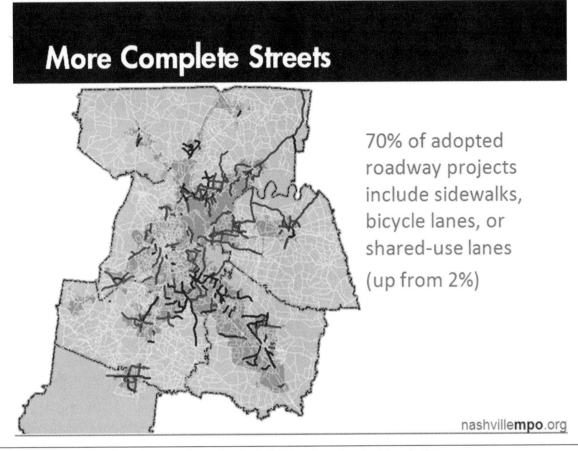

Figure 38.4 Adopted roadway projects that include bicycle and pedestrian facilities.
Reprinted, by permission, from Nashville Area Metropolitan Planning Organization.

ing stakeholders and community members to create a vision for a vibrant and thriving community. These stakeholders included representatives from various sectors such as land use planning, engineering, parks, schools, health, law enforcement, economic development, housing, tourism, and others. From the vision, a series of goals and objectives were created by staff for how transportation could support the vision. The goals and objectives were in turn translated into the scoring criteria, which were presented to the public for feedback and endorsed by the MPO executive board. By starting with a vision and not specific projects, and by engaging community members and stakeholders throughout the process, the MPO was able to develop policies based on the community character and transportation components

that residents and stakeholders envisioned for their communities. The MPO also developed priorities first and determined which funding source best fit the priorities, rather than starting with the estimated amount from a funding source and determining which projects should receive the funding. This approach allowed the MPO to ensure that top priorities were funded first and allowed staff to think creatively about how to make funding sources fit the needs of the region.

One of challenges faced by the MPO was a lack of data on populations with health disparities and high rates of chronic diseases such as asthma, diabetes, and heart disease at a subregional level. To address this, the MPO has collected health data as part of a regional household travel survey.

Next Steps: Gathering Data and Benchmarking Progress

The MPO is conducting the Middle Tennessee Transportation and Health Study to survey 6,000 households on travel behavior, health habits, and overall health of household members. The study includes a subset of 600 participants who wore GPS units and accelerometers to collect data on their transportation trips and rates of physical activity. These participants also completed a survey that asks questions about food security, physical activity rates, and prevalence of chronic diseases among household members. The study collected data that are integral to illustrating the relationships among transportation, physical activity, and overall health. These data will be used in the next update of the MPO Regional Transportation Plan to shape additional tools and policies on health outcomes in the regional transportation planning process.

Program Evaluation

The MPO policies recently underwent review by the Centers for Disease Control and Prevention, Division of Nutrition, Physical Activity and Obesity (DNPAO). The review includes an assessment of the MPO's policies related to physical activity and obesity, and as a result the MPO will be promoted throughout the United States as a model that can be replicated by other MPOs for supporting active transportation. The MPO also underwent a review by the CDC-funded Center for Translational Research and Training (TRT) in the Center for Health Promotion and Disease Prevention (Prevention Research Center) at the University of North Carolina, Chapel Hill. The MPO was selected by the Center TRT to be reviewed as an emerging intervention that shows promise for potential public health impact on one or more obesity-related outcomes based on theory and approach. In a separate process, the Center TRT conducted a site visit with the MPO and created an evaluation logic model and process for the MPO to conduct a self-evaluation of the impact of the MPO's policies on health. Should funding become available, the MPO could be a potential candidate for a full evaluation conducted by the CDC.

Summary

The Nashville Area MPO has made a commitment to providing increased opportunities for physical activity through its regional transportation policies and dedicated funding for bicycle and pedestrian facilities. That commitment is expected to affect positively the health of a large number of people over the next several decades by increasing the availability of active transportation infrastructure and community awareness about the importance of a transportation system that includes adequate transit, bikeways, sidewalks, and greenways. Over time, the impacts of the policies may include improved air quality, increased opportunities for physical activity, decreased traffic crashes for all modes, and increased active transportation facilities for all populations. The MPO staff believes that the 2035 Regional Transportation Plan policies represent a paradigm shift in transportation policy and take important steps to link transportation with health outcomes to increase opportunities for physical activity as part of the regional transportation system. This shift broadens the conversation around public policy to emphasize that issues such as public health and physical activity are the responsibility of all government agencies, including transportation agencies. By engaging with multiple sectors, the MPO is working to create policy that has a positive impact for transportation, land use, environmental and personal health, economic prosperity, and quality of life.

Additional Reading and Resources

2035 Regional Transportation Plan: www.nashvillempo.org/plans_programs/rtp/

MPO's Health and Well-Being Initiatives:

www.nashvillempo.org/regional_plan/health/

Middle Tennessee Transportation and Health Study: www.middletnstudy.com/welcome.aspx

CDC Pre-Evaluation Site Visit Summary Report: www. nashvillempo.org/docs/Health/Nashville%20 MPO%20Summary%20Report_FINAL.pdf

References

Alliance for Biking and Walking. 2010. Bicycling and walking in the U.S.: 2010 benchmarking report. www.peoplepoweredmovement.org/site/index. php/site/memberservices/C529.

Besser, M., and A. Dannenberg. 2005. Walking to public transit: Steps to help meet physical activity recommendations. *Am. J. Prev. Med.* 29(4):273-80.

Centers for Disease Control and Prevention. 2010. Behavioral Risk Factor Surveillance System (BRFSS). http://apps.nccd.cdc.gov/brfss/.

de Hartog, J., H. Boogaard, H. Nijland, and G. Hoek. 2010. Do the health benefits of cycling outweigh the risks? *Environ. Health Perspect.* 118(8):1109-16.

Federal Highway Administration. 2009. National household travel survey—2009. http://nhts.ornl. gov/download.shtml.

Lachapelle, U., and L. Frank. 2009. Transit and health: Mode of transport, employer sponsored public transit pass programs, and physical activity. *J. Public Health Policy* 30:S73-94.

Litman, T. 2010. Evaluating public health transportation benefits. Victoria Policy Institute and the American Public Transit Association. www.apta. com/resources/reportsandpublications/Documents/ APTA_Health_Benefits_Litman.pdf.

Litman, T. 2011. Short and sweet: Analysis of shorter trips using national personal travel survey data. Victoria Transport Policy Institute. www.vtpi.org/ short_sweet.pdf.

MacDonald, J., R. Stokes, D. Cohen, A. Kofner, and K. Ridgeway. 2010. The effect of light rail transit on body mass index and physical activity. *Am. J. Prev. Med.* 29(2):105-12. www.ajpmonline.org/article/ S0749-3797(10)00297-7/abstract.

Morabia, A., F.E. Mirer, T.M. Amstislavski, H.M. Eisl, J. WerbeFuentes, J. Gorczynki, et al. 2010. Potential health impact of switching from car to public transportation when commuting to work. *Am. J. Public Health* 100(12):2388-91.

Nashville Area MPO. 2010. 2035 regional transportation plan. www.nashvillempo.org/plans_programs/rtp/.

Pucher, J., R. Buehler, D.R. Bassett,, and A.L. Dannenberg. 2010. Walking and cycling to health: A comparative analysis of city, state and international data. *Am. J. Public Health* 100(10):1986-92.

Surface Transportation Policy Project. 2011. Fact sheet. Transportation and poverty alleviation. www.transact.org/library/factsheets/poverty.asp.

U.S. Department of Health and Human Services. 2001. The Surgeon General's call to action to prevent and decrease overweight and obesity. www.surgeongeneral.gov/topics/obesity/calltoaction/toc.htm.

U.S. Department of Transportation. 1992 Urban transportation planning in the U.S. A historical overview. http://ntl.bts.gov/DOCS/UTP.html.

U.S. Department of Transportation. 2009. National household travel survey: Summary of travel trends. http://nhts.ornl.gov/2009/pub/stt.pdf.

CHAPTER 39

Leveraging Public and Private Relationships to Make Omaha Bicycle Friendly

Kerri R. Peterson, BS, MS
Live Well Omaha Executive Director

Julie T. Harris, BS, MPA
Live Well Omaha Program Coordinator

NPAP Tactics and Strategies Used in This Program

Transportation, Land Use, and Community Design Sector

STRATEGY 1: Increase accountability of project planning and selection to ensure infrastructure supporting active transportation and other forms of physical activity.

STRATEGY 2: Prioritize resources and provide incentives to increase active transportation and other physical activity through community design, infrastructure projects, systems, policies, and initiatives.

STRATEGY 3: Integrate land-use, transportation, community design, and economic development planning with public health planning to increase active transportation and other physical activity.

STRATEGY 4: Increase connectivity and accessibility to essential community destinations to increase active transportation and other physical activity.

In a city where the longest commute is 25 minutes east to west and where the design is intentional for automobiles, the last few years have seen an unprecedented movement toward creating a bikeable community in Omaha. Recognizing the limitations on city and county government in terms of vision and resources, Omaha has reached outside government to leverage private funding streams and "people power" to change the environment. As a result, Omaha has intertwined public and private funding to redefine the vision for Omaha's transportation system, a vision that the city now embraces. In this vision, streets should be designed to move people, not just cars—so that biking, walking, and using mass transit are all safe and convenient; such a design increases connectivity by ensuring access to and use of bicycle facilities, ride parks, green spaces, and trails.

Program Description

Omaha is a classic Midwestern city with a huge sense of community pride. If you ask the average citizen, he or she will say that Omaha is a great city. However, it currently ranks 142 out of 182 in health factors among cities across the United States (indicators measured included physical activity, nutrition, obesity, tobacco use, and binge drinking). Although changing the behaviors that lead to this poor ranking are important, Omaha will not make significant changes until the healthy choice is the easy choice. For that to happen, Omaha must become a place where biking, walking, and using mass transit are safe, convenient, and enjoyable activities that support the needs of all citizens, including children, seniors, and those who either can't afford a car or choose not to own or drive one. Since 1995, Omaha has embraced a collaborative approach to improving the health of the community through a healthy community initiative, Live Well Omaha (LWO).

In 2003, the Robert Wood Johnson Foundation released a grant opportunity called Active Living by Design, offering funding to communities to increase physical activity options for their citizens through community design. By advocating for changes in community design, specifically land use, transportation, parks, trails, and greenways, the Active Living by Design initiative was intended to make it easier for people to be active in their daily routines. The Active Living by Design community action model provided five steps to influence community change: preparation, promotions, programs, policy influences, and physical projects. The 5P model is a comprehensive approach to increasing physical activity through short-, intermediate-, and long-term community changes. This inclusive model facilitated the integration of policy, physical project, and programmatic efforts. In November 2003, Omaha was 1 of 44 communities nationwide (out of more than 800 applicants) that received a five-year, $200,000 grant as part of the Active Living by Design national program (www.activelivingbydesign.org). Through the leadership of Live Well Omaha and its ties in the community, and with the funding from Active Living by Design, the city launched Live Well Omaha: Activate Omaha (LWO: Activate Omaha) to increase levels of active living in the community. ("Active living" is a way of life that integrates physical activity into daily routines in order to accumulate at least 30 minutes of activity each day.)

Local businesses, health-focused organizations, and community planning and urban designers formed an executive leadership committee for LWO: Activate Omaha. The committee and the organization capitalized on existing relationships to reach out to the business community and cultivate buy-in from business leaders. The LWO: Activate Omaha partnership was able to leverage funding from private donors through the philanthropy of these organizations.

To promote awareness of the effort, LWO: Activate Omaha created messaging for various communication channels (e.g., print, radio, television), developed targeted messages for different population segments, and maintained a single brand to represent the initiative. One of the first successes the partnership achieved was launching the Bicycle Commuter Challenge. In 2006, the mayor kicked off the challenge by announcing his support for a bicycle-friendly Omaha. Magazine and newspaper articles and interviews on local television channels promoted the program. In later years, the program incorporated incentives to attract new participants.

The Bicycle Commuter Challenge was very successful. In the first year, more than 300 participants from 27 businesses logged 77,000 miles (124,000 kilometers). Subsequent years saw increases: 109,000 miles (175,000 kilometers) in year 4 and 135,000 miles (217,000 kilometers) in year 5. The LWO: Activate Omaha partnership viewed the program as a way to generate evidence and support for the need for infrastructure change. The partnership did, however, encounter resistance from participants. The city's streets were not conducive to commuting by bicycle: There was only one official mile of bicycle lanes, and drivers were impatient with cyclists.

As a result of that feedback, LWO: Activate Omaha developed a bicycle commuter map for the Omaha–Council Bluffs metro area, using a Robert Wood Johnson Foundation Special Opportunities Grant (figure 39.1). The purpose of the map was to assist commuters in identifying routes to reach their destination safely and conveniently. Participants in the Bicycle Commuter Challenge served on the technical advisory committee that developed and field-tested the map. Five thousand copies were distributed in one month through local bike shops, bike clubs, and libraries. Seeing the high level of interest in the map, the LWO: Activate Omaha partnership pursued a $7,000 grant from the Eastern Nebraska Trails Network to fund printing additional copies.

However, despite the success of the Bicycle Commuter Challenge and interest in the map, a significant problem loomed. Omaha is a city that was designed around a car; it is a point of pride in Omaha that it is so easy to get around the city

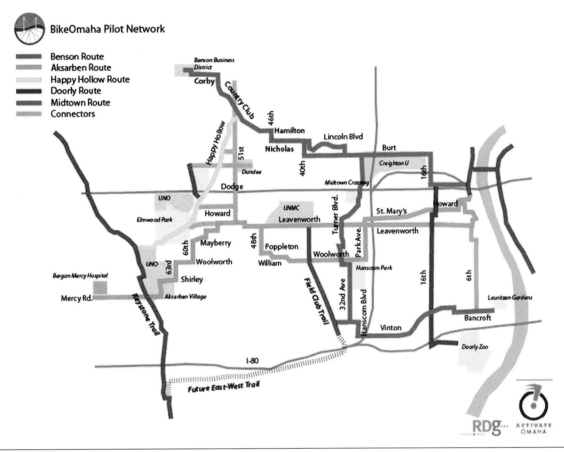

Figure 39.1 Map of Omaha bicycle network.
Reprinted, by permission, from Douglas County Health Department.

by driving. Therefore, promoting and increasing active transportation remained a problem. In addition, Omaha's built environment provided challenges to active living. Omaha has experienced rapid westward growth in recent decades but has been unable to build and expand certain types of infrastructure at the same rate. In 2004, many neighborhoods, both old and new, lacked pavements, and although 60 miles (100 kilometers) of recreational trails existed, they were not well connected. Other factors that limited active living included traffic conditions, aggressive drivers, poor street design, lack of bike lanes, hilly terrain, and harsh winters. Because of these factors, few residents engaged in active living of any kind, including bicycling. Most bicycle trips in Omaha were recreational only, and transportation-related trips were rare. "Our city planner told us his job was to move

cars, not bikes," said Tammie Dodge, former project coordinator of LWO: Activate Omaha.

To educate and influence policy makers and decision makers, LWO: Activate Omaha invited key players in the city to participate in partnership-sponsored events. For example, the partnership invited several community leaders to participate in a trip to Boulder, Colorado, to learn more about successful alternative public transit systems. This trip led to improved relationships and increased participation by policy makers and decision makers in active living efforts.

As enthusiasm for active living grew, the leaders of Live Well Omaha realized that funding for additional changes was not likely to come from city government, which was not driving the change and was constrained by a tight budget. The partnership pursued funding through the Peter Kiewit Foundation and another private funder to develop a 20-mile (32-kilometer) bicycle loop in Omaha as a pilot project to increase physical activity. At an informational meeting with both funders, the leaders of Live Well Omaha went out on a limb and told funders that if the city built it (the bicycle loop), they (bicyclists) would come. The private funders agreed to pay $600,000 to construct the bicycle loop.

The finished system (to be completed in 2014) will be a compilation of *sharrows* (shared-lane markings), new bicycle lanes, existing trail connectors, and changes to existing road lanes. The partnership hoped that the success of the pilot project would encourage the funders to invest additional resources in expanding the loop. By bringing the funding to the city, the partnership created a win-win dynamic: The city could get credit for enhancing the transportation system at little to no cost to city taxpayers. As a result of this pilot work and the emerging cycling infrastructure, the city has since applied for and received an additional $300,000 to put in 10 more miles of bicycle lanes.

Another key to success is to invest in policy work. A local health care system, Alegent Health, funded in part the salary of Omaha's first bicycle and pedestrian transportation coordinator. The city leveraged this funding and funded the remaining salary cost through the local area metro transit budget. This is a huge step for the city's planning department, as it is the first time a staff member has been dedicated to addressing bicycle and pedestrian issues.

Live Well Omaha and the Douglas County Health Department received a grant in 2010 that will be used to address policy that affects the physical environment. From this grant, $300,000 was given to the City of Omaha to update its transportation master plan to include accommodations for bicycles, pedestrians, and transit users. Again, this is an example of how outside funding was leveraged to create sustainable policy change in Omaha. The plan, complete with public input, was completed in 2012 and it will forever affect the design of the city. Advocacy groups such as Mode Shift Omaha and Omaha Bikes are now working to give the city and county grassroots support for the resulting planning decisions.

Program Evaluation

Although no comprehensive evaluation is in place given the lack of funding, LWO is tracking some quantitative measures:

• Use of bike racks: Since the installation of the bike racks on all metro buses, the usage of the bike racks has increased every year—a 150 percent increase from 2008 to 2009, an 8 percent increase from 2009 to 2010, and a 59 percent increase from 2010 to 2011.

• Participation in the Bicycle Commuter Challenge: Every aspect of the commuter challenge has increased in the past two years. The number of teams increased 108 percent, the number of riders increased 62 percent, the number of trips increased 34 percent, and total miles logged increased 22 percent. From 2009 to 2011, in the months of May to August, 444,558 miles (715,446 kilometers) were tracked.

• Use of the pedestrian bridge by bicycles: In May 2011, the Bob Kerry Pedestrian Bridge was observed for three days. Over those days the bridge was visited 5,050 times, and 9.3 percent of the visits were on bikes.

• Bike-friendly businesses: The number of bike-friendly businesses has increased from one in 2009, to seven in 2010, and to nine in 2011.

• Bicycle-Friendly City: In 2011, Omaha applied for and received a Bicycle-Friendly City designation at the bronze level.

• Bike to the Ballpark: In 2011, its first year, Bike to the Ballpark attracted 700 bikes and 50 volunteers. This event was held during the College World Series.

Linkage to the National Physical Activity Plan

The efforts by Live Well Omaha to create a community that supports active living and active transportation are linked to four strategies of the Transportation, Land Use, and Community

Design Sector of the National Physical Activity Plan.

Strategy 1: Increase accountability of project planning and selection to ensure infrastructure supporting active transportation and other forms of physical activity. Live Well Omaha and its partners have consistently provided educational opportunities to planners and engineers to begin to change the decision-making culture in the city's planning department. In addition, the city is updating its transportation master plan so that it focuses on designing for all forms of transportation, not just cars.

Strategy 2: Prioritize resources and provide incentives to increase active transportation and other physical activity through community design, infrastructure projects, systems, policies, and initiatives. Through the updated transportation master plan and community input, the city has developed a priorities list, based on specific criteria. The partnership provides political cover and public support to the city when decisions are made to support multimodal forms of transportation. A dedicated effort is made to leverage funding when public resources are not available.

Strategy 3: Integrate land-use, transportation, community design, and economic development planning with public health planning to increase active transportation and other physical activity. The Douglas County Health Department received a Robert Wood Johnson Foundation grant to conduct three health impact assessments, which Live Well Omaha hopes will be just the beginning of the integration of health impact into planning and designing decisions within the city and county. The head of the city's planning department has joined leadership teams that guide the city's work on obesity prevention.

Strategy 4: Increase connectivity and accessibility to essential community destinations to increase active transportation and other physical activity. Live Well Omaha and its partners are working hard on increasing connectivity. From increasing the miles of existing bicycle lanes to ensuring that essential connectors of the trail system are completed, connectivity requires coordination of many sectors. All metro buses have had bicycle racks installed, which makes it more convenient to merge transit and bicycle users. A shared bicycle system, B-Cycle, is being installed to create connectivity from west to east, focusing on reducing the number of automobile trips that are shorter than two miles (3.2 kilometers).

Evidence Base Used During Program Development

In 2012, the Institute of Medicine released a report titled Accelerating Progress in Obesity Prevention: Solving the Weight of the Nation. The report issued recommendations for accelerating the progress in preventing obesity. One entire goal focuses on making physical activity routine.

Goal 1: Make physical activity an integral and routine part of life.

Recommendation 1: Communities, transportation officials, community planners, health professionals, and governments should make promotion of physical activity a priority by substantially increasing access to places and opportunities for such activity. Strategy 1-1: Enhance the physical and built environment. Communities, organizations, community planners, and public health professionals should encourage physical activity by enhancing the physical and built environment, rethinking community design, and ensuring access to places for such activity. Following are two of the potential actions that have been suggested: Communities, urban planners, architects, developers, and public health professionals should develop and implement sustainable strategies for improving the physical environment of communities that are as large as several square miles, or as small as a few blocks, in ways that encourage and support physical activity. Communities and organizations should develop and maintain sustainable strategies to create or enhance access to places and programs where people can be physically active in a safe and enjoyable way.

Live Well Omaha's comprehensive approach to increasing routine levels of physical activity, using the Robert Wood Johnson's 5P model approach, covers many of the Institute of Medicine's recommendations.

Populations Best Served by the Program

The steps taken by Live Well Omaha and LWO: Activate Omaha are designed to benefit people of all age, socioeconomic, and ethnic and racial groups. Omaha is the largest city in Nebraska, with approximately 430,000 residents, representing more than a quarter of the entire state's population. Like many growing cities, Omaha has a dense, urban section of the city and a sprawling suburban geographic area. Business dominates Omaha's decision-making infrastructure, as it is home to five Fortune 500 companies, including Mutual of Omaha and Con Agra. The city is primarily white (81 percent) with small racial and ethnic populations (11 percent African American, 7 percent Hispanic and Latino). Omaha neighborhoods tend to be defined by race and ethnicity and by income. Omaha has a relatively young population, with 27 percent of residents younger than 18 years and 31 percent between 25 and 44 years old. Omaha also has one of the highest percentages of working mothers in the nation, resulting in a large number of children in full-time daycare. Eighty-five percent of residents have an education level of a high school diploma or greater, and 14 percent live below the poverty level ($22,050 per year for a family of four, U.S. Census). The estimated median household income in 2009 was $46,595. Low-income and minority populations are disparately affected by overweight and obesity.

Lessons Learned

It has taken almost nine years to make the headway that Omaha is beginning to see and experience. The top lessons learned include these:

• Change takes time. In a city that that has focused on moving automobiles in the most

convenient way for the last 30 years, building relationships and educating staff were key elements in taking small steps forward and experiencing success. Patience and compromise led to important changes.

• Come to the table with resources. LWO and its partners brought more than one million dollars to the city for infrastructure and programmatic support. Collectively, LWO has worked in tandem to plan and re-envision what could be for Omaha. LWO also arranged two community site visits (in Boulder and Minneapolis) for key leaders in the city to see first hand how change has occurred.

• Provide political cover when needed. Omaha drivers have been somewhat resistant to the issue of bicyclists on the roads. The city planners are the first to hear the complaints. When possible and appropriate, LWO and its partners publically acknowledge and celebrate the steps the city takes to ensure multimodal forms of transportation.

Tips for Working Across Sectors

Live Well Omaha used several strategies that have contributed to its early successes. The strongest keys to success thus far have been building on a history of partnerships, using media to create awareness and set an agenda for change, and following a planning model in developing programs.

Building on a History of Partnerships

Central to the success of Live Well Omaha to date has been its history of partnering with other organizations in the community and using those partnerships to leverage resources in the community. LWO's network of more than 100 partners and members of Omaha's public and private community engaged in several early collaborations to address obesity and physical activity in the community. Many of these early activities laid the groundwork for LWO's current work.

Using Media to Create Awareness and Set an Agenda for Change

Another key to success is the use of media to engage members of the community with the culture shift that was underway. Residents were not used to seeing bicycles on the road. As a result, LWO launched Omaha's first Share the Road campaign, IRide. LWO built a new website and shared stories in the media about successes (e.g., number of people participating in the Bicycle Commuter Challenge).

Following a Planning Model in Developing Programs

Much of the work was grounded in the Robert Wood Johnson Foundation's 5P model for change (preparation, promotions, programs, policy, and physical). LWO was introduced to this model through its participation in the Robert Wood Johnson Foundation's Active Living by Design community grant program and has used this basic approach with subsequent projects. Using this model provided staff with experience in thinking about policy as a part of change as well as a more holistic framework for thinking about and addressing health issues in the community. By using this model in designing its programs, LWO was better able to strike a balance between working directly on policy change and creating public interest and involvement, which is required for changes in policy to be enacted.

Additional Reading and Resources

Burk, M., with Kurmaskie, J. 2010. *Joyride: Pedaling Toward a Healthier Planet.* Portland, OR: Cadence Press.

Mapes, J. 2009. *Pedaling Revolution: How Cyclists Are Changing American Cities.* Corvallis, OR: Oregon State University Press.

Parker, L., A.C. Burns, E. Sanchez, and the Committee on Childhood Obesity Prevention Actions for Local Governments. 2009. *Strategies to Prevent Childhood Obesity.* Washington, DC: Institute of Medicine and National Research Council of the National Academies.

Volunteer and Nonprofit

Colleen Doyle, MS, RD

The data are clear: Americans are not sufficiently physically active, putting their health and their quality of life at risk. Also clear is that facilitating lifelong physical activity will require improvements in the environments in which people live, work, learn, and play and reduction of the barriers to active lifestyles that many people face. To achieve these goals, national, state, and local organizations must work together on activities that result in policy and environmental changes in workplaces, schools, neighborhoods, health care facilities, and faith-based communities, among others. Nonprofit organizations, because of their mission, infrastructure, and unique capabilities, can serve as effective partners in creating and sustaining more physically active lifestyles among all Americans.

Whether a nonprofit organization focuses on disease prevention or health promotion, targets particular audiences of health professionals or consumers, or focuses on particular age groups, these organizations possess many characteristics and competencies that can be leveraged to build capacity to support more physically active lifestyles. They tend to have a broad base of support—volunteers, members, and other constituents—whose passion for advancing the organization's mission can be used to advance policies and systems changes. Many function at multiple levels and can therefore help to coordinate the multilevel strategies needed for maximum impact. Many nonprofit organizations are leaders in promoting legislation and in building the capacity of communities to advocate for legislative priorities. Some nonprofits focus their work within specific sectors, but many work across sectors and can act as key conveners of cross-sectoral coalitions and collaborations. Many nonprofits already work through key systems and target their work to particular audiences, including youth, the elderly, racial and ethnic minority populations, and health professionals, and can therefore leverage those existing relationships and efforts. Finally, the mission and infrastructure of some nonprofits may be valuable in helping to advance more applied, community-based physical activity research. All of these characteristics can and should be leveraged to advance physical activity policy and systems change priorities nationwide.

The initiatives that follow exemplify a variety of these unique characteristics and competencies of nonprofit organizations and demonstrate how organizations are leveraging them to help facilitate physical activity among all Americans. You will see how nonprofit organizations have increased capacity at national, state, and local levels to advocate for policy and systems changes through training and technical assistance, development of effective coalitions, and community mobilization; how nonprofits have partnered to create and disseminate an effective physical activity program for a special population group and have reduced organizational barriers that could affect adoption of such a program by individuals; and how a national nonprofit organization identified evidence-based strategies to promote physical activity in a workplace setting, tested and evaluated those strategies in a real-world setting, and used its nationwide infrastructure to disseminate strategies that have resulted in physical activity policy and environmental changes in workplaces throughout the country. These examples should stimulate new ideas, inspire creativity and innovation, and demonstrate the critically important role that nonprofit organizations play in achieving the vision set forth by the National Physical Activity Plan: One day, all Americans will be physically active, and they will live, work, and play in environments that facilitate regular physical activity.

CHAPTER 40

Using Legal and Policy Muscles to Support Physically Active Communities

Manel Kappagoda, JD, MPH
ChangeLab Solutions

Robert Ogilvie, PhD
ChangeLab Solutions

Sara Zimmerman, JD
ChangeLab Solutions

Marice Ashe, JD, MPH
ChangeLab Solutions

NPAP Tactics and Strategies Used in This Program

Overarching Strategies

STRATEGY 1: Advocate to local, state, and national decision makers for policies and system changes identified in the National Physical Activity Plan that promote physical activity.

STRATEGY 2: Convene multisector stakeholders at local, state and national levels in strategic collabora-

tions to advance the goals of the National Physical Activity Plan.

STRATEGY 3: Conduct outreach to nonprofit groups' members, volunteers, and constituents to change their own behaviors and advocate for policy and system changes outlined in the National Physical Activity Plan.

When local government officials in Kansas City, Kansas, passed a Complete Streets resolution pushing for the development of safer and more walkable streets in 2011, the victory offered a powerful example of how nonprofit advocacy and partnerships can create policy successes for physical activity. In celebrating the resolution's passage, Mayor Joe Reardon noted that the process of developing the policy had already forged new partnerships between city engineers and the city's public health department as the staff explored new ways of looking at the health implications of local streets. Using model policies developed by ChangeLab Solutions, advocates from Kansas City Healthy Kids (KCHK) who were living and working in Wyandotte County, Kansas, were able to convince community groups, mayors,

and city council members of the policy's value and feasibility. Since that policy passed, one other county and four other cities in the metro Kansas City area have passed Complete Streets policies. The advocacy of KCHK was instrumental in the policy's passage. In the words of Samara Klein, KCHK's advocacy director, model policies gave advocates and policy makers "a starting-off point," making it easier for busy people to move issues forward effectively. (For more information on Kansas City Healthy Kids, go to www.kchealthykids.org/.)

The purpose of this chapter is to highlight how legal and policy technical assistance can support the efforts of leading organizations that are trying to change the built environment to support physical activity. For the purposes of illustration, this chapter focuses on the work of

ChangeLab Solutions, a nonprofit organization based in Oakland, California. For nearly 15 years, ChangeLab Solutions has helped communities create laws and policies that make the healthy choice the easy choice. Our team of attorneys, city planners, and policy analysts consult with advocates and policy makers on tough legal and policy challenges, develop practical model policies, and train local leaders on specific policy strategies and additional resources. ChangeLab Solutions is one of several organizations that provide specialized legal and policy support on issues that affect the public's health. (See, for example, the Network for Public Health Law: www.networkforphl.org/.) Our approach to policy change was developed through our work on the tobacco control movement, and over the years we have applied the same method to new issues. We take an interdisciplinary approach to physical activity policy, incorporating legal and urban planning expertise to develop policies that make communities more walkable, bikeable, and supportive of physical activity.

Program Description

One of the most effective ways to change the behavior of large numbers of people is by changing the underlying social expectations about the types of behavior that are acceptable or approved—an approach known as "social norm change." A social norm involves the expectations of appropriate and desirable behavior widely shared throughout a community or society (Marshall 1998; Zhang et al. 2010). The goal of a social norm change movement is to change people's behavior, but not by nagging them or educating them about the need for change and not by requiring each individual to act a certain way. Instead, a social norm change movement changes people's behavior indirectly by creating a social environment and legal climate in which harmful conduct becomes less desirable, less acceptable, and less convenient, while healthier behavior becomes the norm (California Department of Health Services 1998).

National nonprofits can serve as a catalyst for social norm change, working in partnership with local, state, and federal policy makers and advocates. This approach to policy development strives to achieve system-level changes in a range of settings, including households, schools, entertainment venues, corporations, and government agencies. The changes are institutionalized informally through cultural expectations and peer pressure and formally through legislation and law enforcement. Of the many movements that have shaped the society we live in today—everything from seatbelt use and recycling to civil rights and disability rights—almost all have taken a social norm change approach.

Regular physical activity plays a critical role in mitigating obesity and other chronic diseases. However, modern life and current social norms make it difficult for the average person to incorporate sufficient physical activity into daily life. By supporting efforts that focus on policy and social norm change, national nonprofits can assist advocates and policy makers on a wide range of issues, from broad land use plans to focused place-based strategies like regulating physical activity in child care settings.

Neighborhoods Designed for Active Living

Increasing evidence demonstrates a strong relationship between our health and the environment in which we live. The way neighborhoods, streets, and homes are designed affects whether children can play outside and walk to school, whether families can easily access healthy food and basic services, whether taking transit to work is a realistic option, and even whether neighbors can socialize and look out for one another (Design Community & Environment 2006; Jackson and Kotchtitzky n.d.).

In an effort to curb growing rates of chronic disease such as diabetes, asthma, and heart disease, planners and public health professionals are combining their resources and expertise, working to design and redevelop neighborhoods so that healthy choices are available. One of the main tools that planners and public health officials have at their disposal for creating healthier communities is the *comprehensive plan*. Comprehensive plans are the primary documents guiding land use development patterns, and they can be used to ensure that future development and redevelopment facilitate physical activity. The American Planning Association recently surveyed the interaction between planners and public health departments around the United States, finding that only 27 percent had adopted comprehensive plans that explicitly address health; thus, there is much work to be done (American Planning Association 2011).

A wide range of communities, such as King County, Washington; Chino, California; and Port Towns, Maryland, are beginning to revise their comprehensive plans to address residents' health. Legal and policy assistance from nonprofits such as ChangeLab Solutions is key to enabling jurisdictions to effectively identify areas of improvement such as increasing access to recreational facilities, calling for future developments to be designed to encourage daily physical activity, and building accessibly so that seniors can age comfortably in place. National nonprofits can also work with communities on revising zoning and subdivision codes to promote health and on adopting ordinances and regulations that support bicycles and pedestrians.

Complete Streets

Over the last four decades, transportation planning has increasingly focused on the rapid movement of large numbers of motor vehicles—the result being that today's streets are often dangerous and inconvenient for pedestrians and bicyclists. In contrast, Complete Streets are streets designed and operated to be safe, comfortable, and convenient for all users—pedestrians, bicyclists, motorists, and transit riders of all ages and abilities (National Complete Streets Coalition 2010). Putting a local Complete Streets policy into place ensures that transportation agencies routinely design and operate the entire right of way to enable safe access for everyone (National Complete Streets Coalition 2010). Complete Streets policies can take a variety of forms, including ordinances and resolutions, revisions of design manuals, inclusion in comprehensive plans, and executive orders from elected officials. Communities across the nation are working to make their streets complete, from Kentucky to Washington to New York. Model policies and implementation assistance can be crucial in making these campaigns successful.

Safe Routes to School

Like Complete Streets, Safe Routes to School (SRTS) is a policy approach that focuses on reinstating walking and bicycling as common ways for children and adults to get around. Research shows that children who walk or bicycle to school have higher daily levels of physical activity and better cardiovascular fitness than do children who do not actively commute to school (Davison et al. 2008). SRTS advocates may work with their school district to pass a district policy that promotes and supports SRTS or work with their municipal or county government to incorporate SRTS concepts in the comprehensive plan (National Policy & Legal Analysis Network 2010).

Communities often need to clarify questions about legal issues that arise in connection with SRTS programs. For example, when Nita Mizushima, president of the Nevada City School Board, encountered liability concerns as she was setting up the district's first walk-to-school week, she consulted with a staff attorney at ChangeLab Solutions to explore various issues that had emerged. Could school employees participate? Were waivers necessary? Did the district have built-in protections from liability? With the ability to easily access expertise in this area, she quickly found answers that allowed her to move forward with clarity and assurance.

School Siting

Forty years ago, almost half of all students walked or biked to school (U.S. Department of Transportation 2008); now only 13 percent do so (McDonald et al. 2011). The biggest reason for this change is because today's schools are located too far from children's homes for walking or biking to be practical (Martin et al. 2007). In recent decades, in response to a variety of pressures, schools have increasingly been built on the outskirts of communities (Martin et al. 2007). The consequence is that two thirds of today's schools are located far from where children live (U.S. Department of Health and Human Services 2008). Since 1980, obesity rates in children and adolescents have more than tripled, and currently almost one-third of children are overweight or obese.(Ogden et al. 2008).

But school locations can be an important factor in students' health. When schools are located close to where students live, not only can children get regular physical activity on the way to school through SRTS programs, but also they may be able to take advantage of school playgrounds and facilities outside of school hours (see section titled Joint Use Agreements). To ensure that schools are located near where students live, districts must do two things: (1) retain existing schools that are centrally located, and (2) look within communities instead of on their outskirts when building new schools. By prioritizing proximity of schools to students' homes, school districts can ensure the educational success, physical health, and overall well-being of students and their community.

School districts and community advocates benefit from access to national resources on school siting issues. In Billings, Montana, for instance, a school board member searched in vain for examples of strong school siting policies from state or national school board associations, ultimately contacting ChangeLab Solutions. As our staff attorneys began drafting model policies for the district to use, they participated in meetings involving the Montana School Board Association and a diverse group of personnel from planning departments, transit agencies, school districts, and smart growth organizations, as well as developers, architects, advocates of safe routes to schools, and others. This wide range of perspectives informed the work, and the Billings School Board hopes to be the first school board in the nation to adopt the model policies.

Joint Use Agreements

Many communities, particularly urban low-income and rural communities, lack access to open space, parks, and recreation facilities where residents can play and exercise safely. But almost all communities have schools with a variety of recreational facilities, like gymnasiums, playgrounds, fields, courts, and tracks. These facilities could potentially provide community members with opportunities for exercise after school hours and on weekends, if only they were open to the public. Most states have laws that encourage or even require schools to open their facilities to the community for recreation or other civic uses, but too often these are ignored by school officials who are worried about exposure to liability and about the extra maintenance and operations expenses that could be incurred.

Despite these valid concerns, many school districts around the United States routinely partner with local government agencies and nonprofit and civic organizations through what are known as "joint use" (or "shared use") agreements—formal agreements, often between a school district and a city or county agency or a local nonprofit organization, that set forth the terms and conditions for the shared use of their properties. (Note that joint use agreements can be used for more than just opening up recreational facilities. Such agreements can be used to share all kinds of governmental and community assets including libraries, theaters, and kitchens.) Commonly, these agreements address access to the recreational facilities of the partners, but often they go beyond that to provide access to kitchens for meal programs, land for community gardens, and rights of way for recreational trails. In Spokane, Washington, where the parks and recreation department owns no indoor facilities and the school district has few outdoor facilities, a joint use agreement has been in place since the early 1930s giving each partner access to the other's property as needed, sharing maintenance expenses, and indemnifying each partner from legal action. Assistance by national nonprofits is invaluable for communities across the United States looking to implement new agreements or improve existing ones; this assistance can take the form of toolkits that provide guidance on negotiating joint use agreements, a selection of sample and model contracts, or one-on-one legal and policy support.

Physical Activity in Child Care Settings

Children under the age of five are a particularly important target population for physical activity policy strategies. At this early stage of life, regular physical activity is critical not only to prevent excess weight gain and avoid chronic health problems but also to promote optimal physical, social, and psychological development (Institute of Medicine 2011). The child care setting presents an ideal opportunity to promote physical activity and the early development of healthy behaviors. The Institute of Medicine (2011) recommends that children in child care settings be given the opportunity to engage in at least 15 minutes of light, moderate, or vigorous physical activity every hour while they are in care.

Few states set physical activity requirements for child care. Only three states require that child care settings provide a specified number of minutes of physical activity per day (Benjamin et al. 2008). In Florida, the Miami-Dade County Health Department decided to work on improving standards related to physical activity, nutrition, and screen time in child care settings. Local experts on the Miami-Dade County Child Care Task Force developed model standards for child care providers. The standards are now used as a voluntary training tool for county providers, offering the potential to make a huge difference for thousands of Florida's children.

Linkage to National Physical Activity Plan

The overarching strategies of the NPAP call for a cross-sector approach that works at all levels of government and includes, at its core, a grassroots advocacy effort to create policy change. Legal and policy technical assistance can facilitate efforts to promote physical activity policy via the three strategies laid out in the NPAP recommendations for volunteer and nonprofit organizations. In table 40.1, we set out a number of examples of community-based policy change, identifying linkages to additional aspects of the NPAP.

Strategy 1: Advocate to local, state, and national decision makers for policies and system changes identified in the National Physical Activity Plan that promote physical activity. State and local government agencies—including public health departments, planning departments, parks and recreation agencies, and transportation agencies—have important roles to play in implementing and improving laws and policies related to physical activity, active transportation, and access to recreational facilities. These agencies craft and implement regulations that flesh out the laws on the books. For nonprofit actors to influence agency actions, they need to understand legal and policy issues that may arise during policy implementation and the relationships that must be in place for the policy initiative to flourish.

Community advocates can use legal technical assistance to address barriers to policy change. One example comes from New York State, involving an incident that occurred when Janette Kaddo Marino and her son biked to his middle school one day. When they arrived at the school, they were turned back by school administrators and a state trooper, who told them that they were in violation of a school policy prohibiting bicycling to school. Janette was ordered to return to campus immediately in a car to pick up her son's bike (Yusko 2009). Janette was outraged by this policy, which she believed violated common sense. Working with the Safe Routes to School National Partnership (SRTSNP), she pushed to get the policy changed. Through SRTSNP, she was connected to an attorney who explained that by regulating how students get to and from school, the school district likely exceeded the authority granted to it by the state and may have even violated parents' constitutional rights. The school board subsequently reversed this rule, instituting a new policy that allows children to walk and bike to school.

Strategy 2: Convene multisector stakeholders at local, state and national levels in strategic

Table 40.1 Examples of Community-Based Physical Activity Policy

Community action	NPAP sector and strategy	Policy area
Community advocates in a small rural community with no parks pushed the school district to allow community access to a vacant lot owned by the district. The district and the town entered into a joint use agreement in 2011 that shares the costs and responsibilities of opening the plot of land to the community. *Location: Earlimart, CA*	Education Strategy 3 Develop partnerships with other sectors for the purpose of linking youth with physical activity opportunities in schools and communities	Joint use agreements
A community-based child care task force developed physical activity and nutrition policies for child care settings and provided a policy analysis of nutrition, physical activity, and screen time regulations to state legislators to encourage the adoption of state-level policy. *Location: Miami-Dade County, FL*	Education Strategy 4 Ensure that early childhood education settings for children ages 0 to 5 years promote and facilitate physical activity	Physical activity standards in child care settings
A mother wanted her son to be able to bike to school so she petitioned her local school board to change district policy prohibiting students from biking to school. After months of concerted effort, she convinced the school board to change its policy. *Location: Saratoga Springs, NY*	Education Strategy 5 Provide access to and opportunities for physical activity before and after school	Safe Routes to School policy
A school board wanted to work more closely with the municipal planning department to encourage better land use decisions. The board worked with ChangeLab Solutions to develop school siting policies for the district and a list of 10 fundamental aspects of smart school siting for school districts and local government. *Location: Billings, MT*	Transportation Strategy 2 Prioritize resources and provide incentives to increase active transportation and other physical activity through community design, infrastructure projects, systems, policies, and initiatives	School siting policy
The City of Longmont has a program called Live Well Longmont, which facilitates healthy choices related to food and physical activity. The local collaborative focused on developing a health element for the city's comprehensive plan that promoted active transportation and opportunities for physical opportunity. *Location: Longmont, CO*	Transportation Strategy 3 Integrate land use, transportation, community design, and economic development planning with public health planning to increase active transportation	Land use planning and design for active living
The Cascade Land Conservancy spearheaded a coalition that wanted to get Complete Streets policies in place in the city of Edmonds, Washington. After over a year of determined advocacy, the council approved a Complete Streets ordinance in June 2011. *Location: Edmonds, WA*	Transportation Strategy 4 Increase connectivity and accessibility to essential community destinations to increase active transportation and other physical activity	Complete Streets policy

Technical assistance resources related to each policy area are available on the ChangeLab Solutions website: www.changelabsolutions.org.

collaborations to advance the goals of the National Physical Activity Plan. For some types of policy change, layer upon layer of interlocking, mutually supportive efforts by stakeholders are necessary. One such area involves the promotion of joint use, where many partners are involved in determining state and local policies and practices. The Strategic Alliance Promoting Healthy Food and Activity Environments is a network of stakeholders at the city, county, and state levels who develop and advance cutting-edge policies to improve healthy eating and physical activity opportunities for Californians. The Strategic Alliance was formed in 2001 by the Prevention Institute, a national nonprofit that promotes policies and collaborative efforts to improve health and quality of life. Because of the importance of joint use agreements as a strategy for promoting physical activity, the Strategic Alliance developed a Joint Use Stakeholders Task Force. The leadership and coordination of the Strategic Alliance have helped put joint use agreements into action in communities across the state. For more information, visit the website of the Strategic Alliance: http://preventioninstitute.org/strategic-alliance.

Strategy 3: Conduct outreach to nonprofit groups' members, volunteers, and constituents to change their own behaviors and advocate for policy and system changes outlined in the National Physical Activity Plan. A strong and vibrant network of groups and funders across the United States are working on physical activity policy. The diverse but complementary initiatives include the California Endowment's California Convergence (Lee et al. 2008), the Robert Wood Johnson Foundation's Childhood Obesity Prevention initiative (Strom 2007), and the U.S. Centers for Disease Control's Community Transformation Grants (U.S. Centers for Disease Control and Prevention 2012). Other national groups play leadership roles in specific spheres, like the American Planning Association, the Safe Routes to Schools National Partnership, and the National School Boards Association. The diverse range of organizations working on this issue reflects the myriad ways that physical activity needs to be incorporated into policy development.

Evidence Base Used During Program Development

The tobacco-control movement in the United States provides evidence that the law is an important driver of social norm change in the public health arena. The results have been staggeringly impressive. The state achieved a 35 percent reduction in adult smoking rates between 1988 and 2005: from 22.7 percent to 14 percent (California Department of Health Services 2006). This evidence of success has pointed to the potential for a similar social norm change approach to chronic disease prevention, including physical activity policy.

One of the most prominent initiatives building the evidence base for physical activity policy is Active Living Research (ALR), a program funded by the Robert Wood Johnson Foundation (RWJF). This program supports research examining how environments and policies affect physical activity, especially among children of color and those living in low-income communities. ALR encourages a wide array of experts—in fields as diverse as public health, public administration, law, economics, transportation, medicine, and architecture—to work together to identify promising approaches for increasing physical activity and preventing obesity among children and families. For more information about Active Living Research, go to http://activelivingresearch.org.

Given that research developing the evidence base for active living policy is ongoing, many policy strategies are being tested before science has confirmed their effectiveness. Significantly, our legal system accommodates the reality that public health interventions evolve in concert with our understanding of public health problems. Generally, there need only be a "rational basis" for laws promoting public health, rather than scientific certainty. This means that policy makers can take action to prevent obesity before the scientific community coalesces around the most effective interventions. In fact, states and localities contribute to the obesity-prevention evidence base by passing novel policies and working with researchers to evaluate the health effects of these policies. For a detailed explanation of the concept of rational basis, see Gostin (2008).

Populations Best Served by Program

Changing social norms regarding physical activity works best with strong support at the local level. As a result, legal and policy technical assistance efforts target local policy makers and agency staff as well as community-based organizations. It is important to pay particular attention to underserved communities by writing health equity language directly into a policy whenever possible. Nonprofits should incorporate tenets of the civil rights movement into their work. For example, while working on school siting policies that promote walking and biking to neighborhood schools, we identified a potential tension between these policies and desegregation efforts; in response, we asked national civil rights groups to serve as expert advisors as we worked to design policies that support schools that are walkable *and* diverse.

Lessons Learned

From our work over the past 15 years, we have identified the following key lessons for changing social norms to encourage increased physical activity:

• Take a multijurisdictional approach, paying special attention to capacity-building at the local level. When RWJF made its $500 million commitment to reverse the childhood obesity epidemic, it placed a major focus on local policy change. RWJF recognized that localities, in collaboration with states, wield significant power over how land is used, how restaurants operate, how transit is laid out, how schools function, and many other details of the built and social environment. Public health movements can build momentum at the local level through local policy change, and this local momentum can be very influential at the state and federal level.

• Invest in training and support for interagency collaboration. It is crucial to identify the links among a multitude of issues, build-

ing bridges between the policy makers who can jointly have a profound impact. City planners, public health departments, parks and recreation staff, and redevelopment agencies may not understand how and why to work together. Translating the jargon and specialized knowledge across disciplines and engaging with nontraditional partners is critical if healthier places are to be built.

• Ensure that partners at all levels understand the distinction between a physical activity program and a physical activity policy. A public health *program* is a plan that an agency implements to provide a service. A public health *policy*, in contrast, refers to a law enacted by a government at the local, state, or federal level. As interventions, policies have important advantages over programs because they have broader reach and longer-lasting impact. Through policy we can influence systems and the environment in which programs and individuals operate, affecting many more individuals and reaching them earlier. Additionally, policies are generally longer-lasting because they codify change and survive individual leadership transitions.

Summary

The time is ripe for using policy and legal strategies to change social norms and increase physical activity—particularly with growing momentum toward "Health in All Policies," an approach that requires government agencies to collaborate with each other to ensure that health is considered when policies are developed. (See, for example, California Executive Order S-04-10 [2010], which establishes a Health in All Policies Task Force.) With continued research connecting physical activity to policy strategies, as well as advocates' increasingly tenacious strategic efforts, the need for specialized legal and policy support and innovation will only become more critical in campaigns to promote physical activity in communities nationwide.

References

American Planning Association, Planning and Community Health Research Center. 2011. Comprehensive planning for public health: Results of the planning and community health research center survey. www.planning.org/research/publichealth/pdf/surveyreport.pdf.

Benjamin, S., A. Cradock, E.M. Walker, M. Slining, and M.W. Gillman. 2008. Obesity prevention in child care: A review of US state regulations. *BMC Public Health* 8(188):4-5. www.biomedcentral.com/content/pdf/1471-2458-8-188.pdf.

California Department of Health Services, Tobacco Control Section. 1998. A model for change: The California experience in tobacco control. Sacramento, CA: Department of Health Services. www.cdph.ca.gov/programs/tobacco/Documents/CTCPmodelforchange1998.pdf.

California Department of Health Services, Tobacco Control Section. 2006. Adult smoking prevalence. Sacramento, CA: Department of Health Services. www.cdph.ca.gov/programs/tobacco/Documents/CTCPAdultSmoking06.pdf.

California Executive Order S-04-10. 2010. http://sgc.ca.gov/hiap/docs/about/Executive_Order_S-04-10.pdf.

Davison, K., J. Werder, and C. Lawson. 2008. Children's active commuting to school: Current knowledge and future directions. *Prev. Chronic Dis.* 5(3):1-3.

Design Community & Environment. 2006. Understanding the relationship between public health and the built environment: A report prepared for the LEED-ND Core Committee. www.usgbc.org/ShowFile.aspx?DocumentID = 1736.

Gostin, L. 2008. *Public Health Law: Power, Duty, Restraint*. Berkeley, CA: University of California Press.

Institute of Medicine. 2001. Early childhood obesity prevention policies. www.iom.edu/Reports/2011/Early-Childhood-Obesity-Prevention-Policies.aspx.

Jackson, R., and C. Kotchtitzky. n.d. Creating a healthy environment: The impact of the built environment on public health. Washington, DC: Centers for Disease Control and Prevention. Sprawl Watch Clearinghouse. www.bvsde.paho.org/bvsacd/cd53/creating.pdf.

Lee, V., L. Mikkelsen, J. Srikantharajah, and L. Cohen. 2008. Strategies for enhancing the built environment to support healthy eating and active living.

Convergence Partnership. www.calendow.org/uploadedFiles/Publications/Publications_Stories/builtenvironment.pdf.

Marshall, G., Ed. 1998. A dictionary of sociology. Oxford, UK: Oxford University Press. www.encyclopedia.com/doc/1O88-norm.html.

Martin, S., S. Lee, and R. Lowry. 2007. National prevalence and correlates of walking and bicycling to school. *Am. J. Prev. Med.* 33(2):98-105.

McDonald, N., A. Brown, L. Marchetti, and M. Pedroso. 2011. U.S. school travel 2009: An assessment of trends. *Am. J. Prev. Med.* 41(2):146.

National Complete Streets Coalition. Complete Streets FAQ. 2010. www.completestreets.org/complete-streets-fundamentals/complete-streets-faq.

National Policy & Legal Analysis Network to Prevent Childhood Obesity. 2010. Resources on safe routes to school programs. Oakland, CA: ChangeLab Solutions. http://changelabsolutions.org/childhood-obesity/safe-routes-schools.

Ogden, C.L., M.D. Carroll, and K.M. Flegal. 2008. High body mass index for age among US children and adolescents, 2003-2006. *JAMA.* 299(20):2401-5.

Strom, S. 2007, April 4. $500 million pledged to fight childhood obesity. *New York Times.* www.nytimes.com/2007/04/04/health/04obesity.html.

U.S. Centers for Disease Control and Prevention. 2012. Community transformation grants. www.cdc.gov/communitytransformation/index.htm.

U.S. Department of Health and Human Services, Centers for Disease Control and Prevention. 2008. KidsWalk: Then and now—barriers and solutions. www.cdc.gov/nccdphp/dnpa/kidswalk/then_and_now.htm.

U.S. Department of Transportation. 2008. National Household Travel Survey. Travel to school: The distance factor. www.saferoutesinfo.org/program-tools/travel-school-distance-factor.

Yusko, D. 2009, September 29. School district could backpedal on policy. *The Times Union.* www.timesunion.com/local/article/School-district-could-backpedal-on-policy-557196.php#ixzz1aJzX5pMb.

Zhang, X., D. Cowling, and H. Tang. 2010. The impact of social norm change strategies on smokers' quitting behaviours. *Tobacco Control* 19(Suppl. 1):i51. http://tobaccocontrol.bmj.com/content/19/Suppl_1/i51.full.pdf.

CHAPTER 41

Reducing Barriers to Activity Among Special Populations
LIVESTRONG at the YMCA

Haley Justice-Gardiner, MPH, CHES
The LIVESTRONG Foundation

Ann-Hilary Heston, MPA
YMCA of the USA

NPAP Tactics and Strategies Used in This Program

Health Care Sector

STRATEGY 1: Expand research that identifies and evaluates best practices for physical activity in health care, particularly those effective in population segments at high risk of physical inactivity. Disseminate current best-practice guidelines for promoting physical activity in high-risk subpopulations. Include approaches relevant to primary, secondary, and tertiary prevention.

Public Health Sector

STRATEGY 2: Create, maintain, and leverage cross-sector partnerships and coalitions that implement effective strategies to promote physical activity.

Parks, Recreation, Fitness, and Sports Sector

STRATEGY 1: Promote programs and facilities where people work, learn, live, play, and worship (i.e., workplace, public, private, and nonprofit recreational sites) to provide easy access to safe and affordable physical activity opportunities.

This chapter describes a collaboration between two national nonprofit organizations that developed an initiative designed to improve physical activity among cancer survivors by building the capacity of fitness professionals and creating safe and supportive environments in which survivors can exercise.

LIVE**STRONG** at the YMCA is a 12-week, small-group program designed for adult cancer survivors. The program supports the increasing number of cancer survivors who are seeking physical activity programs to help them cope with the emotional and physical effects of cancer treatment. The program is conducted outside of medical facilities to emphasize that LIVE**STRONG** at the YMCA is about health, not disease. The goal of the program is to help participants build muscle mass and strength, increase flexibility and endurance, and improve functional ability. Additional goals include reducing the severity of therapy side effects, preventing unwanted weight changes, and improving energy levels and self-esteem. A final goal of the program is to assist participants in developing their own physical fitness program so they can continue to practice a healthy lifestyle, not only as part of their recovery but as a way of life. In addition to providing physical benefits, the program gives participants a supportive environment and a feeling of community with their fellow survivors and YMCA staff and members. YMCA fitness instructors work with each participant to tailor the program to his or her individual needs. The instructors are trained to provide postrehabilitation exercise and supportive cancer care.

Program Description

LIVE**STRONG** at the YMCA is part of a multiyear collaboration between YMCA of the USA, the national resource office for the Y, and the LIVE**STRONG** Foundation, an organization dedicated to improving the lives of people affected with cancer. The Foundation is known for its powerful brand LIVE**STRONG** and is a leader in the global movement to fight cancer on behalf of 28 million people around the world living with the disease. The Y is one of the leading nonprofits in the United States working to improve health through community-based initiatives that support healthy living. LIVE**STRONG** at the YMCA, launched in 2008, is designed to improve health and day-to-day quality of life for the increasing population of cancer survivors and their families in the United States by providing supportive environments and experiences in a safe setting.

The program evolved from the desire of the LIVE**STRONG** Foundation and the YMCA of the USA to provide support to this growing population and to address the need for safe and effective physical activity options for individuals diagnosed with cancer. According to the National Coalition for Cancer Survivorship, cancer survivorship begins at the point of diagnosis and continues throughout the balance of a person's life. Friends, family members, and caregivers are also considered cancer survivors. Participation in the LIVE**STRONG** at the YMCA program is limited to individuals who have been diagnosed with cancer; however, many Ys extend a free family membership to program participants, providing an opportunity for family members or caregivers access to health-related/physical activity programming. In 2007, the organizations convened a group of experts

in cancer survivorship—researchers, academicians, and public and private practitioners and administrators. These experts helped identify and define a series of gaps in service for cancer survivors that YMCAs could fill:

- Target population: YMCAs should make an effort to understand and reach out to health-seeking cancer survivors in their communities.
- Relationships: YMCAs should look to develop genuine, caring relationships with and among cancer survivors in their communities.
- Program: YMCAs should offer a variety of programs, activities, clubs, and events developed with and for cancer survivors.
- Staff competency: YMCA staff should have a special understanding of and skills to support cancer survivors in their pursuit of health and well-being.
- Environment: YMCA environments should be conducive to cancer survivors' pursuit of health and well-being.
- Partnerships: YMCAs should build partnerships with targeted organizations in the cancer community to better support the cancer survivor population.

In 2008 and 2009, two cohorts of 10 YMCAs sought ways to close these gaps, including piloting physical activity programs for cancer survivors using the Institute for Healthcare Improvement's Breakthrough Series. This series is an evidence-based model designed to help organizations achieve breakthrough innovations to better meet the needs and interests of their constituents. Through this formal learning process, the YMCAs worked at both their local facility and collectively with the other cohort members to develop leading practices and a signature program, LIVE**STRONG** at the YMCA. These leading practices are now a part of a six-month learning and implementation process that YMCAs must commit to in order to offer LIVE**STRONG** at the YMCA.

YMCAs chosen to participate in this learning and implementation process must meet minimum criteria, demonstrating their capacity and willingness to develop and sustain LIVE**STRONG** at the YMCA. After selection,

YMCAs engage in activities to close the previously listed gaps, including creating and enhancing partnerships in the oncology community, training program leaders, and modifying the environments in their YMCAs. Participating YMCAs must agree to follow program standards, including ensuring required staff competencies and offering LIVE**STRONG** at the YMCA at no charge to participants.

LIVE**STRONG** at the YMCA engages cancer survivors through an approach that focuses on the whole person. Survivors work with trained Y staff to build muscle mass and strength, increase flexibility and endurance, and improve functional ability. In addition to providing physical benefits, the program focuses on the emotional well-being of survivors and their families by providing a supportive community environment where people affected by cancer can connect during treatment and beyond. As a result of their commitment to and focus on cancer survivors, YMCAs have achieved some notable organizational changes:

• Program expansion to additional YMCA branches within the association: Many YMCAs are associations, made up of several branches. Most YMCAs initially engage one to three branches in the learning and implementation process. Upon seeing the success of their colleagues, leaders at nonparticipating branches often seek to become involved, expanding the program throughout the YMCA's service area.

• Development of programs: Recognizing that they could meet additional needs, wants, and interests of cancer survivors and their loved ones, many YMCAs increased their program offerings. Several, like YMCA of the Treasure Valley in Boise, Idaho, now offer a menu of cancer survivorship programs, including yoga, aquatics, a family cancer program, a cancer lecture series, a support group for caregivers, and cancer screening events.

• Partnership growth: Although the YMCA has long been a key community member, it had never before been seen as a credible player in the field of cancer survivorship resources and support. Having developed partnerships with local hospitals, oncology centers, and cancer service organizations like the American Cancer Society, the YMCA is becoming known in local communities as a valued and respected partner in the long-term care of cancer survivors.

• Increased volunteerism: Many who participate in LIVE**STRONG** at the YMCA seek to give back to the program that has meant so much to them.

• Membership conversion: The majority of LIVE**STRONG** at the YMCA participants are nonmembers, many never having been regular exercisers. Following their participation in the program, many elect to continue their health and well-being journey with the YMCA and become members.

• Laying the basis for work with other special populations: Having proved their ability to address the needs, wants, and interests of cancer survivors, YMCAs are now being invited to translate their expertise to other special populations, including those with diabetes, multiple sclerosis, heart disease, and stroke, all of whom can benefit from physically active lifestyles.

The number of YMCAs around the United States offering the LIVE**STRONG** at the YMCA program continues to increase. By the end of 2012, LIVE**STRONG** at the YMCA was offered at more than 250 Ys around the country. To date, approximately 13,000 cancer survivors have participated in the program nationwide. YMCA of the USA and the LIVE**STRONG** Foundation will continue to engage YMCAs in the six-month learning process in order to deliver LIVE**STRONG** at the YMCA to additional communities. With YMCAs in more than 2,600 locations, serving more than 10,000 communities, the YMCA and the Foundation are poised to make a real difference in the lives of cancer survivors throughout the country.

Linkage to the National Physical Activity Plan

LIVE**STRONG** at the YMCA advances a variety of strategies and tactics of the National Physical Activity Plan, including those within the sectors of health care; public health; and parks, recreation, fitness, and sports. These include the following:

Health Care Strategy 1: Expand research that identifies and evaluates best practices for physical activity in health care, particularly those effective in population segments at high risk of physical inactivity. Disseminate current best-practice guidelines for promoting physical activity in high-risk subpopulations. Include approaches relevant to primary, secondary, and tertiary prevention. Evidence suggests the importance of a physically active lifestyle for individuals undergoing cancer treatment as well as for those who have finished treatment. LIVE**STRONG** at the YMCA sought to expand existing research showing that physical activity was not only safe but feasible, during and after treatment, and to disseminate an effective program through the nationwide Y network. Individuals who have been diagnosed with cancer are important audiences for such a program, as many are at high risk of physical inactivity, and inactivity may increase the risk of recurrence as well as the risk of developing other types of cancer.

Public Health Sector Strategy 2: Create, maintain, and leverage cross-sector partnerships and coalitions that implement effective strategies to promote physical activity. Working with multiple partners, representing researchers, academicians, and public and private practitioners and administrators, the Y and the LIVE**STRONG** Foundation collaborated to create, evaluate, and disseminate an effective physical activity program. The program has resulted in additional local partnerships that further support healthy, active lifestyles among individuals who have been diagnosed with cancer.

Parks, Recreation, Fitness, and Sports Strategy 1: Promote programs and facilities where people work, learn, live, play, and worship (i.e., workplace, public, private, and nonprofit recreational sites) to provide easy access to safe and affordable physical activity opportunities. The Y has worked extensively with national and local partners to promote LIVE**STRONG** at the YMCA (figure 41.1).

Evidence Base Used During Program Development

Current cancer treatments, although increasingly efficacious for improving survival, are toxic in numerous ways and produce negative short- and long-term physiological and psychological effects, including pain, decreased cardiorespiratory capacity, cancer-related fatigue, reduced quality of life, and suppressed immune function (Courneya and Freidenreich 2001).

Since the first research study on cancer patients and exercise was conducted in 1986, a growing body of evidence has demonstrated that exercise during and after cancer treatment is safe and minimizes the adverse effects of treatment. However, clinicians have historically advised cancer survivors to rest and to avoid activity.

In 2009, the American College of Sports Medicine (ACSM) assembled a roundtable of experts to review the body of evidence supporting the benefits of exercise among cancer survivors and to develop guidelines that could be used by fitness instructors and trainers. The ACSM recommendations for cancer survivors are the same as those from the U.S. Department of Health and Human Services Physical Activity Guidelines for Americans (age-appropriate) as well as those from the American Cancer Society:

Undertake 150 minutes per week of moderate to intense exercise or 75 minutes per week of vigorous exercise.

Engage in strength training 2 or 3 times a week, completing 8 to 10 exercises of 10 to 15 repetitions per set, with at least one set per session.

Avoid inactivity.

Return to normal daily activities as quickly as possible.

Continue normal daily activities and exercise as much as possible during and after non-surgical treatments.

When making modifications to exercise regimens, practitioners must assess an individual's cancer type, treatment, and side effects. The LIVE**STRONG** at the YMCA program was developed to respond to the need for exercise

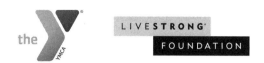

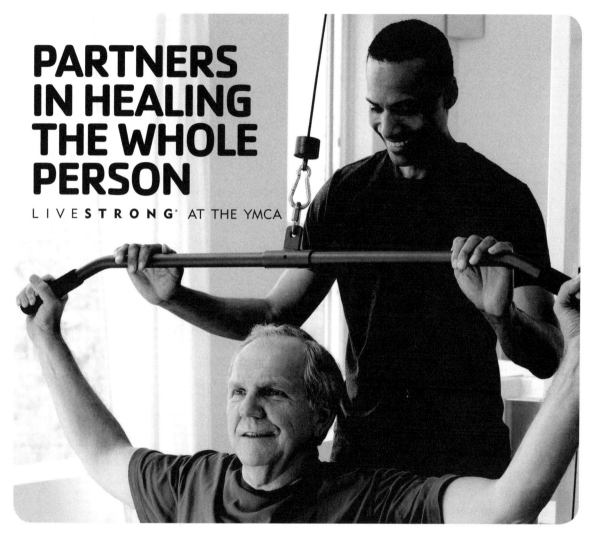

**PARTNERS
IN HEALING
THE WHOLE
PERSON**

LIVE**STRONG** AT THE YMCA

Cancer is a life-changing disease that takes a tremendous physical and emotional toll on those affected. The Y and LIVESTRONG have joined together to create LIVESTRONG at the YMCA, a research-based physical activity and well-being program designed to help adult cancer survivors reclaim their total health.

Participants work with Y staff trained in supportive cancer care to safely achieve their goals such as building muscle mass and strength; increasing flexibility and endurance; and improving confidence and self-esteem. By focusing on the whole person and not the disease, LIVESTRONG at the YMCA is helping people move beyond cancer in spirit, mind and body.

To learn more about LIVESTRONG at the YMCA,
contact: WWW.LIVESTRONG.ORG/YMCA

Figure 41.1 LIVE**STRONG** at the YMCA flier.

opportunities for cancer survivors and adheres to the ACSM cancer exercise guidelines.

Lessons Learned

Through its national dissemination of LIVE**STRONG** at the YMCA, the Y and the LIVE**STRONG** Foundation have learned many lessons that have helped strengthen the program model and aid in program expansion. An initial, important lesson was that successful programming requires staff who have a deep understanding and empathy for cancer survivors in their communities.

Although the process of developing and delivering LIVE**STRONG** at the YMCA has evolved from experimental to more prescriptive, implementation of the program in individual communities and environments requires Ys to be flexible and adaptable to meet the wants, needs, and interests of cancer survivors in their community. To that end, Ys must listen to and learn from cancer survivors, via one-on-one interviews and focus groups, before launching programs and services. This period of discovery not only is foundational to staff awareness but also builds and deepens staff empathy, a key competency for those who will connect and engage with cancer survivors.

A second lesson learned was that Ys must earn credibility with cancer survivors in their communities. Although the YMCA is uniquely suited to provide this program because of its commitment to community outreach and focus on those who need support to gain or regain health, the YMCA has had to establish its credibility as an organization with expertise in cancer survivorship. In a national survey of cancer survivors, the majority believed that a physical activity program at the Y was a good idea, but they wanted to know that it had the backing of their physician or local oncology center and that the instructors were well qualified. Offering the program at no charge was an important factor for often cash-strapped survivors. The Y and the LIVE**STRONG** Foundation have worked hard to ensure that LIVE**STRONG** at the YMCA meets these criteria, building

active partnerships with local agencies that serve cancer survivors, creating a rigorous staff training process, and providing programs at low or no cost to cancer survivors.

A final lesson learned was that before offering the physical activity program, Ys must ensure that their environments are safe and supportive for cancer survivors. Staff of each participating Y must be sure that its atmosphere supports cancer survivors' physical, social, and emotional needs. This insight has led to a variety of changes in facilities: shortening the distance cancer survivors must travel to get into or through the building; installing handrails in hallways and stairways; providing hand gel sanitizer dispensers throughout the facility; having a "resting" or "support" chair in workout areas and changing areas; providing an area where private conversations can be held; and enlisting members in ensuring facilities are clean and germ-free for cancer survivor participants.

Populations Best Served by the Program

The National Cancer Institute estimates that there are more than 13 million cancer survivors living in the United States today. With 1 in 2 men and 1 in 3 women predicted to be diagnosed with cancer in their lifetimes, the need for services that focus on quality of life during and after treatment is increasingly important. Because current evidence suggests that being physically active following diagnosis may reduce the risk of recurrence of some types of cancer, offering programs that encourage and support survivors in living a physically active lifestyle is increasingly important.

LIVE**STRONG** at the YMCA is designed for in-treatment or posttreatment cancer survivors. The program is available in more than 226 cities and more than 250 branches. More than 13,000 individuals have completed the LIVE**STRONG** at the YMCA program, and the LIVE**STRONG** Foundation and the YMCA of the USA are seeking to extend the program to more facilities. The hope is that cancer survivors will have access to a community-based program that is designed to meet their needs, help them establish a healthy lifestyle that will improve their quality of life, and ultimately reduce the risk of cancer recurrence and the development of a second primary cancer.

Program Evaluation

Cancer survivors who participate in LIVE**STRONG** at the YMCA engage in pre- to postprogram functional and quality of life assessments. Functional assessments measure participants' strength, aerobic capacity, balance, and flexibility. Results from a sample 12-week session of LIVE**STRONG** at the YMCA showed the following:

- 56 percent improvement in leg strength
- 45 percent improvement in upper body strength
- 60 percent improvement in aerobic capacity (treadmill or bicycle ergometer time to fatigue)

A 29-question life assessment asks participants to rate their physical functioning, anxiety, depression, fatigue, sleep disturbance, satisfaction with social role, pain interference, and pain intensity. Quality of life assessment scores have not yet been compiled for evaluation.

Participants also complete a post-program survey. A sample of more than 100 of these surveys showed the following:

- 92 percent agree that they have made progress related to their health and well-being goals as a result of their participation in LIVE**STRONG** at the YMCA.
- 86 percent agree that they are part of a supportive community at the YMCA (as defined by four measures).
- 92 percent agree that their program leader has the understanding and skills needed to lead a physical activity program for cancer survivors.
- 93 percent plan to continue their health and well-being journey at the YMCA after the end of the program.

94 percent are highly likely to recommend LIVE**STRONG** at the YMCA to a friend or family member.

The physical benefits are great, but the social and emotional aspects of the program seem to be the most meaningful to cancer survivors. The following quotation is an example of the profound impact that LIVE**STRONG** at the YMCA has had on many cancer survivors' overall well-being:

> This class changed my life. When you get the diagnosis, everything is so bleak—and then they tell you that you can't lift more than five pounds, and it is even more depressing. I felt very alone and then I came to the Y. This class is a community for me. I love it and am happy and thankful that I get to do it. I am so privileged to have had it; I believe it saved my life. This class gave me back my life, my sense of self, hope, and camaraderie and made me a stronger me. It improved my life and my mental outlook.

The program had a positive effect not only on cancer survivors but on YMCA staff members as well. One chief operating officer shared this about his involvement with LIVE**STRONG** at the YMCA:

> At times we can become so overwhelmed with balancing budgets, building facilities, developing marketing tools, and managing staff that we forget why we are part of this mission-driven organization. My involvement with LIVE**STRONG** at the YMCA has allowed me to catch my breath and reconnect with the YMCA mission in a whole new way through the life-changing work that is being done in our YMCAs with cancer survivors.

With YMCAs in more than 10,000 communities across the United States, the potential impact of this program is tremendous. The YMCAs that have engaged in this work describe the experience as game-changing for the YMCA and life-changing for the staff involved. YMCAs are queued up for the chance to invest their own money and six months of their staff time to participate in this program that often transforms the way a YMCA functions and operates.

Additional Reading and Resources

Free Resources

American College of Sports Medicine Cancer Exercise Guidelines: http://journals.lww.com/acsm-msse/Fulltext/2010/07000/American_College_of_Sports_Medicine_Roundtable_on.23.aspxAmerican Cancer Society: www.cancer.org

CA: A Cancer Journal of Clinicians: http://onlinelibrary.wiley.com/doi/10.3322/caac.21142/pdf

The LIVE**STRONG** Foundation: www.LIVE**STRONG**.org/wecanhelp or www.LIVE**STRONG**.org/ymca

National Lymphedema Network: www.lymphnet.org

National Cancer Institute: www.cancer.gov/cancertopics/factsheet/Risk/obesity

www.cancer.gov/cancertopics/pdq/supportivecare/nutrition

www.cancer.gov/cancertopics/chemotherapy-and-you

www.cancer.gov/cancertopics/factsheet/Detection/staging

www.cancer.gov/cancertopics/factsheet/Sites-Types/metastatic

http://riskfactor.cancer.gov/areas/weight/

Journal Articles

Rock, C.L., C. Doyle, W. Demark-Wahnefried, J. Meyerhardt, K.S. Courneya, A.L. Schwartz, E.V. Bandera, K.K. Hamilton, B. Grant, M. McCullough, T. Byers, and T. Gansler. 2012. Nutrition and physical activity guidelines for cancer survivors. *CA: A Cancer Journal for Clinicians.* http://caonline.amcancersoc.org.

Schmitz, K. 2005. Controlled physical activity trials in cancer survivors: A systematic review and meta-analysis. *Cancer Epidemiol. Biomarkers Prev.* 14(7):1588-95. http://cebp.aacrjournals.org/cgi/content/full/14/7/1588?maxtoshow = &HITS = 10 &hits = 10&RESULTFORMAT = &author1 = Schmitz %2C + K&searchid = 1&FIRSTINDEX = 0&resourcetype = HWCIT.

Lawlor, D., K. Fox, and C. Stevinson. 2004. Exercise interventions for cancer patients: Systemic review of controlled trials. *Cancer Causes Control* 15:1035-56. www.jstor.org/pss/3553586.

Textbooks

ACSM's Exercise Management for Persons with Chronic Diseases and Disabilities J. Larry Durstine and Geoffrey Moore. Human Kinetics, Champaign, IL. www.humankinetics.com

Breast Cancer Recovery Exercise Program, 2nd ed. Anna Schwartz & Naomi Aaronson. Desert Southwest Fitness. www.dswfitness.com

Cancer Fitness: Exercise Programs for Patients and Survivors. Anna Schwartz. Simon & Schuster. www.simonsays.com

Exercise and Cancer Recovery. Carol Schneider, Carolyn Dennehy, Susan Carter. Human Kinetics, Champaign, IL. www.humankinetics.com

Handbook of Cancer Survivorship. Michael Feuerstein (Ed). Springer, New York, NY. www.springer.com/public + health/book/978-0-387-34561-1

Cancer Symptom Management, 3rd ed. Connie Henke Yarbro, Margaret Hansen Frogge, Michelle Goodman. Jones and Barlett Publishers, Sudbury, MA. www.jbpub.com/catalog/9780763721428/

Cancer Prevention and Management Through Exercise and Weight Control. Anne McTiernan (Ed). Taylor & Francis Group. www.taylorandfrancis.com

References

Courneya, K.S., and C.M. Freidenreich. 2001. Framework PEACE: An organizational model for examining physical exercise across the cancer experience. *Ann. Behav. Med.* 23:263-72.

CHAPTER 42

New York State Healthy Eating and Physical Activity Alliance

Michael Seserman, MPH, RD
American Cancer Society

Nancy Huehnergarth
*New York State Healthy Eating
and Physical Activity Alliance*

NPAP Tactics and Strategies Used in This Program

Volunteer and Nonprofit Sector

STRATEGY 1: Advocate to local, state, and national decision makers for policies and system changes identified in the National Physical Activity Plan that promote physical activity.

STRATEGY 2: Convene multisector stakeholders at local, state, and national levels in strategic collabora-

tions to advance the goals of the National Physical Activity Plan.

STRATEGY 3: Conduct outreach to nonprofit groups' members, volunteers, and constituents to change their own behaviors and advocate for policy and system changes outlined in the National Physical Activity Plan.

This chapter describes a nonprofit, state-based coalition designed to advance statewide physical activity (and nutrition) policy priorities. The New York State Healthy Eating and Physical Activity Alliance (NYSHEPA) was founded in November 2006 as a statewide partnership dedicated to improving policies and practices that promote healthy eating and physical activity. NYSHEPA is designed to unite like-minded organizations and individuals who are involved in obesity prevention, nutrition, and fitness into one state-level voice in support of the organization's mission. The primary focus of the alliance is policy and environmental changes to support dietary improvement and active living. NYSHEPA's goals are these:

- Enhance communication and coordination among New York State (NYS) organizations and individuals working to improve nutrition and physical activity.

- Increase funding for obesity prevention efforts in NYS.

- Improve NYS policies that promote healthier eating, including those that encourage breastfeeding.

- Improve physical education and physical activity policies and practices in NYS.

Program Description

In 2005, American Cancer Society (ACS) Eastern Division staff met with representatives from the New York State Department of Health's (NYSDOH) obesity prevention program to discuss implementation of the state's obesity prevention plan. Many of the objectives of the plan involved policy changes, and NYSDOH clearly needed the support of the voluntary and nonprofit sector to support plan implementation. ACS had already been a part of the planning group for the obesity prevention plan and had hosted many of the community forums across the state that helped to identify and prioritize the plan's strategies. By the end of the meeting, it became clear to ACS that a state coalition should be developed to support improvements in nutrition and physical activity policies. ACS had experience working with such a coalition; a decade earlier, ACS initiated and continues to spearhead a state tobacco control partnership to advance tobacco policy changes in New York (Coalition for a Healthy NY—originally funded by the Robert Wood Johnson Foundation's SmokeLess States grant).

The following year, ACS staff met with a local volunteer from Westchester who had cofounded a local school health coalition and implemented a successful regional conference on the subject. The volunteer had ambitions of forming a statewide coalition to more aggressively take on the issue of school nutrition and, more broadly, childhood obesity. There was strong agreement that most nutrition and physical activity organizations across New York had little or no influence in Albany, the state capital, where important obesity-related policy decisions needed to be made. Therefore, ACS and the volunteer decided to work together to establish a state policy-focused nutrition and physical activity coalition. The new organization would be based on both the Coalition for a Healthy NY and the Strategic Alliance of California, a successful coalition led by the Prevention Institute.

After many discussions and drafts, a group that consisted of ACS staff and the volunteer drafted a planning document and presentation that could be shared with potential partners. The planning document included a suggested vision, mission, goals, and guiding principles. The group also proposed a simple structure, initial objectives, and a name for the new group: the New York State Healthy Eating and Physical Activity Alliance, or NYSHEPA (nye-shep-a). One of the group's key recommendations was to preserve the coalition's credibility and independence by not accepting funds from the food or beverage industry.

ACS used its position on the planning committee for a NYSDOH Childhood Obesity Summit to be held in November 2006 in Albany to plan a meeting to propose NYSHEPA to other nonprofit, stakeholder organizations. The meeting included a briefing by the director of the Coalition for a Healthy NY on the process and success of that state partnership. Some of the same nonprofit representatives at the meeting also served on the Coalition for a Healthy NY, vouched for the strategy, and helped promote the idea.

All of the groups that attended the meeting agreed on the need for the new group and became the founding steering committee for NYSHEPA. Although the committee made a few minor changes, it accepted the draft mission and planning document. There was no desire to develop bylaws or other complicated rules of governance. The focus was, and continues to be, simply coming together to move statewide policy change forward, to keep constituents informed, and to mobilize those in support of this agenda.

Founding steering committee for NYSHEPA

- American Cancer Society
- American Heart Association
- American Academy of Pediatrics NYS
- NYS PTA
- Be Active New York State
- NYS Nurses Association
- YMCA of New York State
- NYS Dietetic Association
- Schuyler Center for Analysis and Advocacy
- NYS Public Health Association

The volunteer who developed the original vision for a statewide coalition became the director of NYSHEPA and took responsibility for facilitating and coordinating all meetings. ACS became the chair of the steering committee. These leaders established a schedule of monthly meetings or calls to collaborate on the alliance's priorities.

Initial tasks completed to support NYSHEPA included developing an informational website (www.nyshepa.org), creating a comprehensive database of stakeholders and supporters, and prioritizing a list of state and local policies to support.

Since that time, NYSHEPA has been at the forefront of nutrition and physical activity policy change by reaching out to constituents, legislators, and the media to help frame the debate. NYSHEPA representatives have spoken regularly on television and radio and in print about nutrition and physical activity issues and policies. NYSHEPA has generated frequent press releases and held numerous press conferences to increase media coverage of policy options regarding obesity prevention and nutrition and physical activity. Likewise, the NYSHEPA director and steering committee members have generated dozens of letters to the editor and editorials in publications like the *New York Times, Albany Times Union, Buffalo News, Journal News, LI Newsday, Rochester Democrat and Chronicle,* and *Syracuse Post Standard.*

NYSHEPA has created and disseminated fact sheets on numerous nutrition and physical activity policies to assist advocates across the state. The policy documents and other information are distributed via www.nyshepa.org. Regular updates and action alerts on nutrition and physical activity issues and policies also are provided to NYSHEPA members. In 2009, NYSHEPA and the New York State Department of Health received 1 of only 10 grants of its kind from the National Governors Association to work on obesity prevention. As part of that project, NYSHEPA developed an after-school toolkit to improve nutrition and physical activity policies and practices in after-school programs.

Although nutrition policy took the forefront in the early years, more recently NYSHEPA became involved in the campaign to pass Complete Streets legislation. Complete Streets policies require that most new or reconstructed roads be accessible to all users, not just motor vehicles. Another important physical activity–related policy that NYSHEPA supported was the Smart Growth and Public Infrastructure bill. This bill mandates that all state agencies and authorities with funding for infrastructure, such as the Department of Transportation, prioritize their funding and implement decisions using smart growth criteria. Smart growth principles promote more densely populated, multiuse

community designs with a greater emphasis on public transportation, all of which are associated with increases in physical activity.

To date, NYSHEPA has built a statewide coalition and network of more than 800 public health, consumer, and education organizations and individuals dedicated to improving policies and practices that promote healthier eating and physical activity. To that end, NYSHEPA has mobilized and led advocacy efforts across the state. For instance, NYSHEPA organized memos of support for numerous policies, including menu labeling, school nutrition standards, the Green Carts program, Complete Streets, Safe Routes to School funding, the sugar sweetened beverage tax, the Breastfeeding Bill of Rights, and increased funding for obesity prevention.

To further advance a policy agenda that supports active living, NYSHEPA convened a Built Environment Task Force to develop a strategic plan for statewide built environment policy change. A wide range of expert stakeholders participated in the process and produced two documents laying out NYSHEPA's statewide physical activity priorities; one publication was used to educate policy makers and the other to guide and mobilize advocates. The built environment policies identified as priorities included promoting Complete Streets, amending a law that undermines children's walking or bicycling to school, encouraging smart growth, increasing green space, and using health impact assessments.

In 2010, NYSHEPA helped to pass the Smart Growth and Public Infrastructure bill described earlier. During the 2011 legislative session, the Complete Streets bill also was signed into law. Another statewide policy that passed in 2011 has the potential to support physical activity. The Land Bank Act provides localities with new tools to bundle abandoned properties for sale or other uses. As a result, new parks, green space, and other recreation areas could be created by local governments. Access to and promotion of recreational areas have been shown to increase physical activity in a community (Community Preventive Services Task Force 2010).

NYSHEPA also initiated a close working relationship with the NYS Office of the State Comptroller and successfully encouraged the comptroller to audit school compliance with NYS physical education requirements, which are among the toughest in the nation. The results were startling; the comptroller found only 1 of 20 schools audited to be in compliance with state law. NYSHEPA also encouraged the comptroller to audit competitive foods sold in schools. Consequently, in 2009 and 2012, the NYS Office of the State Comptroller released childhood obesity reports that included a recommendation to "take steps necessary to bring physical education programs into compliance with state regulations."

Because of its extensive advocacy work, in 2010 NYSHEPA was awarded the New York Public Health Community Advocacy Award by the Public Health Association of New York City. Despite its successes, however, NYSHEPA has not received consistent funding. A lack of funding for advocacy by state coalitions on nutrition and physical activity is a major barrier to promotion of physical activity policies. A state coalition model focused on physical activity and other public health policies has proven to be an extremely cost-effective strategy and should be replicated in every state.

Program Evaluation

No formal evaluation of NYSHEPA has been conducted. However, since late 2006, when NYSHEPA was created, tremendous progress has taken place in NYS on food- and physical activity–related policy change that exceeds changes in most other states. New York City, where NYSHEPA also has focused, and New York State in general, are now widely recognized nationally as leaders in nutrition and physical activity policy and supportive environments.

Populations Best Served by the Program

The primary target audience for this type of program is policy makers at the state and local level who make decisions regarding physical activity–related policy. NYSHEPA also targets the general public and constituents of health groups across the state to urge them to take

action in support of policies such as Complete Streets legislation. This type of grassroots education or mobilization takes place via letters to the editors in newspapers located in key political districts or by action alerts to NYSHEPA members and member organizations.

Linkage to National Physical Activity Plan

As a nonprofit organization, NYSHEPA has worked with other organizations to advance all of the strategies recommended within the Volunteer and Nonprofit Sector of the National Physical Activity Plan:

Strategy 1: Advocate to local, state, and national decision makers for policies and system changes identified in the National Physical Activity Plan that promote physical activity. NYSHEPA advocated for a Complete Streets bill in the state legislature for three years.

Strategy 2: Convene multisector stakeholders at local, state, and national levels in strategic collaborations to advance the goals of the National Physical Activity Plan. NYSHEPA convened the Built Environment Task Force to collaborate on a strategic plan to advance physical activity in NYS by creating environments that facilitate and support active living. NYSHEPA recruited additional stakeholder nonprofits, such as AARP, Green Options, and Transportation Alternatives, from across the state to join the Task Force.

Strategy 3: Conduct outreach to nonprofit groups' members, volunteers, and constituents to change their own behaviors and advocate for policy and system changes outlined in the National Physical Activity Plan. NYSHEPA organizational members regularly communicate with their own members and constituents to educate them on priority policy issues and encourage them to become involved in policy issues that affect them in their communities.

Evidence Base Used During Program Development

As mentioned previously, the development of NYSHEPA was informed by the SmokeLess

States National Policy Initiative of the Robert Wood Johnson Foundation, which funded state coalitions between 1993 and 2004. A program evaluation released in 2005 reported the following results:

- Coalition policy campaigns, underwritten by matching funds, led to increased excise taxes in 35 SmokeLess States, clean indoor air legislation in 10 states, and ordinances to restrict youth access to tobacco products in 13 states.

- Eight coalitions defeated or blocked pre-emption bills and four states repealed or partially repealed preemption.

- The SmokeLess States grantees secured funds (at least $10 million) for comprehensive tobacco prevention and control programs from the $206 billion Master Settlement Agreement with the tobacco industry, signed in 1998 (Gillespie 2009).

The parallel, peer-reviewed literature from tobacco control also supports a policy-based approach using state and local collaboration. The Centers for Disease Control and Prevention's *Best Practices for Comprehensive Tobacco Control Programs,* originally released in 1999 and updated in 2007, provides ample justification and citations supporting state- and community-level coalitions to facilitate collaboration for social norm and policy change.

In the area of nutrition and physical activity, NYSHEPA was modeled after a successful state coalition in California called the Strategic Alliance, run by the Prevention Institute. Since 2001, when the statewide partnership was created, the Strategic Alliance has led or made major contributions to many state policy achievements. These successes include making California the first state in the country to require menu labeling at chain restaurants; establishing, in 2005, the most rigorous nutrient standards in the nation for foods sold outside of school meals; banning the sale of sodas, K-12, in California's schools; and passing a parks and water quality bond that provided funds for the development of open space and parks in communities that currently lack space for active play (Strategic Alliance n.d.).

Lessons Learned

The NYSHEPA experience in New York illustrates the effectiveness of deliberate and strategic statewide collaboration and coordination among nonprofit health organizations to promote physical activity– and nutrition-related policy interventions. It also demonstrates the advantage of having a lead organization that can facilitate the drafting of legislative support memos and the compilation of signatures across multiple sectors to support a particular bill.

One of the key lessons learned for developing and maintaining a policy-minded coalition is that a strong and committed leader must be identified. As occurs with any collaboration, natural ebbs and flow occur in the levels of involvement, camaraderie, success, and funding. NYSHEPA's experience shows that commitment, determination, and long-term perspective among its leadership and, especially, its director are very important. For example, when funding dries up, someone must take the lead to seek out and apply for new funding sources. Someone must continue to maintain the coalition at a minimal level. In NYSHEPA's case, the director and the American Cancer Society took that role, with some help from other partners.

The coalition leader must possess good communication and negotiation skills in order to gain enough agreement among steering committee members for the coalition to take a position on a bill. Every organization has a representative with an opinion. Some, often the same few, will express that opinion forcefully, but other groups on the steering committee will at times need to be pushed to take a supportive or opposing position on a state issue. Perhaps a local representative of a national organization can't take a position because policy decisions are made by national leadership. Sometimes the issue is simply not a priority or there is not agreement within an organization. For some participants, legislative advocacy beyond supporting their own membership-specific financial interests is not a familiar or comfortable activity. A coalition that is working well will help push organizations outside their comfort zone and move beyond their bureaucratic inertia or traditional focus to take action on an issue.

In New York, coalitions have been most effective and are arguably best suited for educating and advocating for policy change or funding rather than program implementation. Coalition work to change state and local policies is inherently a conflict-driven activity because there are those who support and those who oppose a given proposal. Some health groups shy away from politics and want to focus on health education, but that is not where the greatest public health gains have been realized. It is often easier for organizations to take a controversial position by signing a support letter under the umbrella of a group such as NYSHEPA rather than doing so on their own.

The way NYSHEPA decided to support a particular bill evolved over time. The method used for the past few years has been to take a vote; if a majority of the steering committee members who can take a position are in support, NYSHEPA will work to pass that bill. If only certain members support a policy proposal, an ad hoc group is formed to promote the proposal, and only the names of supporting organizations are included on public documents such as press releases and memos of support.

NYSHEPA's problem of lapsed funding speaks to the need to research and formulate a funding and sustainability strategy from the beginning. On the positive side, NYSHEPA did ensure that there was one organization committed for the long haul to sponsor and support the coalition. However, nonprofit funding is quite limited, so external grants are required; unfortunately, securing funding for policy advocacy is extremely difficult because of restrictions on using foundation and public sector funds for lobbying. Therefore, partnerships like NYSHEPA are frequently forced to divert attention and labor to focus on fundable projects (e.g., programs) that are much less impactful. This funding conundrum is unfortunate and underlies the disadvantage that nonprofits confront when taking on the private sector, which can simply hire lobbyists and mount an ad campaign against a proposal to improve health. Hence, funding mechanisms that do not have lobbying restrictions must be identified to support policy education and action in each state in order to

significantly change our environment and support active living.

If state coalitions are to be successful, regardless of how the coalition is supported, one of the most important elements is to have a full-time, paid director who is adept at using the media to advance the public debate and visibility of an issue. The coalition director should be a very good group facilitator and collaborator, as well as someone who is politically astute and has strong media advocacy skills. Staff turnover is a major threat to a strong coalition. It takes time to rebuild relationships and understand the group dynamics to create a high-performing coalition.

Tips for Working Across Sectors

A critical factor in the success of state coalitions is to include representatives from a variety of sectors within the coalition membership. In the case of NYSHEPA, a mix of organizations that represent health care, education, workplace health promotion, health-related nonprofit organizations, and parents helps to ensure that a variety of policy issues are identified, prioritized, and addressed.

Another important factor is to recognize that not all member organizations may share the same policy agenda or policy priorities. NYSHEPA has successfully navigated this potential challenge by creating the process described previously for determining how, or whether, a bill will be supported by NYSHEPA or by a subset of NYSHEPA members. Anticipating these challenges and creating a plan ahead of time ensures that important issues continue to move forward, despite the fact that the entire coalition does not support each issue.

Additional Reading and Resources

Extensive information on this state coalition model is available on the NYSHEPA website (www.nyshepa.org). The website includes additional information about the coalition's goals, guiding principles, and members as well as its membership process. The site also includes a compilation of both NYSHEPA-specific resources and resources created by other organizations that have been helpful in advancing coalition priorities.

The website provides a few different types of examples of NYSHEPA resources that can be used as models for other state coalitions, such as the following:

Healthy Kids, Healthy New York after-school model guidelines, toolkit, and recognition program (www.nyshepa.org/documents/healthy_kids_healthy_ny_afterschool_toolkit.pdf)

The Healthy Kids, Healthy New York initiative was launched in July 2007, thanks to a grant from the National Governors Association. The goal of the initiative is to fight childhood obesity and create healthy after-school environments. The program focuses on three areas—nutrition, physical activity, and screen time. Model guidelines are provided for each area, which, if followed, will ensure the following:

- Children are served only nutritious snacks and beverages at after-school programs. Children engage in an adequate amount of physical activity in after-school programs.
- Television and recreational screen time are reduced in after-school programs.
- The toolkit, which includes the guidelines, was designed to help after-school

providers implement the program easily. It includes

- a self-assessment instrument, which will help the provider evaluate its current nutrition, physical activity, and screen time environment;
- implementation resources and strategies; and
- materials to help parents support their after-school program in implementing the guidelines and to develop healthier home environments.

References

Centers for Disease Control and Prevention. 2007. *Best Practices for Comprehensive Tobacco Control Programs—2007.* Atlanta, GA: U.S. Department of Health and Human Services, Centers for Disease Control and Prevention, National Center for Chronic Disease Prevention and Health Promotion, Office on Smoking and Health.

Community Preventive Services Task Force. 2010. The community guide. www.thecommunityguide.org/pa/environmental-policy/index.html.

Gillespie, K. 2009. SmokeLess States national tobacco policy initiative. Robert Wood Johnson Foundation. www.rwjf.org/pr/product.jsp?id = 16549.

Strategic Alliance. n.d. Our accomplishments. www.preventioninstitute.org/about-us-sa/our-accomplishments.html.

Index

Note: The italicized *f* and *t* following page numbers refer to figures and tables, respectively.

About the NPAP and NCPPA

The **National Physical Activity Plan Alliance** is a not-for-profit organization committed to ensuring the long-term success of the National Physical Activity Plan (NPAP). The alliance is governed by a board of directors composed of representatives of organizational partners and at-large experts on physical activity and public health. The key objectives of the alliance are to support implementation of the NPAP's strategies and tactics, expand awareness of the NPAP among policy makers and key stakeholders, evaluate the NPAP on an ongoing basis, and periodically revise the NPAP to ensure its effective linkage to the current evidence base.

The **National Coalition for Promoting Physical Activity (NCPPA)** is a blend of associations, health organizations, and private corporations advocating for policies that encourage Americans of all ages to become more physically active. NCPPA spearheads federal policy and advocacy work in support of the National Physical Activity Plan's recommendations, and the organization maintains a strong voice for physical activity in Washington, DC, where NCPPA members and staff work together to encourage federal legislators to make policy changes that promote regular physical activity in all facets of life.

About the Editors

Russell Pate, PhD, is a professor in the department of exercise science at the University of South Carolina at Columbia. Pate led the development of the 2010 U.S. National Physical Activity Plan and served on the 2008 U.S. Physical Activity Guidelines Advisory Committee. He is the chairman of the board of directors of the National Physical Activity Plan Alliance and chairman of the coordinating committee of the National Physical Activity Plan Alliance.

Pate is a past president of the American College of Sports Medicine (ACSM) and served as lead author of the 1995 CDC-ACSM Statement on Physical Activity and Public Health. He is also past president of the National Coalition for Promoting Physical Activity. In 2012, Pate received the Honor Award from the ACSM. He received the Honor Award from the Science Board of the President's Council on Physical Fitness and Sports in 2007.

He resides with his wife in Columbia, where he enjoys running, attending theater performances, and watching collegiate athletics.

David Buchner, MD, MPH, is a Shahid and Ann Carlson Khan professor in applied health sciences in the department of kinesiology and community health at the University of Illinois at Urbana-Champaign. From 2008 to 2013, he directed the master of public health program in his department. He is a board member for the National Physical Activity Plan Alliance. From 1999 to 2008, he was chief of the Physical Activity and Health Branch at the Centers for Disease Control and Prevention. In this role, Buchner chaired the writing group for the *2008 Physical Activity Guidelines for Americans* and participated in numerous public health initiatives to promote physical activity. Buchner's research has focused on physical activity and aging. He has studied the role of physical activity in preventing functional limitations, disability, and falls. His favorite recreational activity is backpacking and hiking with his family.